CHURCHILL'S POCKETBOOK OF

Medicine

For Churchill Livingstone:
Publisher Laurence Hunter
Project Editors Therese Duriez and Barbara Simmons
Production I. Macaulay Hunter
Designer Design Resources Unit
Sales Promotion Executive Marion Pollock

CHURCHILL'S POCKETBOOK OF

Medicine

PETER C. HAYES MRCP MD

Senior Lecturer in Medicine,
Department of Medicine,
Royal Infirmary,
Edinburgh, UK

THOMAS W. MACKAY BSc Hons MRCP

Lecturer in Medicine,
Department of Medicine,
Royal Infirmary,
Edinburgh, UK

Churchill Livingstone

EDINBURGH LONDON MADRID MELBOURNE NEW YORK AND TOKYO 1992

CHURCHILL LIVINGSTONE
Medical Division of Longman Group UK Limited

Distributed in the United States of America by
Churchill Livingstone Inc., 650 Avenue of the Americas,
New York, N.Y., 10011, and by associated companies,
branches and representatives throughout the world.

First published 1992
  Reprinted 1992

ISBN 0-443-04213-6

British Library Cataloguing in Publication Data
A catalogue record for this book is available from the British Library.

Library of Congress Cataloging in Publication Data
Hayes, Peter C.
  Edinburgh pocketbook of medicine/Peter C. Hayes,
Tom W. Mackay.
    p. cm.
  Includes index.
  ISBN 0-443-04213-6
  1. Internal medicine—Handbooks, manuals, etc. I. Mackay,
Tom W. (Thomas W.) II. Title.
  [DNLM: 1. Medicine—handbooks.   WB 39 H418e]
RC55.H39 1992
616—dc20
DNLM/DLC
for Library of Congress   91–8290
                                                              CIP

The
publisher's
policy is to use
**paper manufactured
from sustainable forests**

Produced by Longman Singapore Publishers Pte Ltd
Printed in Singapore

This book is intended to be an invaluable source of reference for final year medical students and house officers working on the wards. Our aim has been to make the information contained within the book as accessible as possible and every part has been designed with this in mind. The book will fit easily into a pocket and the contents are immediately available on the cover with coloured bands directing the reader to the relevant chapter. An index of emergency procedures plus the biochemical reference values are printed inside the covers for quick reference.

The same policy has dictated the contents of the book which emphasize a disease orientated approach. Each disorder is broken down into relevant categories: aetiology, clinical features, investigations and management. Illustrations and tables expand the text where these were felt to be helpful.

This book is not intended to replace more substantive medical texts but to supplement them. By sifting the quantity and diversity of information for quick reference the young doctor will have the information needed on the wards always to hand.

We would like to thank our many colleagues who have helped us in the preparation of the book and the staff of Churchill Livingstone for their help and enthusiasm.

P.C.H
T.W.M
Edinburgh 1992

ABG	arterial blood gases
ACE	angiotensin converting enzyme
ACTH	adrenocorticotrophic hormone
ADH	antidiuretic hormone
APUDO-MAS	amine precursor uptake and decarboxylation — omas
AF	atrial fibrillation
AIDS	acquired immunodeficiency syndrome
ALL	acute lymphoblastic leukaemia
ALT	alanine transaminase
AML	acute myeloid leukaemia
ANF	antinuclear factor
ARDS	adult respiratory distress syndrome
ASD	atrial septal defect
ASO	antistreptolysin O
AST	aspartate transaminase
ATN	acute tubular necrosis
AXR	abdominal X-ray
BBB	bundle branch block
BMT	bone marrow transplant
BTS	blood transfusion service
CABG	coronary artery bypass graft
CAH	chronic active hepatitis
CAPD	chronic ambulatory peritoneal dialysis
CCF	congestive cardiac failure
CCU	coronary care unit
CEA	carcinoembryonic antigen
CLL	chronic lymphatic leukaemia
CML	chronic myeloid leukaemia
CMV	cytomegalovirus
CNS	central nervous system
COLD	chronic obstructive lung disease
CRF	chronic renal failure
CSF	cerebrospinal fluid
CSM	Committee for safety in medicine
CT	computerized tomography
CVA	cerebrovascular accident
CVP	central venous pressure
CVS	cardiovascular system
CXR	chest X-ray
DIC	disseminated intravascular coagulation
DIP	distal interphalangeal
DM	diabetes mellitus
DU	duodenal ulcer
DVT	deep venous thrombosis
EBV	Epstein-Barr virus
ECG	electrocardiogram
EEG	electroencephalogram

ELISA	enzyme-linked immunosorbent enzyme
EMG	electromyography
EMU	early morning urine
ERCP	endoscopic retrograde cholangiopancreatography
ESR	erythocyte sedimentation rate
FBC	full blood count
FDP	fibrin degradation product
FEV_1	forced expiratory volume in 1 second
FFP	fresh frozen plasma
FSH	follicle stimulating hormone
FTA	fluorescent treponemal antibody test
FVC	forced vital capacity
GABA	gamma-aminobutyric acid
GFR	glomerular filtration rate
GGTP	gamma glutamyl transpeptidase
GH	growth hormone
GN	glomerulonephritis
GVH	graft versus host disease
HBV	hepatitis B virus
HDV	hepatitis delta virus
HIV	human immunodeficiency virus
HLA	human leucocyte antigen
HOCM	hypertrophic obstructive cardiomyopathy
HR	heart rate
HSV	herpes simplex virus
IBD	inflammatory bowel disease
ICP	intracranial pressure
IDL	intermediate density lipoprotein
IHD	ischaemic heart disease
IM	infectious mononucleosis
INR	International normalised ratio
ITP	idiopathic thrombocytopenia purpura
IVC	inferior vena cava
IVU	intravenous urography
JVP	jugular venous pressure
KCO	transfer factor for carbon monoxide
LA	left atrium
LAD	left axis deviation
LBBB	left bundle branch block
LDH	lactate dehydrogenase
LDL	low density lipoprotein
LFT	liver function test
LH	lutenizing hormone
LVF	left ventricular failure
MCV	mean cell volume
MEN	multiple endocrine neoplasia
MHC	major histocompatability complex
MI	myocardial infarction
MSU	midstream urine
MTP	metatarsophalangeal
NANB	non-A non-B hepatitis

NMR	nuclear magnetic resonance
NAP	neutrophil alkaline phosphatase
NSAID	non-steroidal anti-inflammatory drugs
OCP	oral contraceptive pill
OGTT	oral glucose tolerance test
PA	pulmonary artery
PABA	para-aminobenzoic acid
PAS	p-aminosalicylic acid
PBC	primary biliary cirrhosis
PCH	paroxysmal cold haemoglobinuria
PCP	pneumocystis carinii pneumonia
PCV	packed cell volume
PDA	patent ductus arteriosus
PEEP	positive end-expiratory pressure
PEFR	peak expiratory flow rate
PIP	proximal interphalangeal
PPD	purified protein derivative
PPS	plasma protein solution
PR	per rectum
PRV	polycythaemia rubra vera
PTH	parathyroid hormone
PT	prothrombin time
PTT	partial thromboplastin time
PTTK	partial thromboplastin time with kaolin
PUO	pyrexia of unknown origin
PUVA	psoralen ultraviolet A
PV	per vagina
RA	rheumatoid arthritis
RAD	right axis deviation
RAG	R antigen
RAST	radio-allergosorbent test
RBBB	right bundle branch block
RCC	red cell concentrate
RF	rheumatoid factor
RIF	right iliac fossa
RTA	renal tubular acidosis
RUQ	right upper quadrant
RVF	right ventricular failure
SACD	subacute combined degeneration
SBE	subacute bacterial endocarditis
SLE	systemic lupus erythematosus
SVC	superior vena cava
SVT	supraventricular tachycardia
TB	tuberculosis
TIA	transient ischaemic attack
TIP	terminal interphalangeal
TPHA	treponema pallidum haemaglutination assay
TPN	total parenteral nutrition
TRH	thyroid releasing hormone
TSH	thyroid stimulating hormone
TURP	transurethral resection of the prostate

U & E	urea and electrolytes
UC	ulcerative colitis
URTI	upper respiratory tract infection
UTI	urinary tract infection
US	ultrasound
VDRL	venereal diseases research laboratory
VF	ventricular fibrillation
VLDL	very low density lipoproteins
VSD	ventricular septal defect
VT	ventricular tachycardia
VWF	von Willebrand factor
WBC	white blood count
WPW	Wolff–Parkinson–White

Addison's disease Primary adrenocortical insufficiency
Alzheimer's disease Senile dementia
Berger's disease IgA nephropathy
Bornholm disease Epidemic myalgia
Budd-Chiari syndrome Hepatic venous outflow obstruction
Buerger's disease Thromboangiitis obliterans
Caisson disease Decompression sickness
Chagas' disease American trypanosomiasis
Charcot-Marie-Tooth syndrome Peroneal muscular atrophy
Christmas disease Factor IX deficiency
Churg-Strauss syndrome Eosinophilic granulomatous vasculitis
Conn's syndrome Primary aldosteronism
Crohn's disease Regional enteritis
Cushing's disease Pituitary dependent adrenocortical hypoplasia
Devic's disease Neuromyelitis optica
Dressler's syndrome Post myocardial infarction syndrome
Eaton-Lambert syndrome Paraneoplastic myasthenia
Erb's paralysis Upper root branchial plexus injury
Fabry's disease Galactosidase-A deficiency
Friedreich's ataxia Spinocerebellar ataxia
Gardner's syndrome Variant of familial adenomatous polyposis
Gelineau's syndrome Narcolepsy
Graves' disease Autoimmune thyrotoxicosis
Guillain-Barre syndrome Acute post-infection polyneuritis
Hanot's disease Primary biliary cirrhosis
Kallman's syndrome Hypogonadotrophic hypogonadism
Klumpke's paralysis Lower root branchial plexus injury
Loeffler's syndrome Simple pulmonary eosinophilia
McArdle's syndrome Type V glycogen storage disease
Marchiafava-Micheli syndrome Paroxysmal nocturnal haemoglobinuria
Meyer-Betz syndrome Paroxysmal myoglobinuria
Osler-Weber-Rendu syndrome Hereditary haemorrhagic telangiectasia
Pickwickian syndrome Obstructive sleep apnoea syndrome
Pott's disease Spinal tuberculosis
Sheehan's syndrome Postpartum hypopituitarism
Sjögren's syndrome Keratoconjunctivitis sicca
Tietze's syndrome Idiopathic costochondritis
Von Recklinghausen's disease Neurofibromatosis
Wilson's disease Hepato-lenticular degeneration

Allelle Alternate forms of a specific gene within the population that are found at a particular chromosomal location.

Clone A unique segment of DNA (which contains a particular gene) that is generated in vitro, usually through the use of restriction enzymes, and reproduced in vivo (in E.coli).

Doppler Usually used in connection with ultrasonography, using the phenomenon of Doppler shift to identify velocity of flow.

Digital subtraction Computer assisted radiology whereby a background image can be removed, principally during angiography, to enhance the angiographic appearance.

Electrophoresis Methods used to separate compounds by means of their movement across an electric field.

Enzyme immunoassay An assay using antibodies to measure the concentration of a specific substance in biological fluids by means of an enzymatic reaction. The method normally requires the use of two antibodies; one raised against the substance to be measured; the second, to which an enzyme is linked, recognizes the first antibody.

Gene A sequence of chromosomal DNA that codes for single protein.

HPLC High performance liquid chromatography. A chromatographic method where compounds are pumped down various columns containing small pore silica and separated depending upon their physical properties.

Hybridization The process whereby fragments of DNA bind specifically to their complementary DNA sequences.

Immunohistochemistry The use of antibodies labelled to visible substances to allow identification of proteins during histology.

In-situ-hybridization A technique used where DNA probes are used to identify the presence of gene messages in cells or tissue.

Monoclonal antibody Identical antibodies produced by hybridizing plasma cells with malignant cells thereby allowing large amounts of a unique antibody with a known specificity to be produced.

NMR Nuclear magnetic resonance scanning provides imaging which depends upon the magnetic spin properties of molecules under a powerful magnetic field. The density of protons in particular, provides image contrast.

Northern blotting   A method to identify and quantify the amount of mRNA encoding a particular protein through the hybridization between a radiolabelled DNA clone and immobilised RNA. The method is similar to Southern blotting but does not involve digestion with restriction endonucleases.

PCR   Polymerase chain reaction. A method that allows the amplification of genes through the use of heat resistant DNA polymerase and oligonucleotide primers specific to either end of the gene that is to be amplified.

Probe   A gene probe is a clone specific sequence of DNA in which nucleotides are radiolabelled.

RFLP   Restriction fragment length polymorphism. This is a means of identifying abnormal alleles, by cleaving DNA into sequences using bacterial restriction endonucleases. Abnormal DNA sequences may be digested into different sized lengths if alterations in the nucleotide sequence occur within the regions recognized by the endonucleases.

Radioimmunoassay   An assay using radiolabelled biochemical (hormone, protein) to quantify the same substance in blood. The method involves competition for binding to an antibody between the radiolabelled substance and an unknown amount of the same compound in blood.

Southern blotting   A method whereby a gene sequence can be identified within a mixture of DNA fragments (that have been separated by electrophoresis and transferred to nitrocellulose paper) by hybridization to a radiolabelled DNA probe and visualization by autoradiography.

SPECT scanning   Single positron emission computerized tomography. This is a computerized imaging technique dependent upon positron emission tomography following the injection of a radioisotope.

Ultra centrifugation   High speed centrifugation used to spin down small intracellular particles.

Western blotting   Use of antibodies to identify specific proteins after their separation by gel electrophoresis and transfer to nitrocellulose paper.

1

History and examination

1

CLINICAL HISTORY

Introduction Introduce oneself and ask permission to interview and examine the patient. Developing rapport with patients is essential for a good interview and this skill comes only with practice ● Ask name and age ● Ask about presenting complaint ● Ask the questions relevant to the system suspected of being involved (→ below).

Past medical and surgical history Specifically ask about jaundice, epilepsy, rheumatic fever, tuberculosis, diabetes mellitus and operations.

Drugs Obtain as much information as possible including those bought over the counter. Allergies to drugs must be sought and any reaction understood.

Smoking history and alcohol consumption Past and present.

Social and family history ● Ask about marital status, occupation, home conditions and social circumstances, health of immediate family and causes of death of parents or siblings ● Any information about illnesses that appear to run in families should be elicited ● Any recent overseas travel should be discussed.

Systemic enquiry (excluding that discussed under history of presenting complaint).

CVS: ● chest pain – site, character, duration, severity, radiation, exacerbating factors, relieving factors, associated features ● breathlessness – onset eg worse on exertion, at night – and relieving factors eg sitting upright, fresh air and any associated wheeze ● palpitations, ask patient to tap out a rhythm ● intermittent claudication ● ankle swelling.

RS: breathlessness ● cough (whether productive and what colour the sputum) ● haemoptysis ● night sweats ● wheeze.

GI: weight (whether increasing, steady or falling) ● appetite ● dysphagia ● dyspepsia (including exacerbating and relieving features) ● nausea and vomiting ● abdominal pain ● bowel habit noting any change from normal ● stool consistency and colour, tendency to float ● faecal incontinence ● rectal bleeding.

UGS: ● urinary frequency ● dysuria ● hesitancy and dribbling ● incontinence ● haematuria or altered colour ● menstrual cycle, noting any change from usual ● post-menopausal bleeding ● impotence ● sexual orientation (if appropriate).

MS: ● mobility ● athralgia ● joint stiffness or swelling.

CNS: ● headache ● eyesight including diplopia ● dizzy spells, faints and falls ● weakness ● numbness ● tremor or involuntary movement ● dysarthria and dysphasia ● sense of taste and smell.

EXAMINATION

GENERAL FEATURES

Well/ill-looking, orientation in time, place and person, agitation, state of hydration, cyanosis (central/peripheral), jaundice, pallor, state of nutrition, lymphadenopathy, breast examination, distribution of body hair, skin, hands and nails (joints, palmar erythema, Dupuytren's contracture, clubbing, splinter haemorrhages), tongue, throat, goitre.

CARDIOVASCULAR SYSTEM

- Pulse (radial) – rate, rhythm, volume, character (normal, slowly rising, collapsing, bisferiens), compare both radial pulses simultaneously to assess synchronicity and check for radial-femoral delay. Tabulate the presence/absence of each radial, brachial, carotid, femoral, popliteal, posterior tibial and dorsalis pedis pulse (→ Table 1.1).

Table 1.1
Tabulation of pulses

	Radial	Brachial	Carotid	Femoral	Popliteal	Posterior tibial	Dorsalis pedis
Right	++	++	++	++	+	–	–
Left	++	++	++	++	+	–	–
key	++	Normal volume					
	+	Diminished volume					
	–	Absent pulse					

- Assess height and character of jugular venous pulse (JVP) with patient sitting comfortably at 45°. Palpate precordium for apex beat (usually in the 5th intercostal space medial to the mid-clavicular line), heaves or thrills.

- Auscultate at the apex (bell), left sternal edge (diaphragm), aortic and pulmonary areas (2nd right and left intercostal spaces respectively using the diaphragm) before listening at the apex with the patient rolled onto their left side (mitral stenosis) and at the lower left sternal edge with the patient sitting forward and the breath held in expiration (aortic incompetence). Pay attention to the character of the first and second heart sounds (normal/fixed/reversed splitting) and for the presence of any additional heart sounds (III or IV) or for any pericardial rubs. Listen for any murmurs and assess their quality, site of origin and maximal intensity and direction of radiation ($\rightarrow$ Fig. 1.1).

● Check for the presence of dependant oedema (ankles/sacrum).

● Always measure the BP (erect and supine if possible) and check for pulsus paradoxus. Auscultate the chest for crackles in LVF.

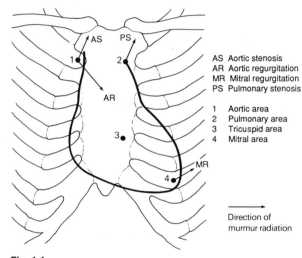

AS Aortic stenosis
AR Aortic regurgitation
MR Mitral regurgitation
PS Pulmonary stenosis

1   Aortic area
2   Pulmonary area
3   Tricuspid area
4   Mitral area

Direction of
murmur radiation

Fig. 1.1
Sites of cardiac auscultation.

RESPIRATORY SYSTEM

● Central and peripheral cyanosis, dyspnoea at rest, digital clubbing, tar staining of fingers, wasting of 1st dorsal interossei muscles in the hand (sign of possible apical lung tumour), signs of carbon dioxide retention (coarse flapping tremor, warm peripheries, bounding pulse, confusion, papilloedema).

● Record respiratory rate (normally 12–14 breaths/min) and breathing pattern (normal/Cheyne-Stokes/Kaussmaul's).

● Always compare both sides of the chest during the examination.

- Observe chest wall movement during both quiet breathing and deep inspiration and expiration. Measure chest expansion in both lateral and anteroposterior directions (should be at least 5 cm). Note presence of intercostal indrawing and the use of accessory muscles of respiration.
- Palpate for subcutaneous emphysema.
- Palpate the position of the trachea.
- Palpate for tactile fremitus.
- Percuss, auscultate and assess vocal resonance/whispering pectoriloquy of both the anterior and posterior aspects of the chest including the apices and in both axillae. Listen to the quality of the breath sounds (normal/absent/bronchial) and for any additional sounds (crackles/wheezes/pleural rubs).
- Always examine any sputum (pink, frothy/purulent/mucoid/ haemoptysis).

GASTROINTESTINAL SYSTEM

- Stigmata of chronic liver disease (leuconychia, palmar erythema, spider telangiectasiae, flapping tremor, lack of secondary sexual hair, jaundice, testicular atrophy, gynaecomastia, caput medusae, ascites, scratch marks).
- Check the appearance of dentition, tongue and fauces.
- Inspect the abdomen (scars, movement with respiration, peristalsis, swellings, cough impulses, herniae).
- Palpate gently and superficially with a warm hand having asked first about any particularly tender areas. Then palpate each area of the abdomen a little deeper. Feel for the liver, spleen and kidneys specifically, and check size by percussion (always percussing in the direction of resonant to dull).
- Percuss gently throughout the abdomen and demonstrate any shifting dullness (ascites).
- Auscultate paying attention to the character of the bowel sounds (normal/diminished/increased in intensity/tinkling in obstruction/absent), and the presence of any bruits.
- Perform a PR and PV examination.

NERVOUS SYSTEM

- Level of consciousness (Glasgow coma scale: best motor response – grades 1–6; best verbal response – grades 1–5; eye opening – grades 1–4: maximum score = 15; table 2.6, p. 21).

- Assess speech (dysphasia, dysarthria, dysphonia).

- Assess gait.

- Check cranial nerves:

  I – smell: test each nostril separately

  II – fundi, visual fields, acuity, direct and consensual pupillary response

  III, IV, VI – external ocular movements, ptosis

  V – motor and sensory components of all three divisions

  VII – motor and sensory components, taste on anterior 1/3 tongue

  VIII – auditory and vestibular components

  IX, X – gag reflex, taste on posterior 2/3 tongue, swallowing reflex

  XI – motor response trapezius and sternocleidomastoid

  XII – tongue movements.

- Check power (grade 1 = flaccid paralysis, grade 5 = normal), tone (normal, decreased, flaccid, increased [spasticity: 'clasp knife' or rigidity: 'lead pipe']), clonus, and coordination of all four limbs. Always compare both sides of the body.

Table 1.2
Reflex root values

Reflex	Root value
Biceps	C5, 6
Triceps	C7, 8
Supinator	C6
Knee	L3, 4
Ankle	S1

- Assess sensation (light, deep touch, proprioception, vibration, temperature appreciation, pain, two point discrimination).

- Perform Romberg's test.

- Check and tabulate reflexes in all four limbs including plantar response (→ Tables 1.2 and 1.3).

Table 1.3
Tabulation of reflexes

	Biceps	Triceps	Supinator	Knee	Ankle	Plantar
Right	++	++	−	++	++	↓
Left	++	++	+	+++	+++	↑

key	+++	Increased reflexes
	++	Normal
	+	Diminished reflexes
	−	Absent reflexes
	↓	Flexor (downgoing) plantar
	↑	Extensor (upgoing) plantar (Babinski response)

2

Common signs and symptoms

Certain signs and symptoms are so common that their recognition and interpretation is part of everyday clinical practice. They are also frequently encountered in examinations: eg 'list the common causes of an enlarged liver in this country', 'what is the difference between a transudate and an exudate?' or 'what are the causes of atrial fibrillation?'. The prudent student will soon realize that there are only a finite number of these commonly encountered signs and symptoms and will spend some time becoming conversant with them.

FINGER CLUBBING

Finger clubbing is an important physical sign and should be sought in all patients. The underlying cause is unclear but arterial hypoxaemia is common and abnormal vascularity, neurogenic factors and/or platelet dysfunction may be involved. The first stage is increased nail-bed fluctuation, which is followed by increased curvature of the long axis of the nail and soft tissue swelling. Associated tenderness of the wrists is characteristic of hypertrophic pulmonary osteoarthropathy which is accompanied by periosteal elevation and new bone formation.

Aetiology   This can be divided into four groups:

Thoracic: bronchial carcinoma, mesothelioma, thymoma, neurofibroma, lymphoma, asbestosis, fibrosing alveolitis, abscess, bronchiectasis, empyema and cystic fibrosis.

Cardiovascular: infective endocarditis, pulmonary a–v malformation, cyanotic heart disease eg, atrial or ventricular septal defect with R–L shunt, Fallot's tetralogy.

Gastrointestinal: cirrhosis eg, PBC or CAH, Crohn's disease, ulcerative colitis, coeliac disease.

Miscellaneous: thyrotoxicosis, brachial a-v malformation, familial.

Clubbing may regress if the underlying disorder eg, bronchial carcinoma, is treated.

CHEST PAIN

Chest pain is one of the most common indications for emergency admission to hospital. Although chest pain can be caused by a large number of conditions, many of which produce similar types of pain, a careful history usually helps in their differentiation. Chest pains can conveniently be divided into those which are focal and those which are poorly localized (→ Table 2.1).

Table 2.1
Types of chest pain

Focal	Poorly localized
Pleurisy	Angina pectoris
Fractured ribs	Myocardial infarction
Herpes zoster	Reflux oesophagitis
Precordial catch	Oesophageal spasm
Tietze's syndrome	Myocarditis
Pericarditis	Hypertrophic obstructive cardiomyopathy
Pulmonary infarct	Aortic dissection

Angina pectoris   This is usually a central, crushing pain or discomfort induced by exercise or excitement, which commonly radiates down the left arm and into the jaw. It is often accompanied by a sense of impending doom. Usually relieved rapidly by nitrates.

Myocardial infarction   This produces a similar pain of longer duration, unrelieved by nitrates, and which often develops at rest or at night. Nausea, sweating and breathlessness are common associated features. The chest pain accompanying an MI may be mild or absent.

Reflux oesophagitis   This often accompanies or follows eating and is made worse by bending, hot drinks or lying supine. Relieved by antacids.

Pleurisy and pulmonary infarction   These produce localized, sharp pain exacerbated by respiration and coughing.

Other causes:

- Cervical spondylosis
- Peptic ulcer
- Biliary colic
- Tracheitis
- Pneumonia
- Mastitis
- Mediastinitis.

ATRIAL FIBRILLATION

Atrial fibrillation may occur in any condition which produces atrial dilatation. It is recognized clinically as an irregularly irregular pulse and absence of the 'a wave' in the JVP. Multiple ventricular ectopics may also cause an irregularly irregular pulse although exercise usually reduces the irregularity unlike atrial fibrillation. The diagnosis is confirmed by a absence of P waves on the ECG. In recent atrial fibrillation the small f waves on the ECG should be differentiated from P waves.

Aetiology:

- Ischaemic heart disease
- Mitral stenosis
- Hypertension
- Thyrotoxicosis
- Cardiomyopathy
- Constrictive pericarditis
- Digoxin
- Sick sinus syndrome
- Pneumonia
- Idiopathic.

12

> *Management* If the underlying cause can be removed (eg thyrotoxicosis) then sinus rhythm usually returns. If not, and the cause has been removed, then cardioversion is indicated. If, however, the underlying cause cannot be removed then the arrhythmia is best treated with digoxin to decrease the ventricular rate. In some patients digoxin treatment alone may not control the rate sufficiently and adding a small dose of a β-blocker or verapamil may be useful. In patients with atrial fibrillation complicating the Wolff-Parkinson-White syndrome digoxin should not be used. In some patients with paroxysmal atrial fibrillation other antiarrhythmics such as disopyramide, quinidine and amiodarone may be indicated.
>
> The risk of strokes in patients with atrial fibrillation is increased but anticoagulation is usually only indicated in mitral valve disease and paroxysmal atrial fibrillation. Many of the strokes in other patients are due to coexistent atherosclerosis and are not influenced by warfarin treatment, which has its own inherent risks.

JAUNDICE

Jaundice occurs when the serum bilirubin exceeds 50 μmol/l. Yellow pigmentation is also present in hypercarotenaemia, but yellow discolouration of the sclera is absent. Bilirubin is derived by breakdown of haemoglobin, with a small component from myoglobin and enzymes. It is carried in the blood bound to albumin and conjugated in the liver by glucuronyl transferase, to bilirubin diglucuronide, which is water soluble and excreted in the bile. In the colon the bilirubin is converted to urobilinogen and excreted in the faeces or reabsorbed and excreted in the urine.

Jaundice occurs for three reasons: ● excess production of bilirubin ● abnormal metabolism and ● impaired excretion. The first two result in increases in unconjugated bilirubin and the latter in conjugated hyperbilirubinaemia (→ Table 2.2).

Table 2.2
Causes of jaundice

Unconjugated	Conjugated
Haemolysis	Hepatitis
Haematoma resorption	Cirrhosis
Gilbert's syndrome	Drug induced cholestasis
Sepsis	Sepsis
Cardiac failure	Dubin-Johnson syndrome
Crigler-Najjar syndrome	Rotor's syndrome
Drugs (rifampicin)	Biliary cirrhosis
	Bile duct obstruction (stones, stricture, tumour)

Gilbert's syndrome is a benign, asymptomatic condition which affects approximately 5% of the population and is characterized by an increase in unconjugated bilirubin which rises with fasting, stress, nicotinic acid administration and alcohol intake. In practice an abnormal bilirubin associated with otherwise normal LFTs in a healthy individual with no evidence of haemolysis (ie. normal haptoglobin levels and no reticulocytosis) implies Gilbert's syndrome and further investigation is not indicated.

In practice patients with jaundice, rather than being divided into those with conjugated or unconjugated hyperbilirubinaemia, are usually categorized into cholestatic or hepatitic groups. This distinction is usually made initially from abnormality of other LFTs (→ Fig. 2.1, p 14), especially the alkaline phosphatase and the aminotransferases: the former implying cholestasis and the latter hepatocellular damage.

Investigation of jaundice (→ Fig. 2.1, p 14)

HEPATOMEGALY

A liver edge that is palpable is not always enlarged and may be due to displacement in patients with pulmonary hyperinflation. It is therefore essential to identify the upper border of the liver by percussion, which is usually at the 5th rib or 5th intercostal space. Hepatomegaly can be defined as a liver with a span of more than 12 cm in the mid-clavicular line. Confirmation of the size of the liver can be obtained by ultrasonography or isotope scanning. The commonest causes of hepatomegaly in the UK are cirrhosis, cardiac failure and cancer (→ Table 2.3).

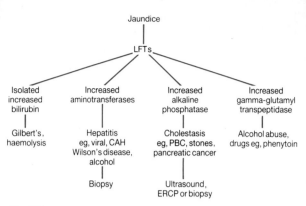

Fig. 2.1
Investigation of jaundice.

As well as the size of the liver its shape, texture and tenderness should be recorded. Pulsation or bruit over the liver should also be sought, the former occurring in tricuspid regurgitation and the latter in hepatitis and primary or secondary malignancy.

Table 2.3 Causes of hepatomegaly		
Process	Disease	Associated features
Congestion	CCF	Peripheral oedema, ↑ JVP
	Budd Chiari	Acute ascites, RUQ pain
Infective	Viral	iv drug abuse, contact with jaundiced subjects
	Bacterial	Haematuria (Weil's disease)
	Protozoal	Suggestive history
	Parasites	Association with dogs (hydatid disease)
Malignancy	Hepatoma	Chronic liver disease, HBsAg+ve, ↑ α-fetoprotein
	Metastases	Primary tumour, weight loss
Myeloproliferative disease	Myelofibrosis	Splenomegaly, abnormal FBC
	Leukaemia	Abnormal peripheral WCC

Table 2.3 (*continued*)		
Process	Disease	Associated features
Infiltration	Fatty liver Amyloidosis	Alcoholism, obesity Enlarged tongue (primary)
	Haemochro-matosis	inflammation (secondary) Cardiac failure, diabetes, pigmentation
Biliary obstruction	PBC Pancreatic carcinoma	Xanthelasma, pruritus Weight loss, pruritus, painless jaundice
Fibrosis	Cirrhosis	Varices, bruising, spider naevi

SPLENOMEGALY

The spleen is not essential for life but has at least four functions: ● immunological (largest single organ of the immune system) ● filtering of bacteria and abnormal blood cells ● blood reservoir helping control portal blood flow and ● haemopoiesis in the fetus and disorders with marrow replacement. The spleen is palpable only when it is approximately three times its normal size. Dullness to percussion can normally be demonstrated between the 9–11th ribs. A palpable spleen is always abnormal and a cause should be sought (→ Table 2.4, p 16).

Hypersplenism is the condition where one or more of the formed components of the blood are reduced due to the overactivity of the spleen.

An anatomically or functionally absent spleen occurs with: splenic infarction, splenectomy, coeliac disease, tropical sprue and Fanconi's anaemia. Such an abnormality can be recognized from the blood film by: target cells, schistocytes, Howell-Jolly bodies and burr cells.

LYMPHADENOPATHY

There are many causes of lymphadenopathy and the commonest ones are listed in Table 2.5, p 16.

Table 2.4
Causes of splenomegaly

Process	Disease	Associated features
Infections	Malaria	Abnormal blood film
	Glandular fever	+ve monospot
	SBE	Cardiac murmur, +ve blood cultures, haematuria
Haematological	Leukaemia	Abnormal blood film
	Myelofibrosis	Abnormal blood film
	Haemolytic anaemia	Jaundice, +ve Coomb's test, ↓ haploglobin
	Polycythaemia rubra vera	↑ Hb, pruritus
	Lymphoma	Lymphadenopathy
	Spherocytosis	Abnormal blood film
	ITP	Thrombocytopaenia
Portal hypertension	Cirrhosis	Hepatomegaly, varices
	Portal vein thrombosis	Varices, normal LFTs
Connective tissue disorders	SLE, rheumatoid	+ve serology

Table 2.5
Differential diagnosis of lymphadenopathy

Neoplastic	Haematological Acute leukaemias, lymphomas, CLL, histiocytosis Non-Haematological Carcinoma: lung, breast, kidneys
Infection	Viral EBV, CMV, HIV, hepatitis A, rubella Bacterial TB, syphilis Fungal Histoplasmosis Protozoal Malaria, toxoplasmosis
Immune conditions	SLE, RA
Metabolic	Lipid storage diseases
Others	Sarcoidosis, drugs (eg phenytoin), Histiocytosis X

SKIN LUMPS

Skin lumps are common and frequently are the cause of a patient seeking medical attention.

Skin lesions

Benign

Warts: are viral, most common in children and adolescents and usually situated on the hands, face and feet. Their spread may be venereal in certain cases giving rise to genital lesions. (→ Dermatology, ch. 13, p 279)

Moles (pigmented naevus): usually flat but may be raised. Usually develop early in life and are commoner in tropical climates. Only rarely are they the site of melanoma transformation.

Sebaceous cysts: a slow growing cyst often with a punctum, containing sebaceous material most common on the scalp, face, ears, back and scrotum.

Lipoma: a mobile overgrowth of fatty tissue. Multiple and tender in Dercum's disease.

Capillary angioma (strawberry naevus): vascular lesions, usually in infants, which tend to enlarge in the first few months of life and then resolve spontaneously.

Cavernous angioma: composed of large vascular spaces and rarely involute spontaneously.

Seborrheic keratoses: slowly growing pigmented lesions usually on the trunk or forehead of elderly subjects.

Pyogenic granuloma: a reddy-brown or dark nodule of proliferating capillaries. They grow rapidly initially, often at the site of trauma. They may resolve spontaneously or require excision.

Molluscum contagiosum: a poxvirus infection producing an umbilicated papule which commonly resolves spontaneously after months.

Furuncle (boil): a perifollicular bacterial infection usually on the neck, face, buttocks or breast which are commoner and tend to cluster (carbuncle) in diabetes mellitus.

Premalignant

Actinic keratoses: red scaling areas of skin which left untreated have malignant potential.

Lichen planus: a pale lesion in the mouth which has malignant potential if left untreated.

Lichen sclerosis: in the genital area this lesion is premalignant if untreated.

Leukoplakia: a pale, thickened mucosal abnormality, usually on the lip, oral mucosa or vulva, may transform into squamous carcinoma.

Malignant ($\rightarrow$ Dermatology p 279)

Basal-cell carcinoma (rodent ulcer): the commonest skin malignancy, most frequent on the face and rarely metastasizes. Small, early lesions should be treated by cautery and curettage whilst larger tumours require radiotherapy.

Squamous-cell carcinoma: these are believed to develop in regions of skin already damaged by ultra-violet radiation, trauma or radiation and are most common on the face. They may metastasize early and they have a poor prognosis compared with basal-cell tumours, especially if they arise on the ear.

Malignant melanoma: a minority originate from moles and are not always pigmented. The prognosis is poorer than for other skin tumours and they should be removed as early as possible with a margin of at least 7 cm.

Bowen's disease: an intra-epidermal carcinoma with a red, scaly appearance not dissimilar to psoriasis with malignant potential. An association with arsenic ingestion can sometimes be identified. Associated internal malignancy can be identified in approximately 40% of patients.

Mycosis fungoides: a rare, telangiectatic, scaly tumour which may take years to involve extra-dermal structures.

Kaposi's sarcoma: this tumour was rare until the AIDS epidemic. It presents as purple nodules often on the thorax.

Paget's disease of the nipple: the epidermal spread of intraduct breast carcinoma and results in an eczematous eruption beside the nipple.

Metastases: an internal malignancy may present with skin metastases. The abdominal wall is the commonest site and the tumours involved include: lung, ovary, renal and gastric.

OEDEMA

Oedema is said to exist when soft tissue swelling occurs due to the collection of interstitial fluid. Such fluid collects either when increased formation or impaired reabsorption exists.

Generalized oedema

This occurs when greater than 3 l of interstitial fluid collects and is always associated with renal retention of sodium. The predominant site of collection varies with the underlying disorder; pulmonary and ankle oedema are typical of cardiac failure, periorbital oedema in renal failure and ascites in cirrhosis. The mechanisms involved also vary with the disease.

Cardiac failure: reduced cardiac output, increased venous pressure, reduced renal blood flow and secondary aldosteronism all result in sodium retention.

Cirrhosis: portal venous hypertension, secondary aldosteronism, intra-renal vascular shunting and hypoproteinaemia are believed important.

Renal failure: impaired renal sodium excretion results in oedema if the sodium intake is not regulated.

Nephrotic syndrome: hypoalbuminaemia and reduced plasma volume are important.

Other causes include: pregnancy, idiopathic oedema, angioneurotic oedema, steroid therapy, hypothyroidism and starvation (especially on refeeding).

Localized oedema

The commonest example is unilateral lower limb oedema complicating a deep venous thrombosis. Blockage of large veins elsewhere may produce oedema such as in SVC, IVC or subclavian vein obstruction. Lymphoedema, due to lymphatic obstruction, may be acquired or congenital (eg Milroy's disease). A paralysed limb may also become oedematous. Localized inflammation may result in localized fluid collection in adjacent potential spaces, eg pleural effusion or ascites.

> *Management*   This depends upon the underlying cause. In generalized oedema sodium restriction is generally necessary and diuretics are advocated in most cases. Since in many instances the plasma volume is reduced overvigorous diuresis should be avoided. Intravenous diuretic administration may be necessary when intestinal oedema results in diuretic resistance.

CONFUSION AND COMA

Confusion is an impairment in the thought processes whilst coma and stupor are abnormalities in the level of consciousness. The two patterns of abnormality not infrequently exist in the same patient. Many patients with severe illnesses become confused which commonly makes their assessment and management more difficult. In the elderly relatively minor illnesses may make the patient confused and care must be taken to look for a cause and not label the individual 'demented'. The history from relatives or neighbours is invaluable in the assessment of confused or comatose patients. Treatment of such patients should be made with a clear understanding of the likely underlying disorder and blanket sedation should be avoided.

Confusion

Aetiology

- Infection (may be occult especially in the elderly)
- Alcohol abuse – delirium tremens is the most severe form and is relatively unusual
- Metabolic – hypo- and hyperglycaemia, uraemia, hypo- and hyperthyroidism, hypercalcaemia
- Drugs, especially sedatives
- Hypoxaemia
- Hypotension
- Subdural haematoma
- Night-time disorientation
- Deafness
- Dementia.

Coma

Aetiology

- Hypoglycaemia – sweaty, tachycardia, fits
- Hyperglycaemia – less often comatose, dehydrated, air-hunger
- Head injury
- Post-ictal
- CVA especially cerebral haemorrhage
- Drugs
- Hepatic failure
- Hysteria.

A formal assessment of the level of consciousness should be performed to allow changes to be identified. The Glasgow coma scale is the best known and has prognostic significance ($\rightarrow$ Table 2.6).

**Table 2.6
Glasgow coma scale**

Score	Motor response	Verbal response	Eye opening
6	Obeys simple commands	–	–
5	Attempts to remove source of painful stimuli to head or trunk	Orientated	–
4	Attempts to withdraw from source of pain	Disorientated	Eyes open
3	Flexes arm at elbow and wrist in response to nail bed pressure	Random speech	Open to speech
2	Extends arms at elbow and wrist in response to nail bed pressure	Mumbling	Open to pain
1	No motor response to painful stimuli	No speech	No opening

Add the individual scores: best = 15, worse = 3.

The investigation and treatment of certain of these causes of coma is described under the appropriate section. Irrespective of the cause the adequacy of ventilation should be ensured by ABG and assisted ventilation introduced when necessary.

ABDOMINAL PAIN

Abdominal pain is one of the commonest symptoms in medicine and is experienced by us all at some time or other. In most instances it is of minor importance but occasionally may indicate serious and life-threatening pathology. Differentiation in most cases relies on the history rather than clinical signs and laboratory investigations.

From a practical point of view the causes of abdominal pain can be divided into medical and surgical categories (→ Table 2.7, p 22 and 2.8, p 23). Uncommon causes are listed in Table 2.9 (→ p 23).

Table 2.7
Medical causes of abdominal pain

Disorder	Symptoms/Signs	Diagnosis
Reflux oesophagitis	Retrosternal pain, dyspepsia flatulence	Endoscopy, barium swallow, pH monitoring
Peptic ulcer	Epigastric pain influenced by food	Endoscopy, barium meal
Biliary colic	Severe epigastric or RUQ pain for 10–60 min	US, ERCP, LFTs
Pancreatitis	Severe epigastric pain radiating posteriorly	↑ amylase, US
Irritable bowel syndrome	Abdominal pain, diarrhoea and/or constipation	Typical history, negative investigations
Hepatitis and hepatic congestion	RUQ pain, jaundice, lethargy	LFTs, US, biopsy
Crohn's disease	Colicky pain, diarrhoea	Barium radiology, endoscopy
Renal colic	Loin pain radiating to groin, haematuria	Abdominal X-ray, IVU
Diverticulitis	LIF pain, PR bleeding	Barium enema, ↑ WCC
Cystitis	Suprapubic pain and dysuria	Urinalysis and culture

Table 2.8
Surgical causes of abdominal pain

Disorder	Symptoms/signs	Diagnosis
Cholecystitis	RUQ pain, vomiting fever, Murphy's sign	US, HIDA scan
Perforated viscus	Vomiting, rebound tenderness, shock	Air under diaphragm on erect CXR
Intestinal obstruction	Vomiting, colic, ↑ bowel sounds	Fluid levels and dilated bowel on abdominal X-ray
Appendicitis	Anorexia, nausea, McBurney's point tenderness	↑ WCC, regional ileus on X-ray, often clinical
Ectopic pregnancy	Shock, PV bleeding, shifting dullness, stabbing pain	US, laparoscopy, pregnancy test may be negative

Table 2.9
Uncommon causes of abdominal pain

Metabolic	Respiratory	Miscellaneous
Ketoacidosis	Pneumonia	Migraine
Addison's disease	Pneumothorax	Myocardial infarction
Hypercalcaemia	Pulmonary	Mesenteric ischaemia
Drugs	embolism	Henoch Schönlein
Lead poisoning	Diaphragmatic	purpura
Uraemia	pleurisy	Hepatoma
Hyperlipidaemia		Haemolytic crisis
Acute intermittent		Spinal disease
porphyria		Tabes dorsalis

PRURITUS

Pruritus or itch is an important symptom because it is a common feature of dermatological disease but may also reflect systemic pathology. Localized itch, such as pruritus ani, indicates local disease whilst generalized pruritus has a wide differential diagnosis. Many factors have been implicated in the pathogenesis of itch such as proteases, histamine, prostaglandins, kinins and bile acids but the underlying mechanism in many disorders remains unclear as is the relief obtained by scratching. Diseases which may cause generalized pruritus include:

- Chronic cholestasis (eg PBC)
- Chronic renal failure
- Polycythaemia rubra vera
- Pregnancy
- Hyper- and hypothyroidism
- Myeloproliferative diseases (Hodgkin's disease, leukaemia, myeloma)
- Carcinoid syndrome
- Iron deficiency
- Parasitosis (eg scabies)
- Drug hypersensitivity
- Mastocytosis
- Diabetes mellitus
- Brain tumour (especially fourth ventricle).

The majority of cases of generalized pruritus can be identified by checking the FBC, LFTs, U+Es, T4 and Fe in conjunction with taking the drug history.

HEADACHE

Headache is a common symptom and is usually of little clinical significance. It may however herald serious disease and a diagnosis of the type of headache is essential. Headache may be vascular or muscular in origin, be related to intracranial hypertension or be due to systemic disease ($\rightarrow$ Table 2.10).

DYSPNOEA

Dyspnoea is defined as the uncomfortable subjective awareness of the process of respiration. It is the symptom of many different disorders and the exact processes involved are ill understood. It should not be confused with hyperventilation, the ventilation in excess of metabolic needs; hyperpnoea, increased ventilation in proportion to metabolic needs and tachypnoea, rapid respiration.

Aetiology

Obstruction: any of the airways from the larynx to the small bronchioles. The commonest causes are chronic bronchitis

**Table 2.10
Causes of headache**

Type	Features
Migraine Common	Common, unilateral, often throbbing. Lasts a few hours with nausea but rarely vomiting
Classical	Less common, unilateral, throbbing, nausea and vomiting usual. Visual scotomata and scintillations characteristic
Cluster	Unilateral retro-orbital or temporal, often nocturnal. Commoner in males. Severe pain, usually for less than 60 minutes with conjunctival congestion and lacrimation. Occur in clusters with free periods of months
Tension	Very common, tight or throbbing generalized or bilateral pain. May be associated with stress and uncommon in morning
Trigeminal neuralgia	Severe lancinating pain lasting for seconds. Trigger areas exist and may interfere with eating, washing, shaving etc. Most usually affect the mandibular or maxillary branch of trigeminal nerve
Temporal arteritis	Elderly patient with tender, palpable temporal arteries. Severe, persistent headache with or without stiffness in shoulder girdle muscles. High ESR
Intracranial hypertension	Dull recurrent headache, often present on waking made worse by bending and coughing. Vomiting and papilloedema may be present
Atypical facial pain	Facial pain without clear cranial nerve distribution. May be related to dental pathology in some cases
Benign intracranial hypertension	Usually in young, obese females, associated with vomiting, raised CSF pressure, papilloedema and normal CT scan

and asthma and may occur at rest as well as with exercise. Stridor or rhonchi may be found on examination.

Parenchymal lung diseases: such as fibrosing alveolitis, sarcoidosis or pneumoconiosis initially produce dyspnoea only on exertion. Auscultation usually reveals crackles.

Cardiac disease: causing an increase in the pulmonary capillary wedge pressure. In the early stages it produces only exertional dyspnoea. Examination may reveal other evidence of cardiac disease such as murmurs, ↑ JVP or features on ECG of ischaemia, myocardial infarction or LVH.

Pulmonary vascular disease: due either to acute or recurrent pulmonary emboli or primary pulmonary hypertension. The onset may be acute or insidious depending upon the cause. Evidence of a DVT may be present but often the examination is normal. RVH may be apparent on the ECG.

Chest wall or respiratory muscle abnormality: such as kyphoscoliosis, obesity or myaesthenia gravis. The diagnosis is usually obvious since only severe abnormality produces significant dyspnoea.

Psychogenic dyspnoea: relatively common but a diagnosis which should only be made after other causes have been excluded. Many patients with organic dyspnoea appear anxious. A common complaint in psychogenic dyspnoea is the feeling of being 'unable to take a deep enough breath'.

Physiological dyspnoea: the normal breathlessness that accompanies exercise, the onset of which depends upon the individual's fitness. Factors other than fitness such as altitude or anaemia may be important.

3

Cardiovascular disease

INVESTIGATIONS

All patients suspected of cardiac disease should have a thorough history and physical examination which will often establish the diagnosis. Commonly required investigations include:

CXR This will identify cardiac enlargement and in some instances the cardiac chamber involved and any associated pulmonary congestion or pulmonary oedema ($\rightarrow$ Fig. 4.3, p 58).

ECG This can confirm ischaemic heart disease showing ischaemia at rest or myocardial infarction. However a normal ECG does not exclude IHD and an exercise ECG, under medical supervision, is useful in the assessment of the patient with suspected angina. The ECG is also essential in the diagnosis of cardiac arrhythmias and conduction abnormalities. Characteristic abnormalities may occur in LVH, mitral stenosis, pulmonary embolism, pericarditis, ventricular aneurysm and hypothermia.

Echocardiography 2-dimensional scans have now largely replaced the M-mode echo and allow, in expert hands, visualization of all four chambers, their wall thickness and valves in the heart. Combined with Doppler studies the flow of blood across valves or septal defects can be determined and quantitated.

Angiography This can be used to outline the coronary circulation and is essential in the assessment of coronary atheromatous disease in those who would be candidates for coronary surgery or angioplasty. Cardiac catheterization with contrast studies, pressure measurement and O_2 saturation allows accurate assessment of ventricular size and function, valvular heart disease or intracardiac shunts.

Isotope scans These can be used in the assessment of ventricular function, myocardial ischaemia and myocardial infarction. Pulmonary perfusion scans are commonly used in the diagnosis of pulmonary embolism.

ANGINA

Angina pectoris is the commonest and most important symptom of ischaemic heart disease and is due to an imbalance between the myocardial oxygen supply and demand. Variants of classical angina include Prinzmetal angina, due to coronary artery spasm and unstable angina which increases in severity until occurring at rest and commonly is the forerunner of MI. Conditions other than ischaemic heart disease which may produce angina include cardiomyopathy, coronary artery spasm and aortic stenosis. The major risk factors for IHD are cigarette smoking, hypertension, male sex, age, family history, diabetes mellitus and hypercholesterolaemia.

Clinical features

Symptoms: severe chest pain described variably as gripping, crushing or tight. The pain frequently radiates down the left arm and into the neck and jaw. It is typically induced by exercise and stress and relieved within 1–2 minutes by nitroglycerin.

Signs: Often none. Risk factors such as hypertension or aggravating factors such as anaemia may be identified.

Investigations ● ECG: although this may be entirely normal between attacks, particularly in those without a history of MI, it is usually abnormal during an attack. The classical abnormalities include ST segment depression and T-wave inversion. ST segment elevation occurs in coronary artery spasm (Prinzmetal angina) or myocardial infarction. In patients with a suggestive history but normal resting ECG an exercise test should be undertaken, using either a bicycle or treadmill, providing aortic stenosis and unstable angina have been excluded. This is performed until a required heart rate is reached or the patient becomes symptomatic, develops an arrhythmia or hypotension. Monitoring throughout is essential and should include blood pressure, heart rate, duration of exercise, quantitation and duration of any ECG abnormality ● Radio-isotope thallium scanning may provide additional information ● Coronary angiography is the gold standard in the diagnosis of coronary artery disease and is required in those being considered for coronary artery surgery or angioplasty ie those with refractory angina, those who develop hypotension or more than 2 mm ST depression during mild exercise which indicates high risk of triple or left main stem coronary disease (in whom surgery prolongs life).

Management Recognize and correct risk factors such as hypertension, smoking, obesity and hypercholesterolaemia. Advice regarding exercise and occupation. Adequate investigation to identify those likely to benefit from surgery.

Drug therapy: Nitrates: sublingual for symptomatic relief; oral for prophylaxis, allowing an 8–10-hour interval without therapy to prevent tolerance (eg isosorbide mononitrate 20 mg bd). *β-blockers:* B_1 selective antagonists reduce adverse reactions (eg atenolol 50 mg/day). Titrate dose to achieve a resting heart rate of approximately 60/minute. Particularly indicated post-MI.

Calcium antagonists: eg nifedipine 10 mg tid, diltiazen 60 mg tid for both stable and unstable angina, particularly where coronary artery spasm exists. This latter is suggested by rest pain associated with transient ST segment elevation, which may be identified only by 24-hour ECG monitoring.

Coronary angioplasty: useful and successful in treating proximal arterial stenoses, particularly in those with single vessel disease. Its role shortly after acute myocardial infarction is still controversial.

Coronary artery bypass surgery: indicated in those with severe coronary artery disease ie, triple vessel disease and left main stem stenosis, where surgery prolongs survival. The main indication remains symptomatic relief in those refractory to medical management where bypass is anatomically possible.

Unstable angina

This is defined as angina ● of recent onset which is severe ● present with minimal exertion or at rest ● with recent rapid increase in severity and duration or rapid decrease in exercise tolerance. Aggressive management is indicated to reduce the otherwise high risk of infarction. This includes:

● Bed-rest.

● Aspirin 300 mg daily.

● Removal of exacerbating factors such as cardiac failure, infection, hypertension and arrhythmias.

● Maximal therapy with β-blockers, calcium antagonists and nitrates (often intravenous).

● Intravenous heparin anticoagulation (PTT-2x normal).

● Angiography in those whose pain does not settle, with subsequent options of angioplasty or CABG.

MYOCARDIAL INFARCTION

Myocardial infarction, death of part of the cardiac muscle, is the commonest cause of death in the UK and affects 1 in 200 people per year.

Clinical features

Symptoms: severe crushing, central chest pain, often radiating into the neck and down the arms, which is prolonged and not relieved by nitrates. Commonly associated with sweating, nausea, vomiting and dyspnoea. Many infarcts are associated with lesser or no chest pain, the so-called silent infarct.

Signs: pallor, peripheral shut down, tachycardia, change in BP, cyanosis, 4th heart sound (S_4) and if LVF exists basal crepitations, raised JVP and S_3.

Investigations • ECG: Classical changes are early ST elevation and T-wave inversion followed by Q-wave development • In subendocardial (non Q-wave) infarcts ST depression and T-wave changes only occur • Cardiac enzymes these develop serially: first increases in creatine kinase MB (peaks 18–24 h), then aspartate transaminase (peaks 24 h) and lastly lactate dehydrogenase (peaks 3 d). None of the enzymes are specific for MI but the pattern of change is highly suggestive. The peak of the creatine kinase rise correlates approximately with the size of the infarct. Thrombolysis therapy may modify the pattern of enzyme release causing an earlier, higher peak • In cases where doubt exists 99m Tc-pyrophosphate scanning shows the infarct as a 'hot spot' • CXR is useful in identifying pulmonary oedema and a proportion of aortic dissections. (→ Figs. 3.1, 3.2 & 3.3, p 31, 32.)

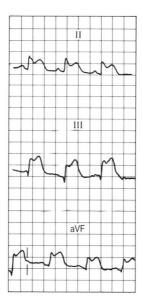

Fig. 3.1
Acute inferior myocardial infarction.

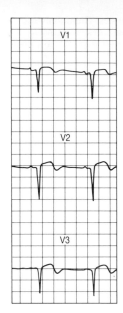

Fig. 3.2
Established anteroseptal myocardial infarction.

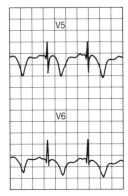

Fig. 3.3
Subendocardial lateral myocardial infarction.

Management

- Adequate pain relief and transfer to CCU.
- Continuous ECG monitoring and iv access.
- Bed-rest and oxygen administration.
- Thrombolytic therapy if within 6 hours of the onset of pain and no contraindications.
- Subcutaneous heparin (5000 IU 8-hourly).
- Look out for complications (→ below).
- Blood for cardiac enzymes.
- Prohibition of smoking.

Complications

Tachyarrhythmias: sinus tachycardia is common and may be a sign of incipient cardiac failure. AF is not uncommon and is usually adequately treated with digoxin. If cardiovascular collapse develops DC cardioversion is indicated. Ventricular tachycardia requires treatment with iv lignocaine 100 mg over 2 minutes followed by 4 mg/minute initially then reducing slowly over 36 hours. Second line agents include mexiletine, disopyramide, flecanide and amiodarone. Cardioversion is indicated for VT if hypotension or heart failure develops and is always immediately indicated for VF.

Bradyarrhythmias: sinus bradycardia and AV block is common following infarction, especially an inferior MI. If it is symptomatic treatment with atropine is usually sufficient, although insertion of a pacemaker is required for resistant and haemodynamically significant bradycardia. Bradyarrhythmias associated with anterior MI signify major myocardial damage and pacing is indicated for any bradycardia associated with hypotension and prophylactically for 2nd degree heart block (Mobitz type II), complete heart block and bifascicular block.

Cardiogenic shock: hypotension with peripheral and renal shut down is a serious prognostic event following MI. A Swan-Ganz catheter should be inserted and the pulmonary wedge pressure maintained between 15–20 mmHg by vasodilator and inotrope therapy. A right ventricular infarct may cause hypotension with a low LA filling pressure and appropriate fluid replacement may reverse the shock. Inotropic agents are important in increasing cardiac output and tissue perfusion. Any arrhythmia which may make the hypotension worse should be reversed.

Pulmonary oedema: this is common and is usually responsive to diuretic therapy. If resistant vasodilators such as iv nitrates should be added and the pulmonary capillary wedge pressure monitored. Occasionally positive pressure ventilation is required.

Pericarditis: this should be suspected in patients complaining of sharp, positional pain in whom a pericardial rub may be heard. It is associated with transmural MI and is treated with NSAID (eg ibuprofen 400 mg tid). Anticoagulants should be used with caution in such patients as haemopericardium is a recognized complication.

Dressler's syndrome: this may follow an MI from 2 weeks onwards and is characterized by fever, pleuritic chest pain and ECG changes of pericarditis ie concave ST segment elevation. It is believed to have an autoimmune basis.

Post infarct VSD or papillary muscle rupture: this should be suspected in patients who suddenly deteriorate with heart failure and a new systolic murmur.

ARRHYTHMIAS

> Cardiac arrhythmias are traditionally divided into supraventricular and ventricular and brady- and tachyarrhythmias.

Supraventricular tachyarrhythmias

Generally these can be recognized from the clinical signs and an ECG showing narrow QRS complexes. Aberrant conduction with widening of the QRS complex is unusual and requires to be differentiated from VT.

Sinus tachycardia Due to increased sympathetic drive as occurs with hypotension, anxiety, exercise, infection, pregnancy, thyrotoxicosis. Treatment should be aimed at the underlying disorder.

Atrial flutter This should be suspected in patients with a regular pulse between 125–160/minute and is associated with IHD, hypertension, mitral stenosis, thyrotoxicosis and MI. The flutter (F) waves occur at 300/minute and AV block usually occurs and can be recognized clinically from the JVP where 'a' waves exceed the pulse rate. Pressure over the carotid sinus increases the AV block and slows the pulse rate whilst pressure is maintained. Treatment is usually with digoxin to slow the ventricular rate although a β-blocker eg atenolol 50–100 mg/day or verapamil 80 mg tid may also be used. In otherwise well patients with new atrial flutter cardioversion should be attempted. If the atrial flutter has been present for some time the patient should be anticoagulated and digoxin withheld before cardioversion.

Atrial fibrillation This should be suspected in an individual with an irregular pulse (→ Fig. 3.4). Carotid sinus compression does not influence the heart rate and the 'a' waves are absent from the JVP. Digoxin is the drug of choice although a β-blocker or verapamil may sometimes be required in combination to control the ventricular rate. If cardioversion is considered the patient should be anticoagulated and digoxin withheld. The risk of cerebral embolism is increased in patients with atrial fibrillation although anticoagulation is usually indicated only in those with mitral valve disease, with intermittent AF and patients under 50 years.

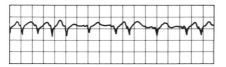

Fig. 3.4
Atrial fibrillation.

Paroxysmal supraventricular tachycardia This disorder is characterized by episodes of atrial or nodal tachycardia, with a heart rate of 140–220/minute, which may be self-limiting or require treatment. There is often a past history of arrhythmias or palpitations. In a minority pre-excitation syndromes such as Wolff-Parkinson-White or Lown-Ganong-Levine (short PR interval without the delta wave) syndrome can be identified. The patient can often be taught to treat their own attacks by the Valsalva manoeuvre. Carotid sinus pressure frequently terminates an attack. In others treatment with intravenous verapamil or β-blocker may be required or, more rarely, cardioversion. Prophylaxis against further attacks may be obtained with verapamil, β-blockers, disopyramide or digoxin.

Wolff-Parkinson-White syndrome This is a pre-excitation syndrome characterized by the presence of a delta wave before the QRS complex thereby shortening the PR interval. Pre-excitation occurs via an accessory AV conduction pathway – the bundle of Kent. It is particularly important to recognize this disorder because the supraventricular arrhythmias which occur (including SVT and AF) should not be treated with digoxin which may worsen the problem. Treatment is by cardioversion if shocked or disopyramide or amiodarone.

Ventricular tachyarrhythmias
Generally these are more sinister arrhythmias recognized by an ECG with wide QRS complexes which usually vary in size and shape from one beat to the next.

Ventricular tachycardia This is a serious arrhythmia usually signifying serious underlying cardiac disease (→ Fig. 3.5, p 36). The heart rate is between 140–220 and carotid sinus pressure has no influence on the rate. The commonest causes include acute MI, cardiomyopathies and ventricular aneurysm. With the exception of an idioventricular rhythm, which arises from an ectopic focus high within the ventricular conducting system and which is common following acute MI, all ventricular tachycardias require urgent treatment. The treatment of choice in those with an adequate BP is intravenous lignocaine (100 mg over 2 min followed by 4 mg/min initially then reducing slowly over 36 h) although disopyramide (2 mg/kg (max 150 mg) slowly) or mexiletine (100–250 mg over 10 min. followed by 250 mg infusion over 60 min) may sometimes be required. In hypotensive patients DC cardioversion followed by iv lignocaine should be carried out urgently. Oral treatment of patients recovering from ventricular arrhythmias is usually indicated with mexiletine (200–250 mg tid/qid) or flecanide (100 mg bd). Long-term treatment, for more than 6 weeks, is controversial.

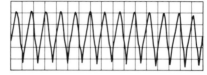

Fig. 3.5
Ventricular tachycardia.

Ventricular fibrillation This is the commonest cause of death following acute MI (→ Fig. 3.6). It is generally a reversible condition with adequate treatment and its recognition is the basis for cardiac monitoring in CCU. Risk factors include hypokalaemia, acid-base imbalance and catecholamines such as iv adrenaline. It should be recognized by cardiovascular collapse and a ECG showing chaotic QRS complexes. Treatment is by immediate DC cardioversion followed by iv lignocaine (100 mg over 2 min) and sodium bicarbonate to reverse the metabolic acidosis which develops after a period of cardiac standstill. Oral therapy to reduce the risk of recurrence is the same as for VT.

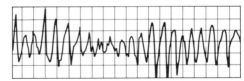

Fig. 3.6
Ventricular fibrillation.

Bradycardias

Sinus bradycardia a heart rate below 60/minute is usually due to increased vagal tone. It occurs in athletes, post inferior MI and with β-blocker treatment. It is rarely symptomatic but if it does require treatment atropine 0.6 mg iv is usually effective.

Sinoatrial block   when this occurs a complete cardiac cycle is missing on the ECG and is a common feature of the sick sinus syndrome. Treatment, when symptomatic, is by pacemaker insertion.

First degree heart block: manifested by a prolongation of the PR interval (>0.2 s) does not produce bradycardia and is an electrocardiographic phenomenon.

Second degree heart block: is divided into two types: Mobitz type I (Wenkebach), where the PR interval progressively lengthens until a beat is omitted and the cycle repeated and Mobitz type II, a more serious disorder, where QRS complexes are dropped every 2, 3 or 4 beats but where the PR interval is constant.

Third degree or complete heart block: exists where there is no association between the p wave and the QRS complexes and the ventricular rate is maintained by an escape rhythm originating in the ventricular conducting system or ventricles ($\rightarrow$ Fig. 3.7). Treatment of second and third degree heart block is by insertion of a temporary or permanent pacemaker.

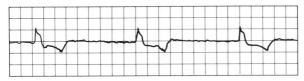

Fig. 3.7
Complete heart block.

CARDIAC AXIS AND BUNDLE BRANCH BLOCK

The cardiac axis is determined using the standard limb leads. The normal axis is between $-30°$ and $+110°$. The lead with equiphasic QRS complexes should be sought and the axis lies at right angles to this. A look at the QRS complexes in the other leads should clarify whether the right angle is clockwise or anticlockwise of the equiphasic lead ie, a tall R wave in I indicating anticlockwise rotation (L axis deviation; LAD) whilst a tall R in III, clockwise rotation (R axis deviation; RAD). The cardiac axis is useful in identifying L or RVH and bifascicular block ($\rightarrow$ below).

Bundle branch block describes the ECG pattern which appears with major interruption of the normal electrical conduction through the Purkinje system. The QRS complex is always greater than 0.12 second. Right bundle branch block (RBBB) (→ Fig. 3.8): a M-shaped QRS complex in V1 and W in V6. This may be congenital but also develops with ischaemic heart disease. Left bundle branch block (LBBB) (→ Fig. 3.9): a W-shaped QRS in V1 and M-shaped in V6. This is usually acquired and associated with ischaemic heart disease. Less commonly BBB may be found in conjunction with atrio-ventricular cushion defects and cardiomyopathy. BBB may be present intermittently in such disorders as paroxysmal atrial tachycardia where incomplete recovery in a bundle occurs due to the rate resulting in aberrant conduction.

Bifascicular block: The combination of marked axis deviation and RBBB suggests a block in two bundles. Hence RBBB and LAD indicates block in the right and left anterior bundle; and LBBB – blockage of both left bundles.

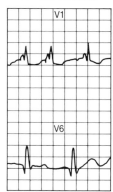

Fig. 3.8
Right bundle branch block.

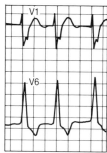

Fig. 3.9
Left bundle branch block.

Trifascicular block: This is said to be present when first degree heart block, RBBB and L anterior or posterior hemiblock coexist or first degree HB and LBBB.

Bifascicular and trifascicular blocks may be found as complications of ischaemic heart disease but are also characteristic of ostium primum ASDs.

HEART FAILURE

> Heart failure exists when the heart pump is unable to pump sufficient blood to satisfy the body's metabolic requirement whilst maintaining normal filling (preload) pressures. Although clinically failure is commonly divided into left or right-sided failure it is rare for these to exist in isolation.

Aetiology The commonest cause of heart failure is ischaemic heart disease (IHD) but it is important to identify the underlying cause in each patient in order to avoid missing correctable disorders. Other causes include: valvular heart disease, hypertension, arrhythmias, pulmonary embolism, anaemia, thyrotoxicosis, myocarditis, infective endocarditis, cardiomyopathy and thiamine deficiency (wet beriberi).

Clinical features

Symptoms: In LVF dyspnoea on exertion, orthopnoea and paroxysmal nocturnal dyspnoea are common. In RVF ankle swelling and RUQ discomfort may occur. In both fatigue and lethargy are usual.

Signs: ankle and sacral oedema, raised JVP, basal crepitations, hepatomegaly and a third and/or fourth heart sound. Table 3.1 shows a classification of heart failure.

Investigation • CXR may show cardiomegaly, pulmonary ve-

Table 3.1 New York Heart Association: Functional classification of heart failure	
Class I:	No limitation
Class II:	Slight limitation of physical activity
Class III:	Marked limitation of physical activity, but comfortable at rest
Class IV:	Symptoms present at rest and inability to perform any physical activity without discomfort

nous distension, Kerley B lines, alveolar oedema, (often in a 'bat's-wing' distribution) and pleural effusions. It may also provide evidence of the underlying cause eg L atrial enlargement in mitral stenosis ● ECG may show LVH often due to chronic hypertension or aortic stenosis, p-mitrale of mitral stenosis or evidence of IHD ● How well the LV is contracting, the chamber size and the state of the valves can be assessed by echocardiography. If no obvious cardiac disorder can be identified high cardiac output states such as thyrotoxicosis and thiamine deficiency should be excluded ● Other causes of pulmonary or peripheral oedema should also be ruled out such as nephrotic syndrome, acute renal failure and liver disease.

Management This should be directed to the cause in such correctable disorders as valvular heart disease and thyrotoxicosis. In most cases, however, usually due to IHD, treatment is purely symptomatic and includes:

● Dietary salt reduction.

● Diuretics, usually a thiazide for mild CCF and loop diuretics in more severe cases.

● Digoxin in patients with associated AF.

● Vasodilators can be used to reduce either pre-load, such as the long-acting nitrates (avoiding tolerance by allowing an 8–10-hour treatment free period daily), or after-load, such as ACE inhibitors, eg captopril or enalapril which have been shown to prolong life in severe heart failure. Other after-load reducers such as hydralazine and prazosin are used less commonly today.

In patients with refractory CCF hospitalization and the administration of iv loop diuretics, vasodilators eg isosorbide dinitrate infusion and inotropes (dopamine, dobutamine) may be required. In young patients with severe, intractable cardiac failure cardiac transplantation is now a viable therapeutic option.

Management of acute LVF:

● Oxygen 40–60%.

● Sedation and pre-load reduction with morphine 10 mg iv.

● iv frusemide 40–120 mg or bumetanide 1–2 mg.

If refractory or severe:

● iv nitrate to reduce pre-load.

● iv inotropes eg dobutamine 2.5–10 µg/kg/minute plus a 'renal' dose of dopamine 2 µg/kg/minute (higher doses of dopamine reduce renal perfusion).

● Venesection and positive pressure ventilation very occasionally required in extreme cases.

HYPERTENSION

It has been recognized for many years that high blood pressure is associated with an increased risk of MI and strokes. However the cut off between normal pressure and hypertension remains controversial. It is generally agreed that individuals less than 60 years with a BP consistently above 140/99 mmHg should be treated as should those older patients with a BP >160/100 mmHg. Clinical trials of treatment of such patients have shown a reduction in deaths from both IHD and strokes although the benefit varies in different studies regarding such factors as sex and smoking.

Screening The majority of individuals with hypertension are asymptomatic and therefore detection depends for a large part on screening. It is important that the blood pressure should be checked on more than one occasion some weeks apart before a diagnosis of hypertension is made.

Aetiology In approximately 90% no obvious cause can be found and the patients are labelled as having essential hypertension. In the remaining minority the cause can be identified as due to: renal disease, such as renal artery stenosis due to fibromuscular dysplasia or atheroma, chronic glomerulonephritis or pyelonephritis, polycystic kidneys or renal vasculitis; endocrine causes including Conn's syndrome, Cushing's syndrome, acromegaly, diabetes mellitus and phaeochromocytoma; other causes including coarctation of the aorta, polycythaemia vera, toxaemia of pregnancy and drugs (eg prednisolone).

Clinical features

Symptoms: usually none, occasionally headache, cardiac failure, MI and renal failure.

Signs: other than high blood pressure, retinopathy, LVF and LV heave. Bruits may be heard in coarctation of the aorta and in renal artery stenosis. Grading severity: four stages according to the retinal findings exist:

- Stage I: arteriolar narrowing

- Stage II: arteriolar irregularity

- Stage III: 'blot' and 'flame' haemorrhages and 'cotton wool' exudates

- Stage IV: papilloedema, associated with malignant hypertension

Investigations • In all patients CXR, ECG (→ Fig. 3.10, p 42), urinalysis and urea, electrolytes and creatinine • In se-

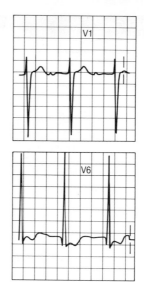

Fig. 3.10
Left ventricular hypertrophy.

lected patients, especially if young or if biochemical or clinical results indicate, IVU, urinary metadrenaline, urinary free cortisol and plasma aldosterone to exclude renal artery stenosis, phaeochromocytoma, Cushing's syndrome and Conn's syndrome respectively.

Management This depends upon the cause. If a correctable lesion is found such as renal artery stenosis or Conn's syndrome treatment for this should be undertaken. For those in whom no cause is identified treatment is along the following lines:

- Reduction of excessive dietary salt intake.

- Reduction of stress, where possible.

- Weight reduction, if appropriate.

- Thiazide (eg bendrofluazide 5 mg) or β-blocker (eg atenolol 50 mg) both have adverse reactions and treatment should be tailored to the individual.

If hypertension remains:

- Add a vasodilator such as a calcium antagonist (eg nifedipine 10–20 mg tid), an ACE-inhibitor (eg captopril 25 mg tid) with a loop diuretic or hydralazine 25–50 mg bd. Again the treatment regimen, which often involves three or more drugs, should be tailored to the patient who may have to take such medications for many years. A close check should be kept on U+Es and creatinine to ensure renal function is not compromised.

In malignant hypertension ie diastolic BP >120 mmHg with symptoms such as encephalopathy, cardiac failure and/or deteriorating renal function, the BP should be reduced as suggested below. However in certain clinical circumstances very high BP may be found transiently, such as occurs with a CVA, where rapid reduction of hypertension may be detrimental.

Treatment of malignant hypertension is essential as the 12-month survival untreated is only 10%. The patient should be admitted to hospital, put on bed-rest and started on oral nifedipine 10–20 mg tid or oral metoprolol 50–100 mg promptly. Intravenous therapy with labetalol 2 mg/minute (max 200 mg) should be administered to those with encephalopathy. Once the BP is controlled oral maintenance therapy (see above) should be commenced.

MITRAL VALVE DISEASE

MITRAL STENOSIS

Aetiology   At one time common but now relatively rare following the falling incidence of rheumatic fever. Since the scarring process on the valves may take many years new cases may still be recognized in the elderly, in whom a history of rheumatic fever may be found in 50%.

Clinical features

Symptoms: breathlessness, particularly during pregnancy, cough and haemoptysis.

Signs: malar flush, peripheral embolism, atrial fibrillation, tapping apex beat, loud first heart sound, opening snap and a low-pitched, rumbling diastolic murmur with presystolic accentuation in patients in sinus rhythm. Endocarditis is uncommon with pure mitral stenosis.

Investigations   ● CXR may show L atrial enlargement and pulmonary congestion ● ECG p-mitrale or atrial fibrillation ● echocardiography is important in both diagnosis and assessing the severity of stenosis by means chamber enlargement, valve motion and doppler studies ● Cardiac catheterization may be used to quantitate the gradient across the valve, the cardiac output and R heart pressures.

Management Many patients because of age or associated medical disorders are treated with diuretics, digoxin for patients in AF and with warfarin because of the risk of peripheral embolism. Definitive treatment is surgical, either by mitral valvulotomy if the stenosis is not accompanied by regurgitation or by valve replacement if regurgitation or heavy calcification exists.

MITRAL REGURGITATION

Aetiology Includes myxomatous degeneration, papillary muscle dysfunction, rheumatic heart disease, mitral valve prolapse, secondary to LV dilatation due to cardiomyopathy or post MI.

Clinical features

Symptoms: fatigue and breathlessness.

Signs: large pulse pressure, LV heave, soft S_1, wide splitting of S_2, S_3, and an apical pansystolic murmur radiating towards the axilla.

Investigations • CXR may show cardiac enlargement and • ECG, LVH and AF • echocardiography may reveal an enlarged LA, LV or abnormal mitral valve and • Doppler studies can be useful in assessing the severity • Cardiac catheterization may be used to quantitate the severity of regurgitation.

Management In many patients treatment is of the associated cardiac failure and controlling associated arrhythmias. In patients with severe mitral regurgitation valve replacement should be considered.

Mitral valve prolapse: This is most often idiopathic and identified in otherwise entirely well young females. Some patients present with atypical chest pain or cardiac arrhythmias. Examination reveals a mid-systolic click and late systolic murmur. The diagnosis is confirmed by echocardiography and no treatment required except prophylaxis against endocarditis ($\rightarrow$ p 47). In a small proportion progressive mitral regurgitation develops.

AORTIC VALVE DISEASE

AORTIC STENOSIS

Aetiology Congenital and rheumatic in younger ages and calcification of congenital bicuspid valve and degenerative in the elderly. Subaortic stenosis may complicate hypertrophic cardiomyopathy and supravalvar stenosis may be associated with infantile hypercalcaemia (often with facial deformity).

Clinical features

Symptoms: dyspnoea, angina, syncope and sudden death (although often asymptomatic).

Signs: plateau pulse, small pulse pressure, heaving apex beat, basal thrill, ejection systolic murmur maximal in the right 2nd intercostal space radiating to the neck, with a quiet 2nd sound and often a 4th sound ($\rightarrow$ Table 3.2). An ejection click may be present and excludes supra- or subaortic stenosis.

Investigation ● ECG: LV (+LA) hypertrophy ● CXR: cardiomegaly and post-stenotic dilatation of the proximal aorta ● Echocardiography: LV hypertrophy, valve orifice size, valve cusp appearance and opening abnormal ● Doppler echogram: useful in predicting gradient across valve.

Complications LVF, arrhythmias (including sudden death), infective endocarditis.

> *Management* Treat cardiac failure and angina avoiding after-load reduction, avoid strenuous exercise. Valve replacement in symptomatic patients with gradient >50 mm Hg. Balloon valvuloplasty in the elderly is controversial. Antibiotic prophylaxis for invasive procedures.

AORTIC REGURGITATION

Aetiology Congenital bicuspid valve, endocarditis, rheumatic. Uncommon: syphilis, connective tissue disease (SLE, ankylosing spondylitis, Reiter's and Behcet's syndrome), Marfan's syndrome, coarctation, aortic dissection and traumatic rupture.

Clinical features

Symptoms: often none, dyspnoea, palpitations, angina uncommon.

Signs: collapsing pulse, wide pulse pressure, cardiac apex displacement, early blowing diastolic murmur maximal at left sternal edge with patient sitting forward in full expiration. Systolic flow murmur common. Diastolic murmur at apex similar to mitral stenosis (Austin Flint). 2nd sound soft and 3rd sound common.

Investigation ● ECG: LV hypertrophy ● CXR: cardiomegaly ● echocardiography: dilated aortic root or valve cusp abnormality and mitral valve fluttering ● Doppler studies aid in quantifying regurgitation.

Complications   Cardiac failure, endocarditis.

> *Management*   Treat cardiac failure and underlying disease if possible. Valve replacement for severe regurgitation in symptomatic patients or those asymptomatic subjects with LV dysfunction or LV end systolic internal diameter >5.5 cm. Antibiotic prophylaxis for invasive procedures.

Table 3.2
Heart murmur characteristics

Lesion	Murmur	Heart sounds	Radiation
MS	Mid-diastolic (patient on L side)	Loud S_1 opening snap	None
MR	Pansystolic	Soft S_1, split S_2 S_3 common	Axilla
AS	Ejection systolic	Soft delayed A_2 S_4 common	Neck
AR	Early diastolic (patient sitting forward)	Soft A_2 S_3 common	L sternal edge

INFECTIVE ENDOCARDITIS

> Infective endocarditis, the infection of cardiac valves, usually by bacteria is a serious but frequently preventable disorder. The valves involved are usually but not invariably abnormal before the infection. Clinically three types are recognized.

Subacute infective endocarditis: which is characterized by an insidious onset, pyrexia, night sweats and fatigue.

Clinical features: include haematuria, retinal infarcts, Osler's nodes, peripheral infarcts, changing murmur, joint pains and splenomegaly. The valve abnormalities at most risk are bicuspid aortic, rheumatic and prosthetic valves, particularly if regurgitant. Other sites of infection include VSD and PDA. The organism most often involved is *Strep. viridans*; others include staphylococci, *Strep. faecalis* and coliforms. Infection with *Strep. bovis* is associated with colonic cancer.

Acute or fulminant endocarditis: is much less common and previously normal valves may be affected. For this reason the diagnosis may be delayed with dire consequences as the disorder is rapidly fatal. *Staph. aureus* is the usual organism. Features include pyrexia, retinal haemorrhages (Roth spots), petechiae and peripheral emboli.

Right-sided endocarditis: presents with pleuritic chest pain, pyrexia, breathlessness and fatigue. Risk factors are iv drug abuse and the presence of central iv lines. The tricuspid valve is most usually involved resulting in multiple pulmonary infarcts, abscesses and severe right-sided cardiac failure.

Investigation • The most important test is numerous sets of blood cultures (at least 4) over a 24–36-hour period • Antibiotics must not be administered before these are taken • Supplementary investigations include echocardiography for vegetations (this may be negative in 30–40%), FBC showing a leukocytosis and a normochromic, normocytic anaemia and elevated ESR • Haematuria containing casts and a reduced serum C3 is common. Approximately 20% of cases are culture negative, either because antibiotics have been administered before blood cultures were taken or the infecting organism is difficult to identify such as fungi or coxiella.

> **Management** This should be tailored to the organism identified and bacteriological advice should be sought. Antibiotics should be administered parenterally for at least two weeks and for longer in many cases. For penicillin sensitive streptococci benzylpenicillin 10–20 million units daily in divided doses along with gentamicin 1 mg/kg tid for 2 weeks followed by amoxycillin 500 mg tid for a further 2 weeks.

Prevention This is vitally important and all patients with abnormal or prosthetic valves and those with VSDs and hypertrophic obstructive cardiomyopathy should receive prophylaxis before procedures likely to produce bacteraemia.

Procedures: dental and oral surgery and bronchoscopy – 3 g oral amoxycillin 1 hour before (oral erythromycin should be used in penicillin sensitive subjects or in those who have taken penicillin within 4 weeks, 1.5 g 1 h before and 0.5 g 6 h later); GI and GU surgery or endoscopy, bladder catheterization – ampicillin 1 g plus gentamicin 1 mg/kg before and ampicillin 500 mg 6 hours later. Prolonged or repeated courses of antibiotic encourage the emergence of antibiotic resistant organisms.

CONGENITAL HEART DISEASE

> Traditionally congenital heart disease is divided into cyanotic (R to L shunt) and acyanotic (L to R, or no shunt).

CYANOTIC

These are uncommon, particularly in adults since mortality without corrective surgery is high. The best known is Fallot's tetralogy which consists of pulmonary stenosis, VSD over which the aorta takes its origin and RVH. Eisenmenger's complex is said to exist when reversal of the L to R shunt in VSD occurs with pulmonary hypertension. The other form of cyanotic congenital heart disease is transposition of the great vessels. This is rapidly fatal without intervention by Rashkind's procedure or surgery.

ACYANOTIC

These include ASD, VSD, patent ductus arteriosus, aortic coarctation and pulmonary stenosis. In those disorders with L to R shunts the development of pulmonary hypertension may result in shunt reversal and cyanosis. Significant pulmonary hypertension is a contraindication to surgery and treatment must aim to prevent its development.

Atrial septal defect
This is often unsuspected until adult life when breathlessness and palpitations present.

Signs: prominent v wave of JVP, L parasternal heave, fixed splitting of S_2 and parasternal systolic and tricuspid diastolic flow murmurs.

Investigations • CXR: prominent pulmonary vasculature and RV • ECG: partial RBBB and RAD (LAD with ostium primum defect, which is less common than secundum defects) • Echocardiography: enlargement of RA and RV. Transatrial and increased pulmonary flow may be detected by • Doppler studies.

> ***Management*** For those with a pulmonary flow 1.5x greater than systemic flow surgery is indicated unless pulmonary hypertension exists.

Ventricular septal defect
These are commonly asymptomatic and may close during childhood.

Clinical features In adults this is with fatigue and breathlessness.

Signs: systolic thrill, loud P_2, S_3, loud pansystolic murmur at lower L sternal border and a diastolic mitral flow murmur.

Investigations • CXR: prominence of pulmonary vasculature • ECG: may be normal, or show LV hypertrophy

• Echocardiography: visualization of VSD in some, LA, RV and LV enlargement in those with large shunts and • Doppler demonstration of L to R flow.

> *Management* As for ASD with same criteria for surgery. Prophylaxis against endocarditis.

Patent ductus arteriosus

The failure of closure of the ductus arteriosus, between the aorta and the pulmonary artery, which is commoner with maternal rubella, may be asymptomatic for years.

Clinical features

Symptoms: This usually presents with fatigue and breathlessness on exertion.

Signs: thrusting apex beat, systolic-diastolic 'machinery' murmur at L upper sternal edge.

Investigations • CXR: prominent pulmonary vasculature, enlarged ascending aorta • ECG, LVH • echocardiography on 2-D echo the patent ductus may be visualized, whilst • Doppler may demonstrate turbulent flow in the PA.

> *Management* Ligation providing pulmonary hypertension has not developed. Prophylaxis against endocarditis.

Coarctation of the aorta

This disorder, a narrowing of the aorta just beyond the L subclavian artery, may be asymptomatic or present with hypertension, heart failure or poor perfusion in the lower limbs.

Signs: hypertension measured in the arm, radial-femoral pulse delay, visible collateral intercostal and periscapular vessels, systolic murmur posterosuperiorly.

Investigation • CXR: rib notching • ECG: LVH.

> *Management* Surgery; prophylaxis against endocarditis.

Other congenital heart disorders

These include: bicuspid aortic valves which usually cause no symptoms until late in life when stenosis may develop, pulmonary stenosis when the patient may occasionally be cyanosed, and dextrocardia which usually cause more problems for the doctor than the patient!

PERICARDITIS

> Pericarditis, inflammation of the pericardium, is common and causes include: MI, viral infection (particularly

coxsackie), malignancy, renal failure, tuberculosis, Dressler's syndrome, connective tissue disorders and trauma.

Clinical features

Symptoms: usually sharp, localized chest pain characteristically relieved by leaning forward. It may occasionally have a pleuritic element, pleuropericarditis.

Signs: pericardial rub at L sternal edge, commonly present only transiently. Evidence of RVF, pulsus paradoxus and a rising JVP on inspiration may accompany a pericardial effusion that is causing cardiac tamponade ($\rightarrow$ Fig. 3.11).

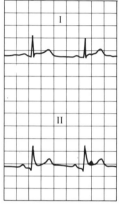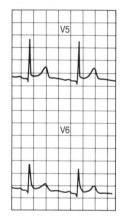

Fig. 3.11
Pericarditis.

Investigations ● ECG ST elevation without reciprocal ST depression ● CXR may show globular cardiac enlargement suggestive of an effusion which should be confirmed by echocardiography.

Management Should be of underlying disorder plus analgesia with NSAIDs. Large pericardial effusions, associated with pulsus paradoxus, RVF and hypotension require aspiration under ECG and echocardiographic monitoring and with cardiac surgical backup. This may also be necessary for diagnostic purposes. The aspirate should be examined biochemically, bacteriologically and by cytology.

CONSTRICTIVE PERICARDITIS

A rigid pericardial sac which limits ventricular filling, may be caused by TB, malignancy, renal failure, viral infection and post cardiac surgery.

Clinical features

Symptoms: These include fatigue, ankle and abdominal swelling and breathlessness.

Signs: raised JVP which rises with inspiration (Kussmaul's sign), tachycardia with low volume pulse, ascites, ankle oedema and occasionally a pericardial knock after S_2.

Investigations • ECG may have low voltage • CXR small cardiac shadow sometimes with peripheral calcification • Echocardiography shows a thickened pericardium and, unlike restrictive cardiomyopathy, a normally contracting ventricle.

Management Surgical resection of the pericardium.

PERIPHERAL VASCULAR DISEASE

ARTERIAL

Large vessel disease

In Western society this is almost invariably due to atherosclerosis. Other rare causes include giant cell arteritis, Buerger's disease and Takayasu's disease. Risk factors for atheroma include hypertension, diabetes mellitus, hyperlipidaemia, smoking, male sex, family history and age. The lower limbs and cerebral vessels are commonly involved whilst the upper limb vessels are usually spared. Cerebrovascular disease is discussed elsewhere (p 149).

Clinical features These depend upon whether the arterial insufficiency develops acutely eg arterial emboli or over a long period.

Symptoms: these depend upon the vessel involved and the speed of onset but the commonest include hemiparesis and intermittent claudication.

Signs: these also vary with the vessel involved and include carotid bruit, hemiplegia, absent peripheral pulses, peripheral ulceration and gangrene, absent digits and cold, cyanosed peripheries..

Investigations • angiography of the implicated vessels is the investigation of choice and will demonstrate the site and severity of the stenosis. Other less invasive tests include • thermography and • Doppler flow studies.

Management All patients with atheromatous disease of medium and large arteries should be strongly advised to stop smoking which is the single most important risk factor. Treatment of hyperlipidaemia and hypertension should also be addressed. Increased perfusion to ischaemic tissues can be realized by reducing blood viscosity and venesection, if the patient is polycythaemic, and iv dextran may be useful. Low dose aspirin therapy (300 mg/d) reduces platelet aggregability and may produce benefit in reducing thrombi but is associated with increased risk of cerebral haemorrhage. Oral anticoagulation with warfarin is of value when cardiac emboli are the cause of ischaemia. Where localized arterial disease is identified surgery offers most benefit in the form of angioplasty and bypass. Endarterectomy, formerly popular for carotid stenosis, has been shown to be of limited value.

Small vessel disease

Disorders which result in disease of, or occlusion of, small vessels include diabetes mellitus, arteritides such as polyarteritis nodosa, rheumatoid disease and SLE, hyperviscosity such as myeloma, Waldenstrom's macroglobulinaemia, polycythaemia and cryoglobulinaemia, and Raynaud's syndrome. Disease or occlusion of arterioles results in clinically apparent lesions in the peripheral circulation (fingers and toes) but also lesions in the circulation to internal organs such as the kidneys, heart, eyes and brain.

Clinical features

Symptoms: these again depend upon the site of disease but common symptoms include cold hands and feet often with pain and changes in colour.

Signs: small infarcts of extremities and ulceration, haematuria, retinal infarcts and haemorrhages and cold peripheries with good peripheral pulses.

Investigations ● For diabetes: fasting blood glucose and HbAlc ● myeloma: immunoelectrophoresis, Bence-Jones proteinuria and serum calcium ● haematological disease: haemoglobin, haematocrit, platelet count and ● connective tissue disease: ESR, ANF, C3 and renal angiography.

Management This depends upon the underlying disease.

VENOUS DISEASE

Two forms of venous thrombosis are recognized, thrombophlebitis, where the endothelium of the vein is inflamed and phlebothrombosis, a primary thrombosis in an otherwise normal vessel which carries a higher risk of pulmonary embolism.

Risk factors include sluggish peripheral circulation, increased viscosity of the blood, damage to the vein, and malignancy (eg pancreatic cancer).

Clinical features Usually pain with accompanying signs of localized inflammation in thrombophlebitis and swelling, superficial venous distension, increased temperature, red discolouration and tenderness in deep venous thrombosis. The differential diagnosis includes musculoskeletal disorders, cellulitis, lymphangitis and a ruptured Baker's cyst.

Investigations ● The diagnosis of thrombophlebitis is usually obvious but deep venous thrombosis is notoriously difficult; diagnosis on the basis of physical signs is erroneous in a large minority whilst signs may be absent in those with venous thrombosis ● The definitive test is venography and is essential for the diagnosis of thrombosis in the pelvic veins. Other tests such as ● thermography and ● radio-labelled fibrinogen scans are useful in the diagnosis of more distal thromboses.

> *Management* Thrombophlebitis usually requires only symptomatic therapy and anticoagulation is not indicated unless the deep veins are also involved. Phlebothrombosis with its accompanying risk of pulmonary emboli and chronic venous insufficiency should be treated initially with iv heparin (approximately 1000 units/h, the dose depending upon the thrombin time), followed by oral anticoagulants, usually warfarin, for at least 4 weeks. Prophylactic measures, such as subcutaneous heparin, should be considered in bed-bound patients at risk of, or with a past history of, DVT.

CARDIOMYOPATHY AND MYOCARDITIS

Cardiomyopathy and myocarditis represent diseases of cardiac muscle excluding IHD. The term cardiomyopathy is used to denote an abnormality of the myocardium capable of producing heart failure whilst myocarditis is applied to those where there is an inflammatory process, most often infective.

CARDIOMYOPATHIES

These can be divided into three main groups:

Dilated: characterized by dilatation of the R and L ventricles and impaired ejection fraction; clinically the apex beat is diffuse and displaced, S1 is often quiet and a gallop rhythm and MR common ● echocardiography is invaluable diagnostically although the clinical history ● ECG and ● coronary angiography are important in excluding alcoholic and IHD; treatment is of the associated cardiac failure and the prognosis poor. Warfarin should be considered because of the risk of systemic emboli.

Hypertrophic: this is commonly familial and characterized by marked hypertrophy of the ventricle and/or interventricular septum; the latter commonly resulting in obstruction to LV outflow, HOCM). Clinical examination may reveal a 'jerky' pulse, double apical impulse and a systolic murmur. ● Echocardiography usually confirms the diagnosis. Treatment is with β-blockers or calcium antagonists to reduce the heart rate and contractility and amiodarone to treat ventricular arrhythmias. Digoxin and vasodilators may increase outflow obstruction and should be avoided. The prognosis is variable and the condition is not infrequently identified at autopsy in young adults with sudden death.

Restrictive: characterized by reduced compliance (or increased stiffness) of the ventricles which reduces ventricular filling. It occurs in endocardial eosinophilia, cardiac amyloid and tropical endomyocardial fibrosis. The diagnosis should be suspected in patients with cardiac failure and normal systolic function. Cardiac biopsy will differentiate pericardial constriction from endocardial disease. Treatment is symptomatic, most usually with diuretics.

MYOCARDITIS

Aetiology Causes include ● infective: viral (influenza and Coxsackie B), bacterial (diphtheria) and protozoal (Chaga's disease) ● metabolic: pregnancy, thyroid disease, haemochromatosis, thiamine deficiency and amyloidosis ● connective tissue disease: SLE ● infiltrative leukaemia and sarcoidosis: ● Neuromuscular: muscular dystrophy and Friedreich's ataxia ● drugs: alcohol, phenothiazines and arsenic ● radiation.

Clinical features May present like IHD of sudden onset with pain, sinus tachycardia with or without a third heart sound, cardiac failure and arrhythmias.

Investigations ● ECG for arrhythmias and to exclude MI ● CXR often reveals cardiomegaly and LVF ● echocardiography to exclude pericardial effusion and mitral stenosis ● Serology to identify recent viral infection or connective tissue disease.

Management This depends upon the underlying cause but in many is symptomatic. Steroid therapy (prednisolone initially 40 mg/d) is indicated in those with connective tissue disease. The prognosis in the majority of patients is good.

4

Respiratory disease

INVESTIGATIONS

Much can be learnt of a patient's respiratory disorder from a thorough history and examination. Common investigations include:

CXR This is the single most important investigation in respiratory medicine and provides essential information concerning the underlying disease process in many patients eg pneumonia, pulmonary fibrosis, tuberculosis, sarcoidosis and carcinoma. Some patients may have serious or advanced respiratory disease with a normal CXR eg asthma. Ideally both a PA and lateral view should be obtained.

Sputum microscopy and culture This is of considerable importance in order to select the appropriate antibiotic. Cytological examination of sputum, especially if repeated on three samples is a reasonably sensitive test for bronchial carcinoma.

Peak expiratory flow rate This is a useful bedside and outpatient method for monitoring the severity of asthma and response to therapy.

Arterial blood gas analysis Because clinical signs such as cyanosis may be unreliable all patients with acute respiratory disease should have PaO_2, $PaCO_2$, $H+$ and HCO_3 concentrations measured in arterial blood.

Spirometry This again is a simple side-room test which allows measurement of the vital capacity and FEV_1 and allows separation of restrictive from obstructive airway disease ($\rightarrow$ Figs 4.1 & 4.2).

Bronchoscopy This allows direct visualization of the proximal bronchial tree with the facility to take cytological specimens and biopsies from bronchi and lung parenchyma. Lavage fluid obtained is useful in the diagnosis of interstitial lung disease and *Pneumocystis carinii*.

Radio-isotopic ventilation and perfusion scans These are important in the diagnosis of pulmonary embolism. Pulmonary angiography is indicated when the results are inconclusive.

Percutaneous pleural biopsy This is useful in the diagnosis of tuberculosis, carcinoma and mesothelioma.

CT scanning This has largely replaced tomography in the accurate localization and staging of pulmonary lesions. It also has a place in the diagnosis of pulmonary fibrosis and bronchiectasis.

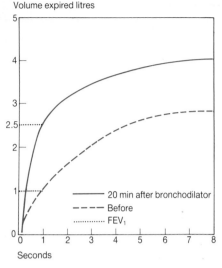

Fig. 4.1
Reversibility test. Forced expiratory manoeuvres before and 20 min. after inhalation of a beta₂ adrenoreceptor agonist. Note the increase in FEV₁ from 1.0 to 2.5 litres.

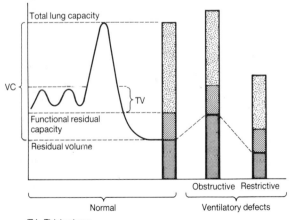

TV: Tidal volume
VC: Vital capacity

Fig. 4.2
Normal lung volumes and the changes which occur in obstructive and restrictive ventilatory defects.

CHEST X-RAY

The chest X-ray is an important part of the investigation of any patient with either cardiac or lung disease. Its examination should be systematic (→ Figs. 4.3 & 4.4):

- Check the name on the film and L and R markers.

- Check whole chest is on film and penetration satisfactory.

- Note trachea is central, mediastinum of normal width and hila position normal (the L hilum may be up to 2 cm higher than the R).

- Assess cardiothoracic ratio (the sum of the maximum width of the heart on either side of the midline divided by the maximum internal diameter of the chest), should be less than 50% in healthy adults on a PA film and is increased in cardiac failure, pericardial effusion, L or R ventricular hypertrophy.

- Pulmonary vessels: plethoric in L to R shunts and hyper-dynamic states; oligaemic in recent pulmonary emboli, cardiac tamponade, RV failure and R to L shunts. In pulmonary hypertension large central arteries rapidly 'prune' to give peripheral oligaemia. Pulmonary venous hypertension, most often due to LV failure, is manifest as distension of upper lobe veins (→ Tables 4.1 & 4.2, p 60).

- Lung fields: identify any obvious abnormality and then move on to comparing the two sides. Look particularly at the lung markings on the two sides and follow them to the lung edge. The apices and costophrenic angles should be closely scrutinized. Lobar collapse is a common finding in bronchial carcinoma (→ Tables 4.3 & 4.4, pp 60–61).

- Bones: these should be systematically studied looking for erosion, notching and fractures.

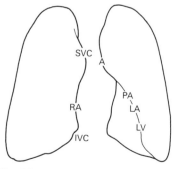

SVC	Superior vena cava
RA	Right atrium
LA	Left atrium
IVC	Inferior vena cava
PA	Pulmonary artery
LV	Left ventricle
A	Aorta

Fig. 4.3
A normal CXR.

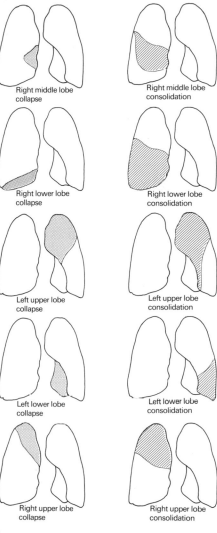

Fig. 4.4
Common CXR abnormalities.

- Soft tissues: surgical emphysema, air in the soft tissues, may be missed if not looked for, as may a mastectomy.

If a CXR in an exam initially looks normal the following should be excluded:

- A small apical pneumothorax.
- A fluid level behind the heart due to a hiatus hernia.
- R middle lobe collapse with loss of clarity of the R heart border.
- L lower lobe collapse with absence of the outline of the L diaphragm behind the heart (sail sign).
- A deviated trachea.
- Paratracheal lymphadenopathy.
- Air beneath the diaphragm.
- Rib notching.
- A mastectomy.
- Dextrocardia with the film reversed.

Table 4.1
Causes of bilateral hilar enlargement

Sarcoidosis
Lymphoma
Tuberculosis
Pulmonary hypertension
Pulmonary embolism
Septal defects
Silicosis

Table 4.2
Causes of unilateral hilar enlargement

Bronchial carcinoma
Tuberculosis
Sarcoidosis
Lymphoma
Pulmonary embolism

Table 4.3
Causes of pulmonary nodules

Bronchial carcinoma
Metastases
Pulmonary infarct
Adenoma/hamartoma
Tuberculoma
Abscesses
Arteriovenous malformation
Rheumatoid nodule
Wegener's granulomatosis
Sequestrated lobule
Fluid in oblique fissure ("vanishing tumour")

Table 4.4
Causes of complete opacification of one lung field

Massive pleural effusion
Pneumonectomy
Complete lung collapse
Complete lung consolidation
Mesothelioma

UPPER RESPIRATORY TRACT INFECTION

The upper respiratory tract extends from the oropharynx to the trachea. This region is the entrance to the lungs and is the boundary between the mouth which contains numerous commensal microorganisms and the sterile pulmonary apparatus. Infections in this region are common but usually self-limiting.

Acute coryza (common cold)
This common disorder is due to infection with rhinoviruses, corona-, entero- and adeno-viruses and respiratory syncytial virus.

Clinical features

Symptoms: usually start acutely with sneezing, dry sore throat, headache and rhinorrhoea. Although usually rapidly self-limiting, complications may occur and include sinusitis, otitis media and pneumonia. Symptoms of coryza which recur frequently during the summer are usually due to allergy rather than persistent viral infection.

Acute sinusitis
This disorder which frequently follows an acute viral upper respiratory tract infection is most often due to *H. influenzae*, *Strep. pneumoniae* or *Strep. pyogenes*.

Clinical features These include localized pain and tenderness over the involved sinus, pyrexia and headaches.

Investigations The diagnosis is usually clinical although X-rays usually demonstrate thickening of the sinus mucosa or a fluid level.

Management Antibiotics eg ampicillin 500 mg qid, nasal vasoconstrictors and if necessary operative drainage. Delayed or unsuccessful treatment may lead to chronic sinusitis, meningitis, venous sinus thrombosis or osteomyelitis.

Acute pharyngitis

This is most often due to viral infection (eg EBV) or *Strep. pyogenes*.

Clinical features   Usually there is only a sore throat but in more severe attacks dysphagia may occur. Examination reveals pharyngeal inflammation, lymphoid hypertrophy and, in some, an exudate.

> **Management**   In most patients no treatment is needed other than some symptomatic relief. Where bacterial infection is suspected a throat swab should be taken before antibiotic therapy is started eg ampicillin 500 mg qid or erythromycin 500 mg qid. Avoid ampicillin with EBV.

Complications   In cases of bacterial pharyngitis complications include peritonsillar and parapharyngeal abscess both of which may require surgical intervention.

Acute laryngitis

This is usually a complication of coryza or an infectious disease such as measles. It is characterized by a sore throat with a hoarse voice accompanied by a non-productive cough and is usually rapidly self-limiting although repeated attacks may predispose to chronic laryngitis.

Acute epiglottitis

This potentially lethal disorder is usually due to *H. influenzae* infection in young children.

Clinical features   These include cough, sore throat without hoarseness. In more severe cases stridor may progress to laryngeal obstruction. Where acute epiglottitis is suspected direct visualization of the epiglottis using tongue depressors should be avoided as such instrumentation may precipitate obstruction of the airway.

> **Management**   This is with oxygen, adequate hydration and iv ampicillin 500 mg qid or chloramphenicol 500 mg qid.

Acute laryngotracheobronchitis (croup)

This disease of young children is caused by viral infection usually with the parainfluenza group. Superinfection with bacteria is not uncommon.

Clinical features   These include bouts of coughing, breathlessness, fever, stridor and cyanosis.

> **Management**   Humidification of the air or oxygen helps breathing and loosens secretions. Antibiotics should be used in cases where bacterial superinfection is suspected.

Occasionally bronchoscopy and/or endotracheal intubation may be required to clear secretions from the upper airways.

Acute bronchitis

This disorder is usually a complication of viral upper respiratory tract infection and is due in most cases to pneumococcal, *H. influenzae* or *Staph. aureus* infection. Risk factors include cigarette smoking and damp or dusty conditions.

Clinical features

Symptoms: include cough, retrosternal pain and wheeze.

Signs: rhonchi and coarse crepitations and then productive sputum from which the infecting organism can be cultured.

Management This is with appropriate antibiotics usually amoxycillin 250 mg tid or ampicillin 500 mg qid.

Influenza

This deserves special mention as a cause of upper respiratory tract infection because of its potential severity. It is caused by a group of myxoviruses, influenza viruses A and B. Different strains of these viral types exist and cause epidemics or pandemics.

Clinical features

Symptoms: include headache, myalgia, anorexia and fever.

Signs: commonly absent other than pharyngitis unless complications develop.

Management Symptomatic for fever, aches and pains and cough. Prevention with vaccines should be sought particularly for the elderly and those with chronic chest problems. Because of the difference in antigenicity between different viral strains no single vaccine can confer immunity for more than one strain.

Complications Secondary bacterial infection eg *Staph. aureus* of the upper and lower respiratory tract is common. Viral encephalitis and demyelinating encephalopathy may occur as may cardiomyopathy. The mortality during epidemics, particularly in the elderly and infirm, may be high.

RESPIRATORY FAILURE

This is defined as a respiratory disorder of such extent that respiratory function is inadequate for the individual's metabolic requirements. It is divided into two types:

Type I: hypoxaemia (PaO_2 < 8.0 kPa) without CO_2 retention

Type II: hypoxaemia and hypercapnia ($PaCO_2$ >6.0 kPa).

Table 4.5
Types and causes of respiratory failure

	Type I		Type II	
	Acute	Chronic	Acute	Chronic
	$PaO_2 \downarrow\downarrow$	$PaO_2 \downarrow$	$PaO_2 \downarrow$	$PaO_2 \downarrow$
	$PaCO_2 \leftrightarrow$	$PaCO_2 \leftrightarrow$	$PaCO_2 \uparrow$	$PaCO_2 \uparrow$
	$pH \leftrightarrow$	$pH \leftrightarrow$	$pH \downarrow$	$pH \downarrow$ or $\leftrightarrow$
	$HCO_3 \leftrightarrow$	$HCO_3 \leftrightarrow$	$HCO_3 \leftrightarrow$	$HCO_3 \uparrow$
	Asthma	Emphysema 'pink puffer'	Acute epiglottitis	Chronic bronchitis 'blue bloater'
	Pul oedema	Thrombo-embolic pul HT	Severe acute asthma	Primary alveolar hypoventilation
	Pul embolus	Lymphatic carcinomatosis	Respiratory muscle paralysis	
	ARDS			
	Pul fibrosis			

Clinical features In both types of respiratory failure hypoxia may be accompanied by central cyanosis, breathlessness and confusion whilst hypercapnia may be associated with a coarse tremor (asterixis), warm peripheries, a bounding pulse, peripheral oedema and papilloedema.

Investigations ● clinical examination ● ABG ● CXR ● PEFR ● spirometry ● FBC and ● sputum culture may help establish the cause.

Management Type I failure treat hypoxia with unrestricted oxygen therapy (35% +) and repeat gases after 20 minutes to ensure correction of PaO_2 and absence of a significant rise in $PaCO_2$. In type II failure 24% or at the most 28% oxygen should be administered and close monitoring of the $PaCO_2$ maintained. Since many patients with COLD maintain adequate ventilation by stimulation from hypoxia rather than the $PaCO_2$ level correction of hypoxia with high flow oxygen may depress respiration resulting in CO_2 narcosis and death. If adequate correction of hypoxia cannot be achieved without worsening hypercapnia mechanical ventilation may be indicated if the underlying pathology is reversible. In those patients where this is not considered appropriate respiratory stimulants such as iv doxapram 1–4 mg/minute have some value. Other treatment depends upon the cause. Physiotherapy is important in the management of exacerbations of COLD as is appropriate antibiotic therapy. Bronchodilators and steroids are indicated if airways obstruction exists.

CHRONIC OBSTRUCTIVE LUNG DISEASE

This term is usually applied to patients with chronic bronchitis or emphysema. Many patients have a mixture of these disorders and classification is often on the basis of the major abnormality. Chronic bronchitis is defined symptomatically as the production of sputum daily for three months of the year for two consecutive years. Emphysema is defined anatomically as the distension of airways distal to the terminal bronchioles accompanied by destruction of alveolar walls.

Classification: 'blue bloaters', patients with cor pulmonale, hypoxia, at risk of CO_2 retention and 'pink puffers', those with hyperinflation, low PaO_2 and frequently low $PaCO_2$ levels.

Aetiology The most important risk factor for COLD is cigarette smoking. Other causes include occupational exposure to irritants such as coal dust. α_1-antitrypsin deficiency predisposes to emphysema. In many patients with subclinical lung disease an acute respiratory infection may precipitate respiratory failure as well as worsen the underlying pulmonary problem.

Clinical features In 'blue bloaters' productive cough and breathlessness are characteristic with signs such as cyanosis, peripheral oedema, coarse crepitations and L parasternal heave. Respiratory failure, cor pulmonale and polycythaemia can all develop. In 'pink puffers' breathlessness is the predominant problem associated with signs of tachypnoea, chest hyperinflation with reduced breath sounds.

Investigations ● A thorough clinical history including risk factors ● CXR ● reduced PEFR ● spirometry revealing an obstructive pattern with increased residual volume ● ABG ● reduced transfer factor ● sputum microscopy and culture and ● ECG.

Management Since exacerbations of COLD are often due to lower respiratory tract infections appropriate antibiotics eg ampicillin 500 mg qid or cotrimoxazole 960 mg bd since the infection is usually due to *Strep. pneumoniae* or *H. influenzae* and physiotherapy are important. Where bronchospasm is present treatment with nebulized salbutamol

5 mg and ipratropium bromide 0.5 mg and slow release aminophylline 225 mg bd may produce symptomatic benefit. In more severe cases steriod therapy eg prednisolone 40 mg/day for 10 days may be indicated. Maintenance steroid therapy is rarely indicated and where used the dose should be kept as low as possible. Some patients with acute respiratory failure are candidates for mechanical ventilation although this should only be considered in those who have sufficient respiratory reserve to be weaned from the ventilator upon recovery. Long-term domicillary oxygen therapy has been shown to improve survival in 'blue bloaters' with cor pulmonale. Exercise programmes may be beneficial but the predominant factor is to persuade the patient to stop smoking.

ASTHMA

Asthma is a disorder of the lower airways characterized by wide variations in the airways calibre either spontaneously or as a result of treatment. The bronchoconstriction is intermittent and reversible and varies from mild to life-threatening.

Aetiology This is incompletely understood but immunological mechanisms are undoubtably important. The increased sensitivity of the distal airways may be to readily recognized antigens such as the house dust mite, animal danders or pollens, non-specific trigger factors such as cold or exercise, drugs such as β-blockers and aspirin or to factors which cannot be pinpointed. Patients can generally be divided into those with extrinsic asthma (atopic) and those with intrinsic asthma (non-atopic). In extrinsic asthma allergens can be identified either by skin or provocation tests and a family history of atopy can frequently be established. In intrinsic asthma such trigger factors cannot be established by such methods and a family history is usually absent.

Clinical features

Symptoms: are usually typical consisting of expiratory wheeze and breathlessness frequently worse at night. The patient may be well aware of any trigger factors. In children cough is often the major symptom.

Signs: during an attack chest hyperinflation, tachypnoea, prolonged expiration and an audible expiratory wheeze are typical. In more severe attacks tachycardia, restlessness, pulsus paradoxus and cyanosis occur. A silent chest especially in a patient too distressed to speak indicates a severe attack and requires urgent treatment. Between attacks the patient may have no signs although nasal polyps, sinusitis and skin rashes should be sought.

Investigation • CXR • PEFR • FEV_1/FVC less than 75% and which improves with bronchodilator administration. The FEV usually falls with exercise • FBC and • sputum examination may reveal an eosinophilia. Curschmann's spirals (casts of small airways) may be found in the sputum • ABG analysis establishes the severity. Hypoxia with a low $PaCO_2$ is common but hypoxia with hypercapnia indicates severe disease and requires aggressive therapy and/or ventilation • Hypersensitivity skin tests are useful in identifying atopic individuals.

Management No smoking and avoid precipitating factors where possible. Hyposensitization injections are potentially dangerous and are rarely performed in the UK. Antihistamine drugs are of no value. Maintenance control of day-to-day symptoms is with bronchodilators eg salbutamol inhaler 2 puffs PRN along with regular inhaled corticosteroid eg beclomethasone 100 ? puffs bd. It is vital to ensure adequate inhaler technique and in those not capable of using inhalers administer the drugs via devices such as 'spacers' or using dry powder preparations eg Ventodisks/Becodisks. Disodium cromoglycate (Intal) 20 mg 4–8 times/day is a prophylactic inhaled medication of value in children and those with exercise-induced asthma. Nocturnal symptoms may be improved by sustained release theophyllines eg Uniphyllin 200–400 mg nocte or Phyllocontin 225–450 mg nocte although adverse reactions are common eg nausea, dyspepsia and occasionally life-threatening from cardiac arrythmias. Their use should be undertaken only when plasma levels are checked regularly. Sustained release bronchodilators eg salbutamol 4–8 mg nocte are useful but commonly associated with adverse reactions such as palpitations and tremor. New long acting inhaled beta-agonists (eg Salmeterol) may be useful in nocturnal asthma, in conjunction with inhaled steroids.

The management of severe acute asthma is outlined in Fig. 4.5 (p 68). This requires urgent assessment and aggressive management as it is life-threatening and approximately 1500 deaths still occur annually in the UK. Indications for mechanical ventilation are indicated in Table 4.6 (p 68).

PNEUMONIA

Infection of the parenchyma of the lung can be divided into primary (specific) pneumonia, due to microorganisms with special pathogenicity for lung or secondary (aspiration)

Table 4.6
Indications for mechanical ventilation in asthma

Do not delay until the patient is moribund
● PaO_2 < 6.5 kPa and falling
● $PaCO_2$ > 6.5 kPa and rising
● pH < 7.3 and falling (H^+ > 50 nmol/l and rising)
● Increasing exhaustion and respiratory distress
● Cardiorespiratory arrest

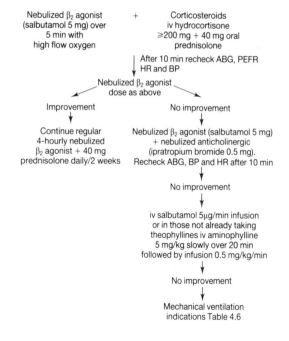

Nebulized β_2 agonist   +   Corticosteroids
(salbutamol 5 mg) over   iv hydrocortisone
5 min with   ≥200 mg + 40 mg oral
high flow oxygen   prednisolone

After 10 min recheck ABG, PEFR
HR and BP

Nebulized β_2 agonist
dose as above

Improvement   No improvement

Continue regular   Nebulized β_2 agonist (salbutamol 5 mg)
4-hourly nebulized   + nebulized anticholinergic
β_2 agonist + 40 mg   (ipratropium bromide 0.5 mg).
prednisolone daily/2 weeks   Recheck ABG, BP and HR after 10 min

No improvement

iv salbutamol 5µg/min infusion
or in those not already taking
theophyllines iv aminophylline
5 mg/kg slowly over 20 min
followed by infusion 0.5 mg/kg/min

No improvement

Mechanical ventilation
indications Table 4.6

Fig 4.5
The management of severe acute asthma.

pneumonia, where organisms affect already damaged lung tissue or where predisposing factors for aspiration exist.

PRIMARY PNEUMONIA

The microorganisms commonly responsible for this are listed in Table 4.7 (p 70). In immunosuppressed patients the number of potential organisms is greatly increased.

Clinical features

Symptoms: Productive cough, rigors, chest pain and breathlessness.

Signs: pyrexia, herpes labialis, reduced chest expansion, dull to percussion, bronchial breathing, crepitations.

Investigations • Leukocytosis • sputum microscopy and culture • blood cultures • CXR showing segmental or lobar consolidation • Serological tests are important in confirming aetiology • Less often bronchoscopy may be indicated when the patient fails to respond to therapy.

> **Management** Antibiotics after blood and sputum taken for culture, initially on a best guess basis and subsequently modified according to the results of culture. Physiotherapy, oxygen and rehydration are required in the majority of cases. Inadequate or delayed treatment predisposes to the formation of lung abscess which invariably results in permanent lung damage, empyema, respiratory failure or septicaemia.

SECONDARY PNEUMONIA

Many of the organisms which can cause pneumonia in healthy lungs are commonly responsible for the infection in those with underlying pulmonary disease. *H. influenzae* and other gram negative and anaerobic organisms may also be responsible. Access to the lungs is usually by aspiration of upper respiratory tract commensals. Predisposing factors include chronic illness, anaesthesia, vomiting, bronchial carcinoma, drugs which suppress cough or respiration, gastro-oesophageal reflux and immunocompromised patients.

Clinical features

Symptoms: Worsening of underlying pulmonary disease such as chronic bronchitis, with cough, increased sputum and rigors.

Signs: pyrexia, cyanosis, basal dullness to percussion, bilateral basal crepitations. Signs of consolidation often absent.

Table 4.7
Microorganisms which cause primary pneumonia and treatment

Organism	Treatment
Streptococcus pneumonia	Benzylpenicillin 1.2 g qid or ampicillin 500 mg qid
Streptococcus pyogenes	Ampicillin 500 mg qid
Staphylococcus aureus	Flucloxacillin 500 mg qid
Klebsiella pneumonia	Mezlocillin or gentamicin
Mycoplasma pneumonia	Tetracycline 500 mg qid or erythromycin 500 mg qid
Chlamydia psittaci	Tetracycline 500 mg qid
Coxiella burnetii	Tetracycline 500 mg qid
Legionella pneumophilia	Erythromycin or rifampicin
Pneumocystis carinii	Cotrimoxazole 1920 mg qid
Influenza viruses A and B	No antibiotic effective

Investigations • Leukocytosis • sputum and blood cultures • CXR looking for patchy, often bilateral, areas of consolidation.

Management Recognition is important as late diagnosis results in lung damage. • Physiotherapy and oxygen therapy should support antibiotics which again should initially be used on a best guess basis with modification according to bacteriological results eg broad spectrum penicillins or cephalosporins such as iv azlocillin 2 g tid or cefuroxime 750 mg tid combined with an aminoglycoside such as gentamicin or tobramycin. Metronidazole 500 mg tid iv or 1 g tid pr should be added when anaerobic infection is possible eg aspiration pneumonia. Prevention of bacterial infection in those with chronic lung disease is better than treatment. Vaccination against influenza is important.

PULMONARY ABSCESS

Pulmonary consolidation with damage to the lung parenchyma may result in abscess formation. Predisposing factors include infection with *Staph aureus* and *Klebsiella pneumoniae*, inhaled foreign bodies, pulmonary infarction, malignancy, TB, fungal infection, aspiration and immunosuppression.

Clinical features

Symptoms: Usually very ill with large volumes of purulent sputum, haemoptysis, rigors and sweating.

Signs: include pyrexia, finger clubbing (which may develop rapidly), signs of consolidation or pleural effusion, pleural rub and metastatic abscesses (eg cerebral).

Investigations • CXR usually confirms the diagnosis with consolidation with cavitation and a fluid level • Chest US is useful in identifying fluid collection and allows diagnostic aspiration • Bronchoscopy is indicated in all patients with evidence of bronchial obstruction to exclude foreign body aspiration and bronchial carcinoma.

Management Surgery is rarely necessary provided appropriate and adequate antibiotic therapy eg 6 weeks treatment with ampicillin 500 mg qid, flucloxacillin 500 mg qid and metronidazole 400 mg tid is instituted. Erythromycin 500 mg qid should be substituted for penicillin in hypersensitive patients. Regional pulmonary fibrosis is an invariable sequela.

BRONCHIECTASIS

Respiratory airways that are permanently damaged and dilated are common sites for recurrent infection due to pooling of secretions. Such infections result in further damage resulting in a spiral of deterioration.

Aetiology Otherwise normal respiratory airways may be damaged by infections such as measles, pertussis or tuberculosis. The airways of patients with cystic fibrosis, bronchopulmonary aspergillosis, Kartagener's syndrome, α_1-antitrypsin deficiency and immunosuppression are susceptible to infection because of impaired airway defence or clearance mechanisms.

Clinical features

Symptoms: Frequent respiratory infections, chronic cough productive of large volumes of purulent sputum, weight loss and haemoptysis. Respiratory failure, pleurisy, empyema and distant abscesses eg cerebral are all recognized complications:

Signs: finger clubbing, rhonchi and coarse crepitations.

Investigations • Sputum culture • CXR showing fibrosis, cysts and tramlines due to bronchial oedema • Spirometry revealing reduced vital capacity and • bronchography showing bronchial irregularity • thin section CT scanning may be useful in certain cases • Proteinuria may develop due to amyloidosis.

Management Physiotherapy with postural drainage and antibiotics eg ampicillin 500 mg qid or cotrimoxazole 960 mg bd for episodes of respiratory infection. In patients with cystic fibrosis *Pseudomonas aeruginosa* infection is common and requires specific therapy eg iv ceftazidime, ciprofloxacin or azlocillin. Bronchodilator therapy and humidifier therapy is useful in those with bronchospasm and thick, tenacious secretions. Prophylactic antibiotics may be useful in reducing the number of infections eg cyclical courses of ampicillin, erythromycin and cotrimaxazole. If the disease is localized surgical resection should be considered.

BRONCHIAL CARCINOMA

This is the commonest tumour in males in Western society and the mortality has continued to increase over the last 30 years. Its prevalence to a large part is due to cigarette smoking. Four main types can be identified: ● squamous ● adenocarcinoma (including alveolar cell) ● large cell and ● small cell. Identification of type is important since treatment regimens vary with pathology.

Clinical features

Symptoms: Cough, sputum, haemoptysis, breathlessness, chest pain, dysphonia, dysphagia, stridor and persistent chest infection.

Signs: include finger clubbing, cachexia, consolidation, cavitation or pleural effusion, Horner's syndrome, SVC obstruction.

Investigations ● CXR, including a lateral, reveals the majority of tumours although those centrally situated may be obscured by the heart or great vessels ● Sputum cytology especially if repeated on at least three samples has a sensitivity of approximately 80% • The investigation of choice, particularly because it allows direct visual conformation as well as histological confirmation in central tumours is fibreoptic bronchoscopy ● Investigations such as FBC, LFTs, abdominal and cranial CT scans, mediastinoscopy and abdominal US may indicate disseminated disease, whilst thoracic CT scans are helpful in determining local invasion ● Small cell tumours (APUDOMAS) may secrete substances such as ACTH, resulting in Cushing's syndrome, or ADH producing hyponatraemia ● Squamous carcinoma may present with hypercalcaemia due to secretion of a PTH-like substance. Before treatment can be considered the extent of the disease must be determined (staging).

Management This depends upon the histological type of tumour. Peripheral small cell tumour may be amenable to resection whilst larger lesions may respond well initially to chemotherapy and/or radiotherapy. Non-small cell tumours if small and localized may be resected whilst larger lesions may respond to radiotherapy. Radiotherapy should be considered for symptomatic metastatic lesions in bone and the CNS, SVC obstruction, haemoptysis or large airway obstruction. Palliation of obstructive lesions by endoscopic laser therapy or radiotherapy should be considered where appropriate.

Prognosis at the time of diagnosis three-quarters of patients have unresectable disease and of the quarter of patients with localized disease only one-third of those will be alive at five years.

SARCOIDOSIS

This is a disease of unknown aetiology characterized by non-caseating granulomas which may affect many organs in the body, particularly the respiratory tree. The granulomata cause fibrosis and damage to the parenchyma of involved organs. The highest incidence occurs in young adults, especially females. Two main clinical types of sarcoidosis are recognized: subacute which is self-limiting and chronic.

Clinical features These depend upon the organ system involved, although weight loss, tiredness and fever are common.

Skin: lupus pernio, subcutaneous nodules, erythema nodosum, maculopapular rashes.

Lungs: this is the most commonly affected organ but is frequently asymptomatic until extensive pulmonary fibrosis exists. In many only hilar lymphadenopathy is found incidentally on CXR (stage 1). Transient pulmonary infiltrates may be recognized in addition to hilar lymphadenopathy (stage 2). Interstitial fibrosis may occur in chronic sarcoidosis (stage 3) and be accompanied by pulmonary hypertension.

Liver: granuloma common (70%) but usually asymptomatic.

Kidneys: nephrocalcinosis related to hypercalcaemia and hypercalciuria.

Eyes: uveitis and corneal calcification.

Nervous system: both the CNS and peripheral nerves may be involved.

Haematological: anaemia and thrombocytopaenia.

Heart: arrhythmias, conduction defects and impaired contractility.

Salivary glands: parotid swelling.

Joints: phalangeal cysts and arthritis.

Investigations ● CXR for hilar lymphadenopathy and pulmonary infiltration ● FBC ● U+Es ● serum calcium ● urinary calcium ● serum ACE, derived from the pulmonary capillaries is often increased and correlates with disease severity ● Mantoux to exclude TB ● Kveim test using antigen from human sacroid spleen, although it takes 6 weeks for a positive result ● Bronchoscopy allows bronchial/transbronchial biopsies and bronchoalveolar lavage which contains increased numbers of lymphocytes ● Isotope gallium scanning reveals lung tissue actively involved ● Reduced vital capacity, lung volumes and CO transfer factor ● Biopsies from skin lesions or the liver may also identify granulomata.

Management Subacute sarcoidosis is self-limiting and treatment usually unnecessary although short courses of steroids may be required to treat skin lesion, uveitis or systemic disturbance such as pyrexia or fatigue. Chronic sarcoidosis commonly requires long-term steroid therapy to control pulmonary and/or eye disease. The initial dose should be prednisolone 40–60 mg/day for 1–2 months followed by a reducing dose to a maintenance level of 10 mg/day. Disease progression should be monitored by serial lung function tests, CXR and ACE levels. The prognosis is good unless extensive pulmonary fibrosis is present.

PULMONARY FIBROSIS

Three types of fibrosis occur within the lung: ● replacement fibrosis secondary to damage caused by disorders like infarction, TB and pneumonia ● focal fibrosis in response to irritants such as coal dust and silica; and ● interstitial fibrosis which occurs in cryptogenic fibrosing alveolitis and extrinsic allergic alveolitis.

FOCAL FIBROSIS

The most common cause for this is occupational lung disease the commoner of which are listed in Table 4.8 (p 76). The fibrogenic dusts involved are inhaled and carried by macrophages to nearby lymphoid tissue where fibrosis starts. The three most important diseases are coal miner's pneumoconiosis, asbestosis and silicosis.

Coal miner's pneumoconiosis
This is caused by the inhalation of coal dust particles most of which are less than 5 μm in diameter and often made worse by

cigarette smoking. The disease can be subdivided into the simple type and progressive massive fibrosis. The former is categorized according to the severity of radiological changes and is non-progressive if dust exposure is halted. Progressive massive fibrosis which is associated with dusts containing high proportions of quartz, is characterized by large often confluent masses predominantly in the upper zones and progresses even if exposure is stopped. The clinical features of coal miner's pneumoconiosis are essentially the same as chronic bronchitis. In certain patients ANF and rheumatoid factor may be found in the serum. In Caplan's syndrome rheumatoid arthritis coexists and fibrotic nodules can be seen within the lung. The diagnosis of coal miner's pneumoconiosis is important since industrial compensation may be available.

Asbestosis

Exposure may occur in such occupations as mining, building trade, pipe-fitting and demolition. The two main types of asbestos involved are chrysotile and crocidolite (blue asbestos). The major medical problems are pulmonary fibrosis and malignancy of the respiratory tract, pleura and peritoneum. The fibrosis is related to the severity and duration of exposure whilst malignancy has a less clear correlation and a longer latency period (15–20 years). Cigarette smoking substantially increases the risk of bronchial carcinoma but has little influence on the development of mesothelioma. Bilateral pleural plaques indicate past exposure to asbestos and have little significance otherwise. Fibrosis tends to be more severe in the lower lung fields and develops in those with heavy exposure.

Silicosis

Exposure to crystalline quartz (silica) occurs in such industries as mining, sand blasting and stone cutting. Two types of silicosis are recognized: acute due to high intensity exposure over a short period (months) and chronic, in those with protracted (10 years+) but limited exposure. The former results in rapidly increasing, severe and frequently fatal pulmonary fibrosis. Chronic silicosis results in fibrosis mainly in the upper zones associated with an increased risk of pulmonary tuberculosis. The CXR shows pulmonary fibrosis and often 'egg shell' calcification of enlarged hilar lymph nodes.

INTERSTITIAL FIBROSIS

Fibrosis of the alveolar walls results in reduced pulmonary compliance and maldistribution of ventilation. The commonest causes include fibrosing alveolitis either idiopathic or related to connective tissue disorders and extrinsic allergic alveolitis.

Table 4.8
Forms of occupational lung disease

Dust	Disease	Tissue reaction
Coal dust	Coal miner's pneumoconiosis	Marked
Asbestos (chrysotile, amosite and crocidolite)	Asbestosis, mesothelioma	Marked
Silica	Silicosis	Marked
Beryllium	Berylliosis	Moderate
Iron oxide	Siderosis	Mild
Tin dioxide	Stannosis	Mild
Aluminium	Aluminosis	Moderate
Barium sulphate	Baritosis	Mild

Fibrosing alveolitis

This results in generalized pulmonary alveolar fibrosis for no identifiable reason (idiopathic) or associated with underlying connective tissue disease eg RA, scleroderma, SLE.

Clinical features

Symptoms: These include progressive exertional breathlessness and a dry cough.

Signs: finger clubbing, tachypnoea, reduced chest expansion and end inspiratory crepitations. Pulmonary hypertension and cor pulmonale may develop.

Investigations ● CXR: widespread lung opacities and elevated diaphragm ● increased FEV_1/FVC, reduced vital capacity, total lung capacity and CO transfer factor ● ABG reveal hypoxia and hypocapnia ● bronchoscopy with lavage containing increased neutrophils and eosinophils ● transbronchial or open lung biopsy allows histological analysis ● rheumatoid factor and ANF positive in some even without evidence of connective tissue disease: the differential diagnosis includes idiopathic pulmonary haemosiderosis, sarcoidosis, extrinsic allergic alveolitis, histiocytosis X and tuberous sclerosis.

> **Management** Steroids effective in 20–30% but requires high doses eg prednisolone 60 mg/day at least initially and response should be monitored by serial pulmonary function tests. Cyclophosphamide 50–150 mg/day may be used as a steroid sparing agent. The overall survival is poor and lung transplantation may be indicated in some.

Extrinsic allergic alveolitis

This is caused by the inhalation of organic dusts which provoke a diffuse immunological reaction within the respiratory tree.

Some of the agents responsible are listed in Table 4.9. Prolonged exposure results in permanent pulmonary damage with fibrosis, leading to pulmonary hypertension, cor pulmonale and eventually death.

Clinical features

Symptoms: 4–12 hours after exposure breathlessness without wheeze, tiredness, fever, sweating and non-productive cough.

Signs: after exposure pyrexia, cyanosis, crepitations.

Investigations ● CXR diffuse reticular fibrosis ● FBC neutrophilia or eosinophilia ● spirometry reduced vital capacity and a restrictive defect ● ABG hypoxia with normal or reduced $PaCO_2$ ● reduced carbon monoxide transfer factor ● serology positive precipitin test or ● provocation test to the suspected antigen ● transbronchial/open lung biopsy.

> **Management** Oxygen and oral steroid therapy for acute attack. Future exposure to the antigen must be eliminated and if this can be achieved the prognosis is good.

**Table 4.9
Causes of extrinsic allergic alveolitis**

Disease	Antigen	Source of antigen
Farmer's lung	*Micropolyspora faeni* *Aspergillus fumigatus* *Thermoactinomyces vulgaris*	Mouldy hay
Maltworker's lung	*Aspergillus clavatus*	Malt, mouldy hay
Birdfancier's lung	Pigeon droppings and feathers	Pigeons, parrots budgerigars
Mushroomworker's lung	*Micropolyspora faeni*	Mushroom compost
Bagassosis	*Thermoactinomyces sacchari*	Mouldy bagasse
Humidifier fever	*Thermophilic actinomycetes, amoeba*	Air humidifiers

PNEUMOTHORAX

Pneumothorax, the presence of air within the pleural cavity, may be due either to a penetrating injury letting air in from the outside or be spontaneous with air leaking from the lung. The primary causes of spontaneous pneumothorax in the UK are rupture of a subpleural bulla or due to a pleural adhesion. Three types of pneumothorax are recognized: closed where the leak spontaneously closes off; open where the communication between the lung and pleural space remains open; and tension where a small communication remains open but only during inspiration so that the volume of air in the pleural space slowly or rapidly increases compressing the adjacent lung.

Clinical features

Symptoms: Rapid onset of sharp chest pain and breathlessness which is seldom severe.

Signs: may be few but include cyanosis, tachypnoea, hyperresonance, reduced expansion and reduced air entry on the affected side. In tension pneumothorax breathlessness may rapidly increase with evidence of mediastinal shift (deviated trachea and apex beat towards the opposite side) causing severe respiratory and CVS embarrassment and death if left untreated.

Investigations ● Inspiratory and expiratory CXR, small leaks may only be identified on the expiratory film ● CXRs may need to be repeated within a short period to assess change in size especially where a tension pneumothorax is considered ● ABG analysis is essential if pre-existing lung disease exists since respiratory failure may be precipitated by even a small pneumothorax.

Management Small closed pneumothoraces should be left unless the patients has compromised respiratory function from underlying lung disease although a repeat CXR is essential if the patient deteriorates. Larger ones require drainage by insertion of a large bore catheter through either the 2nd intercostal space anteriorly or laterally in the 4th or 5th intercostal space which is connected to an underwater drainage system which acts as a one-way valve allowing air out but not in. Open pneumothoraces usually indicate a bronchopleural fistula and are susceptible to infection. Surgical intervention is usually indicated. A tension pneumothorax is a medical emergency and requires rapid treatment ideally with the insertion of an intercostal drain but where not available a large 'intravenous' cannula should be inserted to relieve intrapleural pressure.

In patients who suffer repeated spontaneous pneumo-thoraces pleurodesis is indicated.

This can be achieved by inserting irritant substances such as kaolin which provokes an inflammatory reaction result-ing in adhesions between the two pleural surfaces. Alterna-tively a surgical procedure involving the stripping of one layer of pleura thus obliterating the pleural space can be performed (pleurectomy).

PLEURAL DISEASES

PLEURAL EFFUSION

Fluid within the pleural space, may be due to pleural or sys-temic disease. Traditionally pleural effusions are divided into transudates, with a protein concentration below 30 g/l, and exudates in which the protein concentration is higher than 30 g/l. All pleural effusions should be investigated by diagnostic aspiration and the fluid examined for protein content, bacteria and cell type. A pleural biopsy is useful in the investigation of pleural exudates. Large effusions that are interfering with res-piration may need to be aspirated for symptom relief but no more than 1000 ml should be removed at one sitting.

Aetiology The causes are shown in Table 4.10.

Table 4.10
Causes of pleural effusions

Transudate	Exudate
Cardiac failure	Empyema
Nephrotic syndrome	Pneumonia
Liver failure	Malignancy including mesothelioma
	Pulmonary infarction
	Connective tissue disease
	Subphrenic abscess
	Pancreatitis (L sided with high amylase content)
	Haemothorax
	Tuberculosis

PLEURISY

Inflammation of the pleura, pleurisy, may be due to underlying pneumonia, viral infection, pulmonary infarction, malignancy and tuberculosis. The condition is characterized by pain which is localized, sharp and exacerbated by deep inspiration or coughing. Such pain in the absence of radiological lung disease may occur in pulmonary infarction (haemoptysis common), viral intercostal myalgia (pleurodynia or Bornholm's disease) or rib fractures.

ADULT RESPIRATORY DISTRESS SYNDROME

Adult Respiratory Distress Syndrome, is a common and serious disorder characterized by acute respiratory failure due to pulmonary injury and accompanied by hypoxia and respiratory distress. The precise pathogenesis is unclear but a leaky alveolar epithelial/endothelial membrane develops and is followed by fibrous tissue deposition. Precipitating factors are shown in Table 4.11.

Table 4.11
Causes of ARDS

Infections	Bacteria, fungi, pneumocystis, TB septicaemia
Embolism	Fat, air, amniotic fluid
Hypovolaemia	
Aspiration	Vomit, water
DIC	
Drugs	Opiates, barbiturates, aspirin
Pancreatitis	
High altitude	
Intracerebral haemorrhage	
Smoke inhalation	
High inhaled oxygen concentration	

Clinical features The usual presentation is a few days after the recognition of a serious underlying disease and not uncommonly during convalescence.

Symptoms: include breathlessness and deterioration in clinical condition.

Signs: tachypnoea, cyanosis, intercostal indrawing and hypotension.

Investigations • CXR shows a 'white-out' with sparing of the costophrenic angles in the early stages. This helps in the differentiation from LVF in which a more central infiltration occurs associated with cardiomegaly • ABG, hypoxia with hypocapnia and respiratory alkalosis; the hypoxia is relatively resistant to oxygen administration and progressive.

Management   This can be divided into two parts; treatment of the underlying disorder and treatment of the lung problem.

The underlying disease: this may not obvious. Shock, if present, should be corrected aggressively but once an adequate circulation has been restored fluid administration, particularly crystalloids, must be administered with care as pulmonary oedema develops readily. The use of high dose steroid therapy is controversial particularly in septic shock but is recommended in fat embolism and following aspiration. Sepsis when present should be treated aggressively with intravenous antibiotics and surgical drainage or resection of septic foci. Where large volumes of blood require to be transfused filters to remove particulate material reduce the risk of ARDS.

The pulmonary problem in ARDS: requires mechanical ventilation with sufficient oxygen to maintain an adequate but not increased PaO_2. High concentrations of oxygen may lead to further lung damage. Control of respiration with increased tidal and minute volumes and PEEP are usually required with careful monitoring of the cardiac output and blood pressure. Prevention of pulmonary oedema by careful fluid balance, loop diuretics and salt-poor colloid administration is important.

Early recognition and adequate treatment of ARDS greatly improves survival. The mortality remains around 70% due most often to multi-organ failure and many patients are left with permanent restrictive lung damage.

CYSTIC FIBROSIS

This autosomal recessive condition is the commonest serious inherited disorder occurring in 1:2000 live births being carried as heterozygotes in 5% of the population. It is characterized by a generalised abnormality of all exocrine glands resulting in the production of unusually viscous secretions. The pathogenesis is unclear at present but the gene responsible has recently been identified.

Clinical features   Presentation usually in infancy with meconium ileus, intussusception and failure to thrive. In older children repeated chest infections leading to bronchiectasis and steatorrhoea is usual. In adolescents and adults repeated chest infections, often due to pseudomonas, pneumothorax, haemoptysis, malabsorption, RVF and cirrhosis with portal hypertension are common features. Eventually pulmonary fibrosis leads to death from ventilatory failure or cor pulmonale. Males but not females are infertile.

Investigations ● In children the sweat test reveals a high concentration of sodium in sweat and is diagnostic ● In adolescents the sweat test is unreliable and the diagnosis remains clinical with repeated chest infections and pancreatic insufficiency ● DNA analysis techniques are likely to be available soon.

Management Chest: prompt and adequate treatment of all respiratory tract infections is essential. *H. influenzae* should be treated with ampicillin 500 mg qid or erythromycin 500 mg qid and *Staph. aureas* with flucloxacillin 500 mg qid. *Pseudomonas* colonization is much more troublesome and eradication is seldom possible. Treatment is with aminoglycosides eg gentamicin, tobramycin or netilmicin (the dose depending upon the patient's height, weight and renal function and should be monitored by peak and trough blood levels) in combination with a broad spectrum penicillin eg azlocillin or carbenicillin or with ceftazidime or ciprofloxacin. Intravenous treatment should be for at least 2 weeks. Physiotherapy with breathing exercises and postural drainage of secretions is important. Bronchodilators and/or inhaled saline administered before physiotherapy may be helpful to clear bronchial secretions.

Pancreas: replacement of pancreatic enzymes with such preparations as 'Pancrex V' and 'Creon' reduce malabsorption and improve nutrition.

Prevention Genetic counselling should be given to parents and older cystic fibrosis patients.

PULMONARY VASCULAR DISEASE

The main disorder of the pulmonary vasculature is pulmonary arterial hypertension. This may be acute, as in pulmonary embolism, or chronic.

PULMONARY EMBOLISM / INFARCTION

Thrombi, most often from DVT in the large veins of the upper leg and pelvis, may break off and arrive in the pulmonary artery via the right ventricle. Risk factors for this are the same as for DVTs and include: bed-rest, low cardiac output, polycythaemia and thrombocythaemia. Pulmonary embolism not uncommonly occurs without signs of DVT and it should never be excluded on this basis.

Clinical features In many the signs and symptoms are few and once the diagnosis has been considered it must be excluded urgently since subsequent emboli may be rapidly fatal.

Symptoms: acute breathlessness, pleuritic chest pain, haemoptysis and collapse.

Signs: hypotension, tachycardia, dyspnoea, raised JVP, pleural rub, cyanosis.

Investigations ● CXR may be normal or show atelectasis ● ECG the S_1, Q_3, T_3 pattern may be found with or without R heart strain but often the cardiogram is unhelpful ● If the CXR is normal the isotope perfusion scan is diagnostic demonstrating perfusion defects ● If the CXR is abnormal a paired isotope ventilation and perfusion scan may help to identify mismatched defects which suggest pulmonary embolism. The results of such isotopic scans are often reported as showing low or high probability of embolism ● Where doubt remains pulmonary angiography is required.

Management Prevention is the best cure for both DVT and pulmonary embolism and many methods have been advocated including elastic stockings and iv dextran. The most commonly used prophylaxis is subcutaneous heparin (5000 Units tid) during the period of increased risk eg during bed-rest post MI. Once the diagnosis of pulmonary embolism has been made treatment depends upon its associated haemodynamic effects. If these are minimal treatment with iv heparin (5000 Units bolus followed by an infusion of approximately 1000 Units per hour). The dose should be titrated against the thrombin time at 2–3x normal. For larger emboli treatment with thrombolytic agents such as streptokinase is indicated provided such contraindications as recent CVA or GI bleeding are absent. Following treatment with such intravenous agents oral anticoagulants most often warfarin should be introduced and continued for 3-6 months, the dose being adjusted to maintain the INR 2–4x normal. Surgery and thrombectomy is indicated only for those with massive pulmonary emboli with circulatory collapse. Patients in whom medical management is contraindicated or unsuccessful, particularly if the risk of further emboli is high, may be treated by the insertion of filters in the inferior vena cava.

CHRONIC PULMONARY HYPERTENSION

This may be due to repeated pulmonary emboli, cardiac disease, cor pulmonale or primary pulmonary hypertension. The first three are discussed elsewhere.

Primary pulmonary hypertension

This uncommon and serious disease of unknown aetiology usually affects young females. Fenfluramine, used as an appetite suppressant, may cause pulmonary hypertension.

Clinical features

Symptoms: Fatigue, chest pain, breathlessness and ankle swelling.

Signs: these vary from prominent 'a' waves, R ventricular heave and loud P_2 in the early stages to frank RVF later.

Investigations • CXR prominent central pulmonary vasculature with peripheral pruning • ECG R axis deviation and R sided stain • Echocardiography R atrial and ventricular enlargement • Cardiac catheterization is required to measure pulmonary arterial pressure • Other investigations may be required to exclude other causes of pulmonary hypertension such as chronic pulmonary emboli, valvular disease and chronic lung disease.

> **Management** Once established the disease is incurable and treatment is palliative. Oral anticoagulant therapy if started early may prolong life. Other drugs such as β-blockers and pre-load and after-load reducers may help control symptoms. Cardiopulmonary transplantation currently is the only curative procedure in selected patients.

MEDIASTINAL MASSES

> Many structures and tumours can give rise to mediastinal masses and it is easiest to divide masses according to their position.

Anterosuperior: retrosternal thyroid, aneurysm, thymoma (malignant in 25% and frequently associated with myaesthenia gravis), metastatic carcinoma.

Anteroinferior: dermoid cyst, metastatic carcinoma, teratoma, pericardial cyst, Morgagni hernia.

Middle: lymphoma, bronchial cyst, metastatic carcinoma.

Posterior: ganglioneuroma, lymphoma, enterogenous cyst, Bochdalek hernia, achalasia, aortic aneurysm, paravertebral abscess, hiatus hernia.

Skin or subcutaneous lesions may appear on a single CXR as a thoracic mass but different views and clinical examination reveal their true position. Presentation of mediastinal masses is variable but commonly with vague chest pain, cough, superior vena caval obstruction or incidentally on routine CXR.

5

Gastroenterology

Gallstone disease 116

INVESTIGATIONS

There are probably more investigations available in the diagnosis of gastrointestinal disease than for any other system. The most important are:

Endoscopy Direct visualization of parts of the GI tract and the ability to take biopsies can be achieved by endoscopy. Flexible fibreoptic instruments have largely replaced rigid scopes except for sigmoidoscopy. Disorders in the oesophagus, stomach and proximal duodenum can be investigated with the gastroscope under light sedation. The pancreas and biliary tree can be visualized following the injection of contrast medium into their ducts at endoscopic retrograde cholangiopancreatography (ERCP) which uses a longer endoscope and where the view is from the side of the instrument rather than end-on. The large bowel and terminal ileum can be investigated using the colonoscope although an examination of the whole large bowel is only possible in approximately 85–90% of subjects. Diseases of the rectum can be investigated with the sigmoidoscope. The flexible instrument allows visualization of the sigmoid colon and descending colon. Endoscopy allows, as well as visualization of the bowel, biopsies to be taken, polyps removed, strictures dilated, vessels injected and laser therapy to be administered.

Laparoscopy is a method of inspecting the abdominal organs directly and a fibreoptic system is usually employed. Laparoscopy may be performed under local or general anaesthesia and is particularly useful in the investigation of abdominal pain of unknown cause and in the investigation of liver disease.

Radiology The whole of the GI tract can be investigated radiologically once contrast medium, usually barium, is applied to the appropriate region. The commonest investigations are the barium swallow, meal and enema. The small intestine can be investigated with the barium meal and follow through and the small bowel enema, in which barium is introduced into the proximal small intestine through an oro-duodenal tube.

Crosby capsule This is used to obtain jejunal biopsies usually in the investigation of coeliac disease.

Faecal fat collection The collection of faeces for 3 or 5 days to quantitate the fat content is important in the diagnosis and investigation of malabsorption.

Faecal occult blood The detection of small quantities of blood in faeces can be made by simple bed-side methods which detect haemoglobin.

Breath tests

14C-labelled glycocholic breath test: is based on the fact that many bacteria deconjugate bile acids. If this happens in the small intestine due to bacterial overgrowth 14C-labelled glycine is released, absorbed and metabolized producing $^{14}CO_2$ which is exhaled. Appearance of $^{14}CO_2$ at 2–3 hours is suggestive of bacterial colonization of the small intestine although rapid transit through the intestine to the colon gives false positive results.

Hydrogen breath test: is used to detect disaccharidase deficiency. After an oral 50 g lactose load patients with lactase deficiency exhale more than 20 ppm compared with values of less than 5 ppm in normal subjects.

Pancreatic function tests No ideal test to assay pancreatic exocrine function exists. Traditionally a standard fatty meal (Lundh meal) is given after a tube has been positioned in the 2nd part of the duodenum. Pancreatic secretions are aspirated and enzymes assayed. Tubeless tests have been devised which include: urinary excretion of PABA which results from hydrolysis of administered N-benzoyl-L tyrosyl-PABA and radio-labelled fatty meals with subsequent analysis of serum radioactivity.

Intestinal motility This can be assessed crudely by observing the speed of transit of radio-opaque markers along the GI tract. Apparatus exists which allows accurate measurement of motility of the oesophagus and the anorectal region.

pH monitoring The investigation of gastro-oesophageal reflux has been greatly advanced by the introduction of portable pH probes which are positioned above the gastro-oesophageal junction and connected to a 24-hour recording system.

OESOPHAGITIS

Inflammation of the oesophagus is usually due to reflux of acid from the stomach. The squamous epithelium is not resistant to low pH and inflammation develops. The severity can be graded into 4 categories from mild (grade 1) to ulcerative (grade 4). Other factors which can result in oesophagitis include alcohol, bile and drugs, particularly if their passage is slowed by a stricture. Infection may affect the oesophagus, the commonest being due to herpes simplex and candida. This latter is commoner in immunosuppressed patients due to drug therapy such as steroids, or AIDS. Reflux of acid, the commonest cause of inflammation, occurs in all of us but the frequency and duration of reflux episodes is greater in those with reflux oesophagitis. Predisposing factors include pregnancy, obesity and smoking.

Clinical features

Symptoms: Heart burn, a dull retrosternal ache, is the commonest symptom and is often triggered by food, sometimes particular factors such as coffee or alcohol. This symptom may be indistinguishable from angina pectoris. Less common symptoms include dysphagia or lethargy due to anaemia.

Signs: pallor due to anaemia caused by occult bleeding, haematemesis may complicate ulcerative oesophagitis. Severe reflux may be associated with aspiration accompanied by coarse crepitations at the lung bases.

Investigation ● Upper GI endoscopy is the most sensitive means of diagnosing and grading oesophagitis and may reveal the underlying cause such as hiatus hernia ● Barium swallow may show mucosal changes of inflammation and/or ulceration and may demonstrate reflux and/or aspiration ● Twenty-four hour pH and motility studies may be useful in identifying gastro-oesophageal reflux.

Management Mild symptomatic reflux causing occasional heart burn is commonly treated only with antacids. In many, acid suppressing agents such as cimetidine or ranitidine are required. Omeprazole 20–40 mg daily is useful for those with ulcerative oesophagitis. For those resistant to such therapy the addition of mucosal protecting agents such as alginates or sucralfate are useful. Agents to increase the lower oesophageal sphincter pressure such as metoclopramide are useful in some. In all patients advice regarding loss of weight (where appropriate), smaller meals, avoiding late evening snacks, stopping smoking and sleeping with the head of the bed elevated should be given.

OESOPHAGEAL CARCINOMA

Carcinoma of the oesophagus occurs most frequently in the distal third of the oesophagus either as adenocarcinoma, from gastric type epithelium, or squamous carcinoma. More proximal tumours are usually squamous. Risk factors include: alcohol abuse, smoking, achalasia, Barrett's oesophagitis, Plummer-Vinson syndrome, tylosis and radiation exposure. It is commoner in males in whom it is the fifth commonest tumour. It is especially common in certain regions as China and Iran.

Clinical features

Symptoms: Dysphagia, initially for solids; weight loss; chest pain, cough and hoarseness.

Signs: include cough, anaemia and pulmonary signs due to aspiration.

Investigations ● Upper GI endoscopy will identify the stricture and enable biopsies and brushings to be taken ● Barium
swallow reveals an irregular stricture.

Management Cure is only possible for those with localized disease. If localized, squamous carcinoma of the upper
and middle thirds of the oesophagus should be treated with
radiotherapy whilst for tumours of the lower third oesoph-
agogastrectomy is indicated. In extensive malignancies,
where cure is not possible, palliation of dysphagia should
be sought by either surgical or endoscopic means. The
insertion of prosthetic tubes allows the patient to swallow
semi-solid foods. Laser therapy and endoscopic ethanol
injection also improves swallowing. Radiotherapy or surgery may offer the best palliation in certain cases.

Prognosis The 5-year survival is less than 10% and palliation, particularly to avoid the distressing inability to swallow
saliva, is the goal in many patients.

DYSPHAGIA

Difficulty in swallowing is a relatively common complaint
and should always be treated seriously and investigated,
usually initially with a barium swallow followed by endoscopy where appropriate. The most frequent causes follow.

Benign stricture
This is usually a complication of peptic ulcerative oesophagitis.
Patients may however have complained little of heartburn until
the dysphagia develops, which is usually for solids initially.
Endoscopy is necessary to confirm the diagnosis histologically
and in many cases to allow endoscopic dilatation. This latter
may have to be repeated regularly.

Oesophageal carcinoma (→ p 89)

Achalasia
This is due to a failure of the lower oesophageal sphincter to
relax. The cause is probably due to abnormal innervation of
the lower oesophagus and resembles closely Chaga's disease.
Dysphagia is invariable and is present for liquids as well as
solids. Chest pain and pulmonary aspiration are common
complications. The barium swallow gives a highly characteristic appearance with proximal dilatation and distal smooth
tapering. Endoscopy is necessary to exclude carcinoma and to
allow hydrostatic or pneumatic dilatation. Alternative treatment is a surgical cardiomyotomy (Heller's operation). Both
methods of treatment may be followed by gastro-oesophageal
reflux.

Oesophageal spasm

This is relatively uncommon. It usually affects the elderly and is associated with muscular hypertrophy of the lower oesophagus. It is accompanied by chest pain which may mimic angina pectoris. Barium swallow shows abnormal peristalsis with uncoordinated contractions which can be confirmed by manometry. Treatment is with muscle relaxants such as isosorbide mononitrate 10–20 mg bd and nifedipine 10–20 mg tid and advice regarding avoiding such factors which may provoke spasm such as hot or cold liquids.

Miscellaneous

Other causes of dysphagia include stomatitis, tonsillitis, head, neck and mediastinal tumours, pharyngeal pouch, scleroderma, Plummer-Vinson syndrome and bulbar or pseudobulbar palsy, neuromuscular incoordination and globus hystericus.

PEPTIC ULCERATION

Peptic ulcers are divided into two main categories, gastric and duodenal ulcers. Ulcers form when there is an imbalance between damaging (acid) and protecting factors. In both types acid secretion is important and when acid is neutralized or secretion inhibited ulcers heal. Over-secretion of acid is associated with duodenal ulcer disease whilst for gastric ulcers impaired mucosal protection is important. Other factors recognized as being important include heredity, stress, NSAID, smoking and infection with *Helicobacter pylori*. This latter has recently been recognized as being important particularly for duodenal ulceration and gastritis but less so for gastric ulcers.

Clinical features   Ulcers may be truely asymptomatic, cause mild discomfort or severe abdominal pain. Most common is localized epigastric pain and the patient may be able to point to the site of maximum pain. Some association with eating is recognised, DUs tending to give rise to pain between meals and during the night whilst GUs often give rise to pain whilst eating.

Symptoms: tend to wax and wane over a period of weeks or months. Exacerbations may occur at times of stress or be triggered by such factors as drugs or alcohol.

Signs: Localized epigastric tenderness is common but not invariable. Anaemia may be obvious in those who have had a recent bleed. A succussion splash may be elicited in those with gastric outlet obstruction due to prepyloric oedema or scarring.

Investigation   ● GUs may be malignant and should always be biopsied ● If identified on a barium meal an endoscopy with biopsies must follow and a further endoscopy after treatment to ensure healing. DUs on the other hand are almost never the site of malignancy and biopsies are not usually necessary. The diagnosis can therefore be made by either barium meal or endoscopy and a follow-up endoscopy to ensure healing after treatment if the patient has become asymmptomatic is usually unnecessary ● In certain patients with numerous or difficult to treat ulcers serum gastrin levels should be checked to exclude Zollinger-Ellison syndrome ● Acid-output studies are not commonly required except to assess the success or otherwise of surgical procedures to reduce acid production ● More recently tests to identify *H. pylori* either by biopsy, breath tests or serum antibody levels have been advocated in the investigation of peptic ulcer disease.

Management   This can be divided into medical and surgical.

Medical: although there are numerous drugs available which heal ulcers they can be separated into those which neutralize or inhibit acid and those that increase mucosal resistance to acid. Antacids if given in sufficient quantities will heal ulcers. H_2-antagonists, the best known of which are cimetidine 400 mg bd or 800 mg nocte and ranitidine 150 mg bd or 300 mg nocte, inhibit the acid secretion that is under vagal-histamine control. They are effective in healing both GUs and DUs but relapse of DUs is common once treatment is stopped, possibly because of the continued existence of *H pylori*. Long-term maintenance therapy is therefore required for many patients. A newer agent omeprazole 20 mg once daily reduces acid secretion by inhibition of the hydrogen potassium ATPase pump and results in a more complete blockage of acid production than H_2-antagonists and may be useful in treating those ulcers resistant to conventional therapy.

Mucosal protecting agents include sucralfate 1 g qid and colloidal bisthmus (De-nol) 240 mg bd. This latter agent also has a bacteriocidal effect on *H pylori* and probably results in a lower incidence of relapse after a course of treatment. Combination therapy with antibiotics eg ampicillin and metronidazole increase bacterial clearance. As well as drug treatment the patient should be given advice regarding stopping smoking, avoiding NSAID and reducing stress where possible.

Surgical: operations are indicated only in those patients resistant to medical treatment and those who have suffered complications such as perforation or haemorrhage. Cutting the vagal nerves at the level of the lower oesophagus effectively reduces acid secretion but frequently is followed by adverse reactions such as post-prandial hypoglycaemia (late dumping) or dizziness and lethargy soon after eating, due to the osmotic effect of large volumes of food in the proximal small intestine (early dumping). These adverse reactions can be largely overcome by a highly selective vagotomy where the nerve supply to the pylorus is left intact removing the need for a drainage procedure such as pyloroplasty or gastroenterostomy. Ulcer relapse after highly selective vagotomy is, however, higher than after truncal vagotomy.

UPPER GASTROINTESTINAL HAEMORRHAGE

Presentation haematemesis, melaena (with bleeding in GI tract down to ascending colon), iron deficiency anaemia.

Aetiology ($\rightarrow$ Table 5.1.) Other causes include: swallowed blood from epistaxis, blood dyscrasia, haemorrhagic telangiectasia, pseudoxanthoma elasticum, Ehlers-Danlos syndrome, Ménétrier's disease, a-v malformations and haemobilia.

Table 5.1
Causes of gastrointestinal bleeding

	%
Duodenal ulcer	40
Gastric ulcer	15
Erosions	10
Varices	10
Oesophagitis	5
Mallory-Weiss	5
Carcinoma	5
Other	10

Assessment and investigation

Clinical features:

Symptoms: ask about dyspepsia, alcohol abuse, analgesic ingestion, family history, syncope, dizziness and antecedent retching.

Signs: blood pressure (systolic BP < 100 = >30% blood volume reduction), heart rate, pallor, sweating and stigmata of liver disease.

Investigations:

Haematology: haemoglobin and haematocrit (may be normal until haemodilution occurs), leukocytosis and thrombocythaemia common.

Biochemistry: raised urea (protein load), abnormal LFTs in liver disease, serum iron, transferrin.

Nasogastric: aspirate: if history of bleeding unclear (some false negatives).

Endoscopy: allows identification of cause in >90% and means of treatment of varices by sclerotherapy. Sclerotherapy may also be useful in stopping bleeding from some peptic ulcers. Risk of rebleeding higher if a 'visible vessel' is seen in ulcer crater.

Barium radiology: identifies bleeding site in 80%. Useful in convalescent phase or with chronic blood loss.

Angiography: useful if bleeding still active but site unknown.

Radiolabelled RBCs: useful in determining low-grade bleeding from GI tract, especially if the pathology is out of reach of the endoscope.

Management An iv line should be established in all patients and blood transfusion given to those with a systolic BP < 100 or HR > 100. The majority of patients stop bleeding spontaneously. Those who continue to bleed, identified by persistent hypotension or continuous transfusion requirement, should be referred for surgery except where variceal bleeding is considered when urgent endoscopy and sclerotherapy is indicated. Those in whom bleeding has stopped should undergo endoscopy on the next available list. Ulcers with adherent clot or a visible vessel at its base are at increased risk of rebleeding and should be treated by sclerotherapy where available. Those who rebleed should be referred for surgery.

Ulcers without stigmata associated with a high risk of rebleeding or where sources such as erosions are found should receive H_2-antagonists eg ranitidine 300 mg bd orally and remain in hospital for 4–7 days. Those with Mallory-Weiss tears require no specific therapy and can be discharged early.

Prognosis the overall mortality from acute upper GI haemorrhage remains unchanged over the last 40 years at around 10%. Adverse prognostic factors include old age, shock at presentation, rebleeding and varices. Early and aggressive resuscitation and treatment, particularly of the at-risk group, is essential.

COELIAC DISEASE

Coeliac disease is characterized by mucosal villous atrophy which improves after gluten withdrawal from the diet. Gluten has two main components, glutenin and gliadin. It is components of the latter which are believed to be antigenic leading to immunologically mediated injury. Genetic association exists with a high prevalence of HLA B8 and DR3 although environmental influences are also important.

Clinical features   Usually children of 1–5 years.

Symptoms: diarrhoea, steatorrhoea, weight loss and failure to thrive. Abdominal pain, irritability and delayed puberty are recognized. Presentation in adulthood occurs usually with diarrhoea or consequences of malabsorption such as anaemia.

Signs: mouth ulcers, peripheral oedema, muscle wasting, skin pigmentation and dermatitis herpetiformis (→ below).

Investigations   ● FBC showing anaemia and Howell-Jolly bodies (hyposplenism) ● LFTs may reveal hypoalbuminaemia ● The xylose tolerance test is usually abnormal ● A jejunal or distal duodenal biopsy is essential and demonstrates subtotal or total villous atrophy along with a chronic inflammatory cell infiltrate.

Management   Gluten withdrawal and dietary education. All barley, wheat, oats and rye containing foods are potentially harmful. A useful booklet containing diets and recipes can be obtained from the Coeliac Society (PO Box 220, High Wycombe, Bucks).

Complications   An increased incidence of intestinal lymphoma and adenocarcinoma as well as oesophageal and pharyngeal tumours exists. Intestinal ulceration and stricture formation are recognized.

Dermatitis herpetiformis
This condition with an itchy, blistering skin eruption is also associated with jejunal villous atrophy which responds to a gluten-free diet. Dapsone is effective in treating the skin rash.

Idiopathic mucosal enteropathy
This disorder presents in middle age with diarrhoea, weight loss and abdominal pain. Jejunal biopsy reveals villous atrophy unresponsive to dietary gluten withdrawal. Other diseases to be excluded include: Crohn's disease, tuberculosis, actinomycosis, typhoid, polyarteritis nodosa and Zollinger-Ellison syndrome.

CROHN'S DISEASE

This is a chronic inflammatory disease of any part of the GI tract the cause of which is unknown. An interplay between an infective agent and an abnormal immune response is currently believed important. The inflammation, unlike UC, affects the entire thickness of the bowel wall. The terminal ileum and proximal colon are the most commonly affected sites.

Epidemiology The annual incidence in the UK is approximately 5/100 000 with an equal sex distribution occurring most commonly between 15–35 years. Familial clustering occurs and involves UC as well as Crohn's disease.

Clinical features It is a chronic, relapsing and remitting disease with symptomatology depending upon the site of involvement in the GI tract.

Symptoms: include malaise, anorexia, nausea, weight loss, fever, abdominal pain, diarrhoea, arthralgia and rectal bleeding.

Signs: pallor, malnutrition, oral ulcers, abdominal mass, perianal abscesses and fistulae, finger clubbing, erythema nodosum, pyoderma gangrenosum and uveitis.

Investigations ● FBC: anaemia due to blood loss and/or folate or vitamin B_{12} deficiency, leukocytosis, increased platelet count which correlates with disease activity ● ESR: elevated ● Biochemistry: hyponatraemia, hypokalaemia, acidosis, hypoalbuminaemia, abnormal LFTs if associated CAH ● Elevated levels of C-reactive protein correlate with disease activity ● Radiology: plain abdominal film may show obstruction, toxic dilatation or perforation. Barium meal, follow-through and enema are useful both in making the diagnosis and in assessing its extent and severity ● US is useful in detecting abscesses ● Endoscopy: both upper and lower GI endoscopy allows direct visualization and biopsies to be taken. Strictures within reach of the endoscope may be treated by balloon dilatation in selected cases ● Radionuclide scanning; technetium and indium-labelled WBC scans may be useful in detecting areas of disease activity ● Histology: the diagnosis of Crohn's disease should, where possible, have histological confirmation; features of Crohn's disease include full thickness inflammation, non-caseating granulomata, fissuring, ulceration and erosions.

Complications Malnutrition, stricture formation, perianal disease, severe haemorrhage, toxic dilatation, abscess formation, fistulae, renal calculi, gallstones and psychological problems. The risk of developing small or large bowel cancer is increased slightly.

Management Symptoms due to inflammation usually respond to medical measures whilst those due to strictures require surgical intervention.

Medical: general measures include replacement of fluid and electrolytes, haematinics if required, nutritional supplements and advice and psychological support. Drugs: corticosteroids, usually prednisolone 40 mg/day, are effective in controlling acute exacerbations in the majority. Large doses should be used for as short a time as possible to reduce adverse reactions and maintenance steroid therapy should be avoided as it does not reduce the frequency of relapse. Sulphasalazine 3–6 g/day is helpful in active colonic Crohn's disease and may reduce the frequency of relapse. Other immunosuppressive drugs such as azathioprine and 6-mercaptopurine may be useful as steroid sparing agents in selected cases. Antibiotics should be used where there is sepsis and when bacterial overgrowth is suspected.

Dietary therapy: important for maintaining adequate nutrition; elemental diets have been shown to induce remission in many cases. Its use is particularly indicated in children to reduce the adverse effects of steroids on growth.

Surgical indications:

● Intractable disease with persistent ill-health despite drug therapy.

● Intestinal obstruction not settling medically.

● Perforation and abscess or external fistula formation.

● Toxic dilatation of the colon.

● Ureteric obstruction due to periureteric inflammation.

Prognosis Acute ileitis is atypical in that it does not recur unlike all other forms of Crohn's disease. Patients with colonic Crohn's disease usually respond well to medical treatment although 50% will require surgery at some time. 70% of those with both large and small bowel disease require surgery at some time. Conservative surgery such as stricturoplasty should be undertaken whenever possible. The overall mortality in patients with Crohn's disease is approximately twice that of the general population due to complications of active disease.

ULCERATIVE COLITIS

This is a chronic inflammatory disease of either part or the whole of the colon. The inflammation is confined to the mucosa almost invariably affecting the rectum and extending proximally to varying degrees in a continuous fashion. The cause is unknown but immunological, dietary, genetic and psychological factors have all been implicated.

Epidemiology The sex distribution is approximately equal, the majority presenting between 25–35 years with an annual incidence of 4–7/100 000. As for Crohn's disease familial clustering is recognized.

Clinical features The clinical course may be acute fulminating, relapsing-remitting or chronic continuous.

Symptoms: include diarrhoea, rectal bleeding, mild abdominal pains, fever and weight loss.

Signs: pallor, mouth ulcers, dehydration, abdominal tenderness, erythema nodosum, pyoderma gangrenosum, arthritis and uveitis. Severe colitis should be recognized when there is bloody diarrhoea >6x/day, tachycardia, fever and anaemia.

Investigations ● FBC: anaemia due to blood loss, leukocytosis ● ESR: increased correlating with disease severity ● Biochemistry: hyponatraemia, hypokalaemia, acidosis, hypocalcaemia and hypomagnesaemia, abnormal LFTs due to associated CAH (↑ ALT) or sclerosing cholangitis (↑ alk phos) ● Radiology: the plain abdominal film is essential in severe acute attacks to exclude toxic dilatation (>5.5 cm in diameter), The double contrast barium enema is useful in the diagnosis and determining the extent and severity of disease, it is contraindicated in those at risk of toxic dilatation ● Colonoscopy: this allows direct visualization and biopsies to be taken which is essential both for the diagnosis and for surveillance of colonic cancer in patients with chronic disease; again contraindicated in those at risk of toxic dilatation ● Histology: the diagnosis of UC should be supported by histological evidence although the appearances are not usually pathognomonic.

Complications (→ Table 5.2)

Table 5.2 Complications of ulcerative colitis	
Local	Extra-colonic
Haemorrhage	Seronegative arthritis
Strictures	Uveitis
Rupture	Chronic liver disease eg CAH, sclerosing cholangitis
Carcinoma	

Management *Medical:* acute severe colitis should be managed with iv fluids, blood transfusion and parenteral nutrition where indicated and high dose parenteral steroids (hydrocortisone 100 mg qid). The commoner relapsing/ remitting course should be treated with high dose steroids (40 mg prednisolone daily) to control symptoms followed by their rapid withdrawal over 2–3 weeks once remission occurs. Sulphasalazine (2–4 g/d) or 5-amino salicylic acid preparations eg mesalazine 6 tabs/day in divided doses should be used to reduce the frequency of relapse. Distal colitis and proctitis may be adequately controlled without systemic steroids but with steroid enemata for relapses and salazopyrine for maintenance.

Surgical indications for surgery are:

• Acute UC not responding to medical management.

• Relapsing/remitting disease responding poorly to drug therapy.

• Long-standing disease where severe dysplasia or carcinoma has been identified.

The commonest operation is pancolectomy with ileostomy. Ileorectal anastomosis is preferred by some although continued disease activity may occur in the retained rectum and long-term surveillance of the rectum for malignancy is required. More recently ileoanal pouch operations have become more popular but are not without their problems.

Cancer surveillance The risk of developing colorectal cancer in UC is well recognized. This depends upon the extent of the disease and duration. In pancolitis the risk is increased after 10 years to 1%, after 20 years to 13% and after 30 years to 34%. Left-sided colitis is associated with a lower but still significant increased risk after 20 years. It is believed that neoplasms in patients with UC are preceded by initially mild and later severe dysplasia of the colonic epithelium and the aim of surveillance is to identify such premalignant changes. Colonoscopy with multiple biopsies should be performed every 18–24 months and more frequently once early dysplasia is recognized.

GASTRIC CARCINOMA

The frequency of gastric cancer is decreasing although it still remains a relatively common and lethal tumour. Sixty percent involve the prepyloric region and antrum but spread into the duodenum is very rare. The cause is unknown but dietary factors and N-nitroso compound ingestion are believed important. It is particularly common in certain countries such as Japan and Chile and is more frequent in individuals with blood group A. Other predisposing factors include atrophic gastritis, pernicious anaemia and previous gastric surgery. It is now not believed that benign gastric ulcer can become malignant and that malignant ulcers are malignant from the outset even though they may initially appear to heal with drug therapy.

Clinical features

Symptoms: These develop late and include epigastric pain, weight loss, dysphagia (tumours in the cardia), vomiting (tumours in the antrum).

Signs: epigastric mass, haematemesis, melaena, pallor, acanthosis nigricans, succussion splash, ascites, supraclavicular lymphadenopathy (Virchow's node, Troisier's sign) and hepatomegaly (due to metastatic spread).

Investigation ● Barium meal commonly shows an irregular ulcer or filling defect. Occasionally a thick wall contracted stomach without peristalsis is identified (linitus plastica); this latter may be missed both at endoscopy and with endoscopic biopsies as the tumour infiltrates deep to the mucosa ● Gastroscopy is the investigation of choice allowing visualization, biopsies and cytology ● US is useful both to exclude hepatic spread but may identify thickening of the gastric wall ● CT scanning may be needed for staging.

Management Surgery offers the only hope of cure but unfortunately only for small localized tumours. The vast majority of gastric cancers diagnosed in Western society do not fall within this category having already spread. This is not true for Japan where screening programmes exist and early diagnosis and treatment is common.

Even for patients where curative resection is not possible surgery offers the best form of palliation, particularly for antral tumours where gastric outlet obstruction is a complication and for cardial lesions which may result in complete dysphagia. The patient's clinical condition should be optimized prior to surgery by blood transfusion, correction of biochemical derangements and parenteral nutrition, if indicated. Radiotherapy is of no value whilst chemotherapy may produce remission in a minority.

Prognosis This depends upon the tumour stage. The 5-year survival for early gastric cancer is over 75% but less than 10% for the later and commoner lesion. Screening programmes for high-risk groups such as post-gastric surgery and pernicious anaemia are advocated by some. Early endoscopy should be considered in all patients over 35 years with dyspepsia.

IRRITABLE BOWEL SYNDROME

Irritable bowel syndrome (IBS) is the commonest gastro-intestinal disorder affecting females more often than males and commonest in the 4–6th decades. The principle symptoms of change in bowel habit associated with abdominal pain and bloating may closely resemble other GI pathology and a diagnosis by exclusion is common.

Pathogenesis Abnormalities in muscular tone of the GI tract are present and are responsible for the symptoms. A family history is common and a diet deficient in fibre is believed important. Emotional and pyschological factors are often important.

Clinical features

Symptoms: Poorly localized abdominal pain most commonly in the L iliac fossa or epigastrium. The pain may be exacerbated by eating, stress and pre-menstrually and relieved by defaecation. Abdominal bloating is common. Alternating diarrhoea, often on rising in the morning, and constipation is characteristic although one usually predominates. The passage of mucus is common but rectal bleeding is *not* a feature and should never be attributed to IBS.

Signs: usually few but include abdominal distension, tenderness over the colon and mucus on PR examination.

Investigation • No diagnostic tests are available although in the young the diagnosis can be confidently made in those with a characteristic history • Sigmoidoscopy • barium enema and • upper GI endoscopy are required in many subjects to exclude such disorders as peptic ulceration and colorectal cancer. In many subjects with IBS such common disorders as gallstones or diverticular disease may be identified and symptoms should not necessarily be attributed to these.

Management An adequate explanation of the disorder is essential and some patients benefit greatly from psychotherapy. Dietary manipulation to gradually increase the fibre content to approximately 7 g may be useful particularly in those with constipation and foods which exacerbate symptoms should be identified and omitted. Drug therapy is not necessary in many patients and where used is directed at symptoms – antispasmodics such as anticholinergics and Colpermin for pain, drugs such as loperamide for diarrhoea and bulking agents such as hydrophilic colloids for constipation. In a small number of patients antidepressants are of value whereas sedatives such as benzodiazepines should not be used.

INFECTIVE BOWEL DISEASE

These can be divided into those which produce acute diarrhoea and specific GI infections and infestations.

ACUTE INFECTIOUS DIARRHOEA

Three clinical syndromes are recognized: (→ also p 253.)

Acute food poisoning: this is characterized by vomiting and diarrhoea within 24 hours of ingesting contaminated food and is due to a bacterial toxin within the food. The commonest organisms are toxin-producing strains of *Staph. aureus, C. perfringens* and *Bacillus cereus.* A rare and atypical cause, *C. botulinum,* the toxin of which causes progressive paralysis.

Acute watery diarrhoea: is due to enterotoxin-producing or invasive organisms transmitted via contaminated water or food or occasionally from person to person. Pathogens include enterotoxin-producing *E. coli* and *V. cholerae:* invasive organisms include Rotavirus, *Salmonella, E. coli,* Norwalk virus and *Giardia lamblia.*

Bloody diarrhoea: the organisms causing this form of diarrhoea in which blood is obvious within the faeces include both invasive and enterotoxin-producing forms such as *Salmonella, Shigella, Campylobacter jejuni, Y. enterocolitica, E. coli* and *E. histolytica. Cl. difficile* may cause pseudomembranous colitis after antibiotic therapy due to toxin production. Antibiotics most frequently implicated are ampicillin, clindamycin and lincomycin. In those where the organism is commensal the cytotoxin is not present.

Investigations ● Faecal culture and parasite screen will identify many organisms although jejunal aspiration may be necessary to identify *Giardia* ● Numerous WBC in the faeces identified by methylene blue staining is suggestive of colonic inflammation of either infective or inflammatory origin ● Sigmoidoscopy and biopsy is useful in the diagnosis of amoebiasis and excluding inflammatory bowel disease and pseudomembranous colitis ● Serological tests are available for *Salmonella, Campylobacter* and *Versinia* infections as well as *E. histolytica.*

Management This consists of rehydration, where indicated by such features as tachycardia, postural hypotension, reduced skin tugor and ocular pressure and oliguria. Replacement can usually be oral using fluids containing sodium, potassium, bicarbonate, chloride and glucose.

Intravenous fluids are indicated in those with persistent vomiting. No restriction on food intake is generally indicated although temporary milk intolerance may occur due to secondary lactase deficiency. Anti-diarrhoeal drugs such as codeine phosphate, diphenoxylate or loperamide may be useful in controlling symptoms but should be avoided in moderate to severe cases as they prolong infection. Antibiotics are listed in Table 5.3.

Table 5.3
Antibiotics for infective bowel disease

Pathogen	Antibiotic	Indication
Salmonella	Ampicillin Chloramphenicol Cotrimoxazole	Only if bacteraemic
Shigella	Cotrimoxazole	Symptomatic cases
Yersinia	Tetracycline	Symptomatic cases
Campylobacter	Erythromycin Tetracycline	Severe or persistent cases
Clostridium difficile	Vancomycin Metronidazole	Only when cytotoxin present
Giardia lamblia	Metronidazole Mepacrine	Repeated courses may be necessary

SPECIFIC INFECTIONS

Intestinal tuberculosis

This is an uncommon disorder in the UK but still prevalent world-wide. Infection of the GI tract with *Mycobacterium tuberculosis* most often affects the ileocaecal region and is usually identified in patients under investigation for suspected malignancy or inflammatory bowel disease.

Clinical features

Symptoms: Abdominal pain, fever, weight loss and diarrhoea.

Signs: RIF mass, splenomegaly and signs of associated pulmonary TB.

Investigation • CXR to identify current or previous TB • Positive Mantoux test and examination of sputum, urine, faeces and gastric aspirates • Barium studies of large and small bowel to identify wall thickening, ulceration and stricture formation similar to Crohn's disease • Colonoscopy and biopsy where appropriate • Laparotomy may be required to confirm the diagnosis.

Management 6 months' therapy with isoniazid and rifampicin. Ethambutol and pyrazinamide should be included for the first 2 months (see p 244).

Surgery is indicated for perforation, abscess formation, major haemorrhage and intestinal obstruction.

Traveller's diarrhoea

This is common in travellers to developing countries due to ingestion of contaminated food or water. The most frequent pathogens are: enterotoxigenic *E. coli*, *Shigella*, *Salmonella* and *Campylobacter*. Prophylactic treatment with cotrimoxazole or tetracycline reduces the incidence of infective traveller's diarrhoea. Less severe episodes of diarrhoea in travellers may just be due to a change in the bacterial flora and not truly infective.

Sexually transmitted intestinal infection

This is becoming more common and affects principally homosexuals and women practising receptive anal intercourse ($\rightarrow$ Table 5.4).

Table 5.4
Sexually transmitted intestinal infections

Problem	Cause
Anal lesions	Herpes simplex, secondary syphilis
Proctitis	Neisseria gonorrhoeae, Chlamydia trachomatis, herpes simplex, syphilis
Proctocolitis	Chlamydia trachomatis, Shigella, Salmonella, Campylobacter

In patients with AIDS other GI problems include enterocolitis due to *Giardia*, *Strongyloides* and *Cryptosporidia*; oesophagitis due to *Candida*, cytomegalovirus and Herpes simplex; cytomegalovirus vasculitis of the colon and Kaposi's sarcoma (p 258).

HELMINTH INFESTATIONS

Although relatively uncommon in the UK they represent a major health problem in many areas of the world.

Nematodes (roundworms)

Ascariasis Usually due to *Ascaris lumbricoides* is the commonest worm infestation in man. The adult worm resides in the upper small intestine and releases eggs which pass in the faeces. Infection is via the faecal-oral route. Ingested eggs release larvae which penetrate the intestinal wall and migrate to the lungs where they are coughed up and swallowed. Complications include anaemia, biliary obstruction, pancreatitis and appendicitis. *Treatment:* mebendazole 100 mg bd for 3 days.

Enterobiasis (threadworm) Infestation with *Enterobius vermicularis* is the commonest infestation in the UK. The adult worm resides in the caecum although the female worm migrates to the anus to lay eggs. Transmission is via the faecal-oral route with children often reinfecting themselves as a consequence of pruritus ani. *Treatment:* mebendazole.

Hookworms Most often **Ancylcostoma duodenale** and **Necator americanus** The adult worm resides in the upper small intestine and eggs are released and pass out in the faeces. These hatch outside the body and the larvae infect man by penetrating the skin (eg soles of feet). They pass then to the lungs, are coughed up and swallowed. *Symptoms* include local or generalized allergic reactions, anaemia and abdominal pain. *Treatment:* mebendazole.

Trichuriasis (whip worm) The adult *Trichuris trichuira* worm resides in the lower intestine and releases eggs which pass in the faeces. These are ingested and the eggs hatch within the GI tract. No visceral stage exists. *Clinical features* include abdominal pain, diarrhoea, eosinophilia and appendicitis. *Treatment:* mebendazole.

Strongyloides stercoralis The larvae of this worm may invade the host tissues especially in the immunosuppressed. *Clinical features* include colitis, malabsorption, pulmonary disease and neurological symptoms. *Treatment:* thiabendazole 25 mg/kg bd for 2–3 days.

Cestodes (tapeworms)

The commonest in man are *Taenia saginata* (beef tapeworm), *T. solium* (pork tapeworm), *Hymenolepis nana* (dwarf tapeworm) and *Diphyllobothrium latum* (fish tapeworm). The adult worm attaches to the intestinal wall by its head (scolex) and the fertilized eggs are passed in the faeces. The intermediate host ingests these and the larvae invade their viscera. Human infestation follows ingestion of poorly cooked or raw tissue from the intermediate host. *Cliniclal features* include nutritional deficiency, abdominal pain, pruritus ani, intestinal obstruction or perforation. *Treatment:* praziquantel.

Hydatid disease This is due to *Echinococcus granulosis* (or less often *E. multilocularis* or *E. oligarthus*) infection. Man is an intermediate host with the dog being the definitive host. Ova from dog faeces are ingested and pass to the liver via the portal vein and there develop into hydatid cysts. *Clinical features* include abdominal pain, hepatomegaly, cholangitis, cough and allergic reaction including anaphylaxis.

Diagnosis: • abdominal X-ray may reveal the calcified rim of the cyst although US is more sensitive • Serological tests and the Casoni skin test are available but may be negative in those where cyst leakage has not occurred. *Treatment:* surgical resection where possible, otherwise mebendazole.

Trematodes (flukes)

These are responsible for Schistosomiasis (bilhaziasis), liver flukes (Clonorchis) and *Fasciola hepatica* infestation ($\rightarrow$ p 128).

MALABSORPTION

> Malabsorption is the term used to describe the presence of nutrients, usually absorbed, in the faeces. In clinical practice it is usually only the fat content of the faeces that is measured. As well as abnormalities of absorption disorders of digestion and intestinal transit are usually included.

Aetiology

Mucosal: coeliac disease, tropical sprue, Whipple's disease, abetalipoproteinaemia.

Structural: intestinal resection, Crohn's disease, amyloidosis, intestinal ischaemia, lymphangiectasia, lymphoma.

Infective: acute enteritis, parasites eg giardia, bacterial overgrowth, TB.

Maldigestion: pancreatic insufficiency, biliary obstruction.

Systemic disease: hyper/hypothyroidism, diabetes mellitus, Addison's disease, dermatitis herpetiformis, connective tissue disease.

Investigations These can be divided into tests of • nutrient malabsorption • mucosal disease and • structural abnormality.

Fat malabsorption: the commonest test of malabsorption is the 3-day faecal fat collection during which the patient must be taking a normal fat diet of approximately 100 g/day. The ^{14}C triolein breath test is based on the release of $^{14}CO_2$ after metabolism of absorbed ^{14}C-labelled oleic acid. Gross steatorrhoea is suggestive of pancreatic disease.

Carbohydrate malabsorption: impairment of absorption of monosaccharides can be tested by the glucose and xylose tolerance tests. Disaccharide malabsorption: lactose tolerance test with normal giving a rise in blood glucose of >1 mmol/l, sucrose tolerance test abnormal in isomaltase deficiency. Radiological studies mixing the appropriate sugar with barium demonstrates intestinal hurry and dilatation.

Protein malabsorption: true malabsorption very rare. Excessive dietary protein catabolism occurs in bacterial overgrowth identified by the ^{14}C-glycocholate breath test. Protein losing enteropathy can be identified by faecal loss of ^{51}Cr-labelled albumin.

Bile salt malabsorption: detected by ^{14}C glycocholate breath test which is abnormal with terminal ileal disease and bacterial overgrowth. The ^{75}SeHAT test is also abnormal with terminal ileal disease but normal with bacterial overgrowth.

Vitamin B$_{12}$ malabsorption: the Schilling test using dual isotopes can differentiate between pernicious anaemia and ileal disease.

Radiology: Malabsorption may give abnormal appearances on the small bowel meal which include: barium flocculation, rapid transit, strictures or ulceration, oedematous mucosal folds and evidence of previous surgery.

Intestinal histology: ● biopsies of the small intestine can be obtained at endoscopy or with a Crosby capsule ● total villous atrophy – coeliac disease, tropical sprue, severe malnutrition, idiopathic mucosal enteropathy and cows' milk or soya sensitivity ● subtotal villous atrophy – partially teated coeliac disease, bacterial overgrowth, dermatitis herpetiformis, intestinal ischaemia and Zollinger-Ellison syndrome ● non-villous abnormality – Whipple's disease (PAS – positive macrophages), giardiasis, Crohn's disease, lymphoma, radiation enteritis, lymphangiectasia and abetalipoproteinaemia ● intestinal biopsies may be processed to assay brush border enzymes in some laboratories to aid diagnosis of malabsorption due to enzyme deficiency ● duodenal aspirates allow quantitative bacteriological studies to be performed in cases where bacterial overgrowth is suspected.

PANCREATIC CARCINOMA

This is the second commonest tumour of the GI tract causing 5% of all cancer deaths. Two main types occur: exocrine, principally adenocarcinoma and the less common endocrine tumours such as insulinomas and glucagonomas. The cause of pancreatic cancer is unknown but cigarette smoking, chronic pancreatitis and diabetes mellitus have all been incriminated.

Clinical features

Symptoms: Epigastric pain which radiates posteriorly is present in the majority, weight loss, jaundice in tumours involving the head of the pancreas, anorexia, nausea and vomiting. In the rare insulinoma, confusion due to hypoglycamia is characteristic.

Signs: include steatorrhoea, palpable gallbladder (Courvoisier's law) and occasionally thrombophlebitis migrans. In glucagonomas a necrolytic migratory erythematous rash may develop.

Investigations • An increased alkaline phosphatase and bilirubin occur with tumours obstructing the CBD • Impaired glucose tolerance or frank diabetes may be found • CEA levels may be increased in those with hepatic metastases • US and CT scanning are the two most useful tests which identify a pancreatic mass and/or dilatation of the CBD • ERCP may identify a stricture of the CBD or pancreatic duct • A tissue diagnosis should be obtained by US or CT-guided fine needle biopsy.

Management Cure can only be achieved by surgery but this is only applicable for those with small, localized tumours. Radical pancreatoduodenectomy (Whipple's operation) should be considered for such lesions. In the majority of patients, who are usually elderly, curative resection is not possible due to early localized spread. Palliation of jaundice and associated itch can be achieved by endoscopic stenting through the CBD stricture or surgery to create biliary diversion such as cholecystojejunostomy. Enteric bypass may be necessary for vomiting due to duodenal involvement. Pain relief is usually required using opiates and/or coeliac plexus block. The use of chemotherapy remains controversial. Endocrine tumours should be resected if localized. Streptozotocin is useful in the treatment of insulinomas.

Prognosis This is very poor with a one-year survival of less than 10%.

PANCREATITIS

Inflammation of the pancreas can be divided into: acute pancreatitis, including relapsing acute pancreatitis and chronic pancreatitis, including relapsing chronic pancreatitis. Differentiation into these categories, particularly the relapsing type may not be obvious and depends upon the permanency of abnormalities on pancreatic function testing.

Aetiology The causes of acute and chronic pancreatitis overlap ($\rightarrow$ Table 5.5). The pathogenesis of pancreatitis is incompletely understood but interruption of the flow of pancreatic juice and/or reflux of bile into the pancreatic duct may be important. The severity of damage to the pancreas varies from mild inflammation with oedema to haemorrhagic necrosis. In chronic pancreatitis the ongoing inflammation results in fibrosis initially around ducts and acini but latter within the acini.

ACUTE PANCREATITIS

Clinical features

Symptoms: Pain, usually severe, is almost always present and maximal in the epigastrium and radiating to the back. The pain may be relieved by sitting forward. Nausea and vomiting are also common.

Signs: include epigastric tenderness and guarding, abdominal distension, pyrexia, jaundice, peri-umbilical or flank bruising (Cullen's and Grey-Turner's signs respectively), shock and coma.

Table 5.5
Pancreatitis

Acute	Chronic
Alcohol	Alcohol
Gallstones	Obstruction of
Drugs eg thiazides, azathioprine	pancreatic duct
oestrogen, frusemide	Hyperparathyroidism
Trauma	Haemochromatosis
Post-operative, post ERCP	Idiopathic
Pancreatic carcinoma	Hereditary
Hyperparathyroidism	Tropical calcific
Viral infection eg mumps,	pancreatitis
coxsackie, E-B virus.	

Investigation ● Serum amylase levels are high in the vast majority. Normal levels occasionally occur because the patient presents late. In these cases high urinary amylase levels may be detected. Other disorders may give rise to hyperamylasaemia (→ Table 5.6 (p 110)) ● Pancreatic calcification on the abdominal X-ray is characteristic of alcoholic pancreatitis; a sentinel duodenal loop due to regional ileus may be present whilst the ● CXR may show elevation of the L hemidiaphragm with atelectasis and pleural effusion ● FBC often shows a leukocytosis and rise in Hb due to haemoconcentration ● Hyperglycaemia, hypocalcaemia, hypoxaemia and methaemalbuminaemia indicate severe pancreatitis ● Peritoneal lavage reveals fluid with high amylase and transaminase levels in severe pancreatitis ● US scanning may detect swelling of the inflamed gland and may also identify gallstones in the gallbladder or dilatation of the CBD; US is particularly useful in identifying pancreatic pseudocysts, a common complication of acute pancreatitis.

> **Table 5.6**
> **Causes of hyperamylasaemia**
>
> Acute pancreatitis
> Intestinal perforation or obstruction
> Laparotomy
> Morphine
> Posterior penetrating DU
> Renal failure
> Mumps
> Mesenteric ischaemia
> Hepatitis
> Pancreatic cancer
> Burns
> Congenital hyperamylasaemia

Complications   These are common and include shock, pancreatic pseudocysts and abscesses, ARDS, diabetes mellitus, renal and hepatic failure and DIC.

> **Management**   No definitive treatment is available and supportive measures such as correcting electrolyte disturbances, fluid replacement and adequate pain relief are important. Recognition and early treatment of renal and respiratory failure, and infection including abscesses is essential. Other treatment such as reducing pancreatic secretion by nasogastric aspiration or glucagon, early surgery for severe necrotic pancreatitis and early ERCP with sphincterotomy to allow passage of bile duct stones have all been shown in some studies to be beneficial.

Prognosis   The mortality from acute pancreatitis is approximately 15% and acute haemorrhagic pancreatitis has a mortality of over 50%. Predictive factors of a poor prognosis include fever, hypotension, tachycardia and respiratory problems on admission. The later development of hypocalcaemia, hypoxaemia and hyperglycaemia are all poor prognostic indices.

CHRONIC PANCREATITIS

This is a relatively common disease the commonest cause of which is chronic alcohol abuse. The pathophysiology is ill understood but may be related to alcohol-induced change in the composition of pancreatic juice resulting in precipitation and obstructive plug formation. Damage to acini results with fibrosis which often appears to involve nerve fibres. Less common causes include hypercalcaemia, hyperlipidaemia and heredity.

Clinical features

Symptoms: The commonest is epigastric pain which may radiate posteriorly. Weight loss, steatorrhoea, nausea and vomiting are common. Diabetes mellitus, with polydipsia and polyuria is common particularly in calcific pancreatitis.

Signs: are few other than abdominal tenderness. Jaundice may occur if the CBD is obstructed. Splenic vein thrombosis may result in splenomegaly and portal hypertension.

Investigation • Faecal fat, gross steatorrhoea is highly suggestive of pancreatic disease • Blood glucose may confirm diabetes • Pancreatic function tests are necessary to confirm exocrine pancreatic insufficiency; the tubeless tests such as the PABA and the Pancreolauryl test are replacing older tests eg Lundh test meal • Plain abdominal X-ray may reveal pancreatic calcification • US in experienced hands is fairly sensitive and both it and CT scanning are useful excluding pancreatic cancer • ERCP usually shows abnormalities both in the main pancreatic duct and side branches but a normal pancreatogram does not exclude chronic pancreatitis.

> **Management** This revolves around adequate pain relief and treating malabsorption, with dietary manipulation to maintain calorie intake whilst reducing fat, and pancreatic enzymes eg Pancrex Forte or Creon 1–5 tab with food, and controlling diabetes mellitus. Achieving adequate pain relief is often difficult and generally patients become dependant on opiates and suicide is well recognized. Absolute abstinence from alcohol is essential. Surgical procedures advocated to relieve pain where medical means fail include distal pancreatectomy, pancreatoduodenectomy, pancreaticojejunostomy and sphincteroplasty (for sphincter of Oddi disease).

Prognosis This is dependent upon age and continued alcohol intake and overall approximately 25–30% die within 10 years.

APPENDICITIS

> Inflammation of the vermiform appendix is usually due to normal bowel flora and is commonly preceded by obstruction of the appendiceal lumen by lymphoid tissue or faecoliths. Inflammation results in oedema and ischaemia of the wall which may lead to gangrene and perforation. It is commonest in children and young adults and is the most frequent cause for acute surgery in this age group.

Clinical features

Symptoms: Pain which characteristically starts periumbilically and moves to the RIF as visceral and parietal peritoneum respectively are involved. Nausea, vomiting and anorexia are common as is recent constipation.

Signs: fever, tenderness over McBurney's point (1/3 along a line from the anterior superior iliac spine to the umbilicus). Guarding and rebound tenderness suggest parietal peritoneal inflammation. Pain on passive hyperextension of the thigh (psoas sign) may be present, tenderness on rectal examination. Ureteric colic may be simulated by an appendix lying beside the R ureter. A mass in the RIF suggests abscess formation.

Investigations ● A leukocytosis is usually present and ● US may be useful. The diagnosis is essentially a clinical one and a large differential diagnosis exists (→ Table 5.7).

Table 5.7
Differential diagnosis in appendicitis

Diagnosis	Useful features
Mesenteric adenitis	Less guarding and pain
Acute regional ileitis	Diarrhoea cf constipation
Pancreatitis	Hyperamylasaemia
Renal colic	Radio-opaque stone and haematuria
Volvulus/intussusception	Characteristic radiograph
Cholecystitis	HIDA-scanning
Pyelonephritis	Urine microscopy

Management Early surgery is standard treatment. In mild cases or when surgery is contraindicated iv fluids and antibiotics may produce resolution but careful surveillance for deterioration or signs of perforation is essential. A fixed mass indicates abscess formation due to a sealed perforation and conservative treatment with delayed surgery is appropriate. Perforation carries a significant mortality and resolution of an appendix abscess may take several weeks.

COLORECTAL CARCINOMA

This is the second commonest malignancy in the UK and is increasing, particularly those of the right side of the colon.

Aetiology Factors implicated include dietary mutagens, deficiency of dietary anti-mutagens, lack of dietary fibre, low dietary calcium and bile acids. Patients at increased risk include those with IBD (especially UC), previous colonic polyps or tumours, a history of ovarian or breast cancer and a family history of colonic cancer or familial polyposis syndromes such as familial polyposis, Gardner's and Turcot's syndromes.

Clinical features

Symptoms: Abdominal discomfort, rectal bleeding, weight loss and change in bowel habit.

Signs: include pallor, abdominal mass, rectal mass or ulcer on rectal examination and jaundice. Occasionally presentation may be acute with intestinal obstruction or perforation.

Investigations • Rectal examination reveals a palpable mass in less than 50% of cases but when combined with rigid sigmoidoscopy the percentage is significantly increased • These investigations in combination with barium enema will detect the majority of lesions • The sensitivity of colonoscopy by an experienced operator is high and allows histological confirmation. In 20% more than one tumour is identified.

Management This depends upon the size and extent of the tumour. Staging is usually according to Duke's classification (→ Table 5.8).

**Table 5.8
Staging in colorectal carcinoma**

Duke's class	Extent	Percentage of 5-year survival
A	Limited to muscularis propria	95
B	Through wall but not involving regional lymph nodes	70
C_1	Regional lymph nodes involved resection complete	35
C_2	Nodes proximal to resection line involved	15
D	Distant metastases present	5

Small tumours confined to polyps may be removed endoscopically. Surgery is indicated for all other lesions and even in Duke's class D surgical palliation prevents intestinal obstruction. The benefit of adjuvant chemotherapy and radiotherapy is controversial.

DIVERTICULAR DISEASE

This is the commonest structural disorder of the large bowel which affects approximately 50% of the population over the age of 70 years. It is generally asymptomatic unless diverticulitis develops. This latter is a complication caused by obstruction of the diverticular neck by faecal material.

Aetiology   It is commonly believed that deficiency of dietary fibre results in hypertrophy of both the longitudinal and circular muscle of the colon leading to hypersegmentation and increased intraluminal pressure with the development of pulsion diverticulae. The evidence of this theory is however scanty and normal aging of the bowel is probably important.

Clinical features

Symptoms: These are largely if not entirely due to complicating diverticulitis with abdominal pain, fever, nausea and vomiting.

Signs: include LIF tenderness and rectal bleeding. Fistula formation may occur between the colon and bladder, vagina and small bowel presenting with pneumaturia, vaginal discharge and malabsorption respectively. Colonic stricture formation may develop with constipation, colic and later vomiting.

Investigations   ● The diagnosis of diverticular disease is made on barium enema ● Diverticulitis can be presumed in those with diverticular disease associated with fever, leukocytosis and pain. The barium enema may reveal signs of active inflammation. The presence of rectal bleeding or stricture formation requires the exclusion of colorectal cancer ● Colonoscopy with biopsy is useful but may be difficult in those with large diverticulae ● Other diseases which may require exclusion include ischaemic colitis, UC and Crohn's disease.

Management   In those with diverticular disease the risk of developing diverticulitis is reduced by a high fibre diet. Treatment of diverticulitis includes bed-rest, iv fluids and antibiotics, analgesics and antispasmodics. Surgical intervention is required in only a minority and is indicated for peritonitis, fistula formation, pericolic abscess formation, persistent haemorrhage, bowel obstruction and repeated attacks of diverticulitis despite medical therapy.

RECTAL BLEEDING

Rectal bleeding is common and may indicate serious disease and must not just be attributed to haemorrhoids without proper investigation.

Clinical features   The freshness of the blood and whether it is mingled within the faeces should be noted and may be of use in determining the site of bleeding ($\rightarrow$ Table 5.9). Fresh blood streaking the faeces is typical of bleeding from haemorrhoids unlike the mixture of blood and diarrhoea in UC.

Table 5.9
Clinical features of rectal bleeding

Profuse bleeding	Minor bleeding
Ulcerative colitis	All causes of profuse
Haemorrhoids	bleeding
Diverticulitis	Colorectal cancer
Arteriovenous malformation	Infective colitis
	Crohn's disease
	Polyps
	Ischaemic colitis
	Idiopathic colonic
	ulcers

Investigation   ● All patients should undergo sigmoidoscopy which allows identification of active bleeding from haemorrhoids, rectal tumours and UC ● Colonoscopy is the investigation of choice although may be difficult in the face of active bleeding. It does allow histological confirmation of lesions such as colonic tumours and allow treatment of such lesions as polyps by polypectomy and a-v malformations by laser ● Double contrast barium enema also identifies many causes of colonic bleeding but is not useful during active bleeding ● Arteriography may be invaluable in identifying bleeding lesions particularly when active bleeding at a rate of 1–2 ml/minute exists ● Radionuclide studies using radio-labelled erythrocytes may be useful in identifying the site of occult bleeding providing significant bleeding takes place at the time of investigation.

Management   This depends upon the cause although investigation should not be undertaken until the patient has been adequately resuscitated.

GALLSTONE DISEASE

By the sixth decade 20% of women and 10% of men have gallstones and with advancing age the prevalence increases, although always commoner in females. In Western society cholesterol or mixed cholesterol-calcium-bilirubin stones account for the majority of stones. The pathogensis is incompletely understood but factors which may produce lithogenic bile include increased cholesterol content, reduced bile acids and biliary stasis. In the majority of cases gallstones are asymptomatic and only 10% develop symptoms after 5 years. Gallstones are responsible for three main disorders: cholecystitis, biliary colic and choledocholithiasis.

CHOLECYSTITIS

Gallstone impaction in the cystic duct is the commonest cause of cholecystitis. Less common causes include primary infection eg *Salmonella typhi* or *Ascaris lumbricoides,* trauma, surgery, chemotherapy and TPN.

Clinical features

Symptoms: RUQ pain often with radiation to the R shoulder, nausea, vomiting and fever.

Signs: RUQ tenderness, gallbladder tenderness demonstrable on inspiration (Murphy's sign), gallbladder usually impalpable and jaundice in a minority of patients.

Investigations ● FBC usually demonstrates a leukocytosis ● abdominal X-ray reveals radio-opaque stones in a minority and occasionally a sentinel loop or air in the biliary tree ● US demonstrates gallbladder stones and thickening of the mucosa ● Radio-isotopic scanning (HIDA; PIPIDA) is useful in identifying obstruction of the cystic duct.

Complications Empyema, gangrene and gallbladder perforation, pancreatitis, perihepatic abscesses, portal pyaemia and septicaemia.

Management Initially supportive with iv fluids, analgesics and antibiotics eg amoxycillin and tobramycin. Cholecystectomy once the patient is stable is the treatment of choice although the timing of surgery ie early or delayed (interval) cholecystectomy is controversial and depends upon the patients condition and age. Percutaneous cholecystotomy may be indicated in seriously ill patients.

BILIARY COLIC

This is usually due to stone impaction in the cystic duct.

Clinical features

Symptoms: A constant epigastric or RUQ pain which usually increases over 2–3 hours before settling. Pain for more than 6 hours should suggest cholecystitis. Nausea and vomiting are common.

Investigations The diagnosis is largely clinical particularly since gallstones are so prevalent. Many patients with gallstones and dyspepsia are not helped by cholecystectomy and in many the abdominal discomfort is due to IBS (hepatic flexure syndrome) ● Transient increases in bilirubin and alkaline phosphatase support the diagnosis of biliary colic ● Biliary scintigraphy may demonstrate cystic duct obstruction if performed during an attack.

> *Management* Analgesia until the attack has passed. Morphine increases the sphincter of Oddi pressure and should be avoided. Cholecystectomy is indicated for those fit for surgery. In those unfit or who refuse surgery gallstone dissolution therapy with ursodeoxycholic acid is appropriate for those with radiolucent stones less than 1.5 cm in diameter and with a functioning gallbladder on oral cholecystography. Complete dissolution occurs in approximately 30% at 12 months.

CHOLEDOCHOLITHIASIS

Common bile duct stones most commonly arise from gallbladder stones but may form in the bile ducts due to biliary strictures, primary or secondary sclerosing cholangitis or in Caroli's disease.

Clinical features May be asymptomatic.

Symptoms: include biliary colic, intermittent or constant RUQ pain, nausea and vomiting.

Signs: fluctuating jaundice, RUQ tenderness and palpable gallbladder in 15%. Fever and rigors indicate cholangitis.

Investigations ● FBC reveals a leukocytosis and LFTs an increased bilirubin, alkaline phosphatase and gamma GT; a mild elevation of transaminases is not uncommon ● A prolonged PT is common ● Abdominal X-rays may reveal radio-opaque stones or rarely air within the biliary tree ● US may reveal dilatation of the biliary tree but is not sensitive in identifying the stones within the CBD which usually requires ERCP or PTC.

Complications Pancreatitis, cholangitis, septicaemia, hepatic abscess and secondary sclerosing cholangitis or biliary cirrhosis.

Management Initially analgesia, iv fluids and antibiotics (eg amoxycillin or tobramycin). Stone removal is best achieved by ERCP, sphincterotomy and extraction with a Dormia basket or balloon. Large stones may be dissolved or reduced in size chemically with methyl-tert-butyl-ether or mono-octanion administered via a naso-biliary tube. Mechanical fragmentation of stones by lithotripsy may prove to be a useful alternative.

6

Hepatology

119

FBC   A macrocytosis is common in chronic liver disease particularly of alcoholic origin. A reduced platelet count is also common due partly to hypersplenism.

LFTs   These reflect hepatic dysfunction rather than function and are discussed in more depth on page 300.

Serology

- AntiHBsAg – previous HBV infection

- AntiHBcAg – recent HBV infection

- IgM antiHAV – recent hepatitis A infection

- AntiHDV – previous Delta virus infection

- AntiHCV – previous hepatitis C infection

- Antimitochondrial Ab – positive in the vast majority of patients with primary biliary cirrhosis

- ANF and antismooth muscle Ab – positive in many patients with autoimmune CAH

Other blood tests

- α-fetoprotein increased in hepatomas ● low levels of α_1-antitrypsin in patients homozygous for PiZ or PiS

- Caeruloplasmin – low in Wilson's disease ● cholesterol – high in Zieve's syndrome (along with haemolysis and leukocytosis) and chronic cholestasis

- Hypoglycaemia in fulminant hepatic failure and some patients with hepatoma

- Ferritin – very high in haemochromatosis

Radiology   ● The plain abdominal X-ray may reveal air within the biliary tree after sphincterotomy or in patients with gallstone ileus ● US is an important investigation looking both at the liver parenchyma and the diameter of the biliary tree ● ERCP is invaluable in investigating the biliary tree ● PTC is useful in investigating those with dilated intrahepatic ducts ● CT scanning is important in identifying lesions within the hepatic parenchyma ● Angiography of the hepatic artery and, during the venous phase, the portal system, may be essential in investigating those with hepatic tumours or portal hypertension ● A measure of the portal pressure can be obtained by hepatic venous catheterization using a balloon catheter (wedged hepatic venous pressure)

Liver biopsy   Either obtained percutaneously or at laparoscopy is usually required in the diagnosis of most hepatic disorders. In those with coagulopathy or ascites a transjugular route for biopsy may be used reducing the risk of haemorrhage.

ACUTE VIRAL HEPATITIS

Acute viral hepatitis is common and may be caused by a large variety of viruses the best known of which are hepatitis A and B viruses, non-A non-B agents, Delta virus and Epstein-Barr virus. The clinical picture in each may vary from mild anicteric disease to fulminant hepatic failure. Patients may present with acute hepatitis due to other causes which require to be excluded especially where viral serology is negative. Other causes include: drugs such as paracetamol poisoning, isoniazid, allopurinol, halothane, methyldopa, sulphonamides; Wilson's disease, poisons such as Amanita phalloides, Reye's syndrome (in children), lymphoma and Budd-Chiari syndrome.

HEPATITIS A VIRUS

A 27–30 nm, single-stranded RNA virus. Infection never becomes chronic and immunity measured by anti-hepatitis A titres is usually life-long. Active or recent infection diagnosed by IgM anti-HAV.

HEPATITIS B VIRUS

Consists of a central structure, the Dane particle, made up of the core antigen HBcAg (the e antigen, HBeAg, is part of the core antigen) within which is contained DNA-polymerase and double stranded DNA. Surrounding the central particle is the surface antigen, HBsAg. The appearance of the various antigens and antibodies during acute HBV infection is illustrated in Figure 6.1. Anti-pre-S antibodies appear early in the infection.

Infection with HBV in the UK is most commonly venereal or via shared needles in iv drug abusers. Classically infection is followed by the onset of jaundice 2–3 months later accompanied by a serum-sickness-like illness with fever and arthralgia. Acute infection is confirmed by IgM anti-HBc. 10% of patients develop chronic carriage and this is more frequent in males. The population carriage rate in the UK is approximately 0.1%. No specific treatment for acute or chronic HBV infection exists although α interferon holds some promise. Prophylaxis can be obtained in the short term by hepatitis B immune globulin and long term with HBV vaccines.

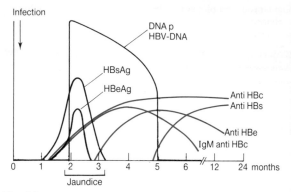

Fig. 6.1
Acute hepatitis B infection.

HEPATITIS D VIRUS

This is a defective virus which requires co-infection with HBV to be pathogenic in man. It is rare in the UK and common in southern Europe. Co-infection with HBV and HDV results in a more severe illness with a higher rate of fulminant hepatic failure. HDV infection in carriers of HBV may result in relapse. Acute infection is diagnosed by IgM anti-Delta antibodies.

NON-A, NON-B VIRUSES

This represents at least three viruses which cause hepatitis which have not yet been characterized. Post-transfusion hepatitis, thought to be due to hepatitis C virus, is the commonest form in the UK. Epidemic infections with non-A, non-B viruses occur and sporadic cases are recognized although the viral aetiology of this latter group is difficult to prove. Chronic liver disease is a recognized sequela of non-A, non-B infection as is fulminant hepatic failure, which seems more likely during pregnancy.

EPSTEIN-BARR INFECTION

Infection results in jaundice in 10–15% and is accompanied by pharyngitis, lymphadenopathy and splenomegaly. The diagnosis is confirmed by atypical lymphocytes in the blood and a positive monospot, although this latter test may be falsely positive in hepatitis A. Chronic liver disease does not occur.

Management No specific treatment exists. Supportive measures include bed-rest, alcohol abstinence and a low fat, high carbohydrate diet. Steroid therapy improves the LFTs in many but does not influence the natural history favourably. Prevention is best and includes the use of immune globulin and vaccines and reducing the risk of transmission by screening blood donors for HBsAg and anti-HBc antibodies and those with elevated serum transaminase levels.

CHRONIC HEPATITIS

This is defined as inflammatory disease of the liver for longer than 6 months. Causes include:

- Chronic HBV infection
- Autoimmune CAH
- Chronic non-A, non-B hepatitis
- Alcohol abuse
- Drugs eg isoniazid, methyldopa, nitrofurantoin
- Metabolic eg Wilson's disease.

CHRONIC HEPATITIS DUE TO HBV CARRIAGE

Approximately 10% of patients, particularly males, with acute HBV infection do not clear the virus by 6 months.

Clinical features Many are asymptomatic and may present only with complications of cirrhosis later. Others may show weight loss, lethargy and hepatomegaly.

Investigations • Serology divides patients into those in the replicative (HBsAg +ve, HBeAg +ve, DNA-polymerase +ve and IgM antiHBc +ve) and non-replicative phase (HBsAg +ve, HBeAg −ve, DNA-polymerase −ve, anti-HBe +ve and IgM anti-HBc −ve). Those in the replicative phase are more often symptomatic and have more active liver disease ie chronic active hepatitis (CAH) rather than chronic persistent hepatitis • Coexistent HDV infection should be excluded.

Management Steroids are not effective and although LFTs may improve viral replication is encouraged. Anti-viral drugs and in particular α-interferon 3–5 million units sc 3 × per week may well be useful particularly in those in the replicative phase of HBV infection.

AUTO-IMMUNE CAH

This is typically a disease of young and middle-aged women, associated with HLA A1, B8, DRW3 and reduced numbers of suppressor T-cells. In most it presents insidiously but may mimic acute viral hepatitis.

Clinical features Spider naevi, amenorrhoea, hepatosplenomegaly. Associated disorders include diabetes mellitus, hypothyroidism, arthropathy, Coomb's positive haemolytic anaemia, fibrosing alveolitis and ulcerative colitis.

Investigations ● HBsAg – ve ● LFTs with 5–10 × increase in transaminases and 2–5 × increase in bilirubin ● Anti-smooth muscle and ANF positive in 70% and antimitochondrial antibodies in 25% ● Liver histology reveals large numbers of lymphocytes in the portal tract infiltrating into the hepatocyte lobules with little fatty change. Cirrhosis develops rapidly without treatment.

> *Management* Prednisolone 30–40 mg daily for one week reducing over next month to maintenance dose of 10 mg/day. If LFTs and liver histology do not normalize add azathioprine (50 mg/d). Continue steroids (and/or azathioprine) for 2 years before slowly withdrawing. Approximately 50% will remain in remission and for those who relapse steroids should be reintroduced.

Prognosis Steroid therapy has greatly improved survival although many patients still develop cirrhosis with its complications of variceal haemorrhage and ascites. Younger patients who develop liver failure should be considered for liver transplantation.

ALCOHOLIC LIVER DISEASE

> Alcohol abuse is increasing in the UK and the incidence of alcoholic cirrhosis, which currently is approximately 10 per 100 000 per year, is also increasing. The threshold beyond which alcoholic liver disease may occur is 21 units (a unit being 10g of alcohol or a 1/2 pint of beer or one measure of spirits) per week for men and 14 units for women.

Aetiology Ethanol is metabolized in the liver mainly by alcohol dehydrogenase to acetaldehyde and hydrogen ions. The latter affects the NADH:NAD ratio in the cell which affects the cell membrane and in conjunction with the toxic effect of acetaldehyde results in cell damage. Other enzyme systems such as the microsomal ethanol oxidising system (MEOS) are also involved particularly in heavy drinkers. Other factors implicated include female sex, associated malnutrition, HLA B8 and DW2 genotype and immunological responses against alcohol induced antigens.

Classification

Fatty liver: this is the mildest form of hepatic injury and is reversible.

Alcoholic hepatitis: with perivenular (zone 3) hepatocellular damage, Mallory's hyaline and an inflammatory cell infiltrate; jaundice, fever and ascites are common.

Perivenular sclerosis with perisinusoidal fibrosis and collagenation of the space of Disse: leads to cirrhosis. It may accompany fatty change resulting in cirrhosis without alcoholic hepatitis.

Cirrhosis: characterized by fibrosis and nodule formation and is irreversible and usually accompanied by portal hypertension.

Clinical features

Symptoms: These include nausea, vomiting, anorexia and fever.

Signs: include spider naevi, hepatomegaly, splenomegaly, ascites, parotitis and macrocytic anaemia.

Investigations ● An accurate history of alcohol intake is essential ● FBC often reveals a macrocytosis ● LFTs an increased GGTP relfects ethanol abuse and an abnormal ALT hepatocellular damage. An AST:ALT ratio of >2 is suggestive of alcoholic damage ● An elevated serum IgA is common and antismooth muscle antibodies may be present.

> ***Management*** Total abstinence of alcohol is the only effective treatment and psychiatric referral may help compliance. In alcoholic hepatitis corticosteroids eg prednisolone 40 mg/day may be beneficial in those with marked cholestasis but improvement in survival is doubtful. Antithyroid drugs eg propylthiouracil has been shown in some trials to be useful in alcoholic hepatitis.

Prognosis This depends upon the stage of the disease and the continued alcohol intake. Alcoholic hepatitis carries a mortality of between 25–60%. In those with cirrhosis who abstain from alcohol the 5-year survival is approximately 70% cf 35% for those who continue to drink. Adverse prognostic features include variceal haemorrhage, ascites and jaundice.

CIRRHOSIS

This is defined as diffuse fibrosis and nodule formation. Classification into macronodular, frequently viral, and micronodular, often alcoholic depends upon the size of the nodules.

Aetiology

Infection: HBV infection, non-A, non-B hepatitis.

Metabolic: alcohol, haemochromatosis, Wilson's disease, α_1-antitrypsin deficiency, galactosaemia.

Immunological: PBC, chronic active hepatitis (CAH).

Drugs: methotrexate, methyldopa, isoniazid.

Vascular: Budd-Chiari syndrome, veno-occlusive disease, constrictive pericarditis.

Miscellaneous: sarcoidosis, prolonged cholestasis, intestinal bypass.

Clinical features

Symptoms: include lethargy, itch (especially PBC), ankle and abdominal swelling.

Signs: hepatomegaly, splenomegaly, bruising, spider naevi, finger clubbing, palmar erythema, parotitis, jaundice, testicular atrophy, ascites, gynaecomastia, reduced body hair and leukonychia.

Investigations These can be divided into those to identify the aetiology ie ● history of alcohol abuse ● high MCV and GGTP, serum ferritin, α_1-antitrypsin, caeruloplasmin ● viral serology ● autoantibodies and those to determine severity ie ● clotting studies albumin, platelets, bilirubin ● US (for spleen and liver size and ascites) ● endoscopy for varices ● portal pressure measurements ● EEG for encephalopathy ● Liver histology is usually required to confirm the diagnosis and disease activity.

Management Cirrhosis is irreversible and no treatment reverses the pathological process. Treatment for certain causes such as steroids for CAH, venesection for haemochromatosis and absolute alcohol abstinence for alcoholic cirrhosis retard disease advancement. The complications of cirrhosis such as ascites, encephalopathy and variceal haemorrhage should be treated appropriately. Propranolol 160 mg LA/day may reduce the risk of variceal haemorrhage and is indicated in those with large varices where no contraindications exist. Hepatic transplantation should be considered for patients with end-stage cirrhosis.

Prognosis This depends upon the cause and severity. For alcoholic cirrhosis the mortality for persistent drinkers is 65% at 5 years cf 30% for those who stop. Assessment of severity can be assessed from the Child's class (→ Table 6.1).

LIVER TUMOURS

> The commonest tumour in the liver is metastatic disease. Two major primary liver tumours exist, hepatocellular carcinoma and cholangiocarcinoma.

HEPATOCELLULAR CARCINOMA

This is a tumour of hepatocytes and is probably the commonest tumour in the world due to the endemic infection of HBV in the Far East.

Aetiology Chronic HBV carriage, cirrhosis of any cause but especially haemochromatosis and α_1-antitrypsin deficiency, toxins such as aflatoxin and drugs such as the contraceptive pill and anabolic steroids.

Clinical features Males 3× commoner than women, abdominal pain, weight loss, ascites, jaundice, fever, hepatomegaly with a bruit. Paraneoplastic syndromes include hypoglycaemia, erythrocytosis, hypercalcaemia and ectopic gonadotrophin production.

Investigations • Increased α-fetoprotein in 85% of cases complicating cirrhosis; much lower frequency in those with

Table 6.1 Child's Classification			
Score	1	2	3
Encephalopathy	None	Mild	Marked
Bilirubin (μmol/l)	<34	34–50	>50
Albumin (g/l)	>35	28–35	<28
PT (s prolonged)	<4	4–6	>6
Ascites	None	Mild	Marked
Bilirubin (In PBC and sclerosing cholangitis)	<68	68–170	>170

Add the individual scores <7 = Child's A, 7–9 = Child's B and >9 = Child's C. The survival for Child's C, the poorest prognostic group, is less than 12 months.

non-cirrhotic livers ● US and CT scanning ● Liver biopsy, often under laparoscopic or US guidance.

> **Management** Resection or liver transplantation currently offers the only hope of cure. Unfortunately early spread and the presence of cirrhosis precludes this in the majority. Chemotherapy with adriamycin or combinations of 5-fluorocytosine, methotrexate, vincristine and cyclophosphamide may be better but are toxic. Perfusion of chemotherapy drugs directly into the hepatic artery or hepatic artery ligation may be appropriate in certain cases. Pain control often requires opiates and/or coeliac plexus block.

CHOLANGIOCARCINOMA

A tumour of the biliary tree, this is much less common.

Aetiology Factors include Thorotrast (an obsolete contrast medium), gallstones and infestation with *Clonorchis sinensis*.

Clinical features Similar to hepatocellular carcinoma although central tumours present with jaundice early.

Investigation (as for hepatocellular carcinoma)

> **Management** Because early spread via the lymphatics occurs resection or liver transplantation is rarely possible. Palliation of jaundice and pruritus may be achieved by surgical bypass or by endoscopic and percutaneous stent insertion.

ACUTE OR FULMINANT HEPATIC FAILURE

> This is defined as the development of encephalopathy within eight weeks of the onset of symptoms in patients without prior liver disease. The commonest causes in the UK are paracetamol poisoning, viral hepatitis due to hepatitis A, B and non-A, non-B viruses and drug toxicity including halothane hepatitis.

Clinical features The most obvious clinical abnormality in fulminant hepatic failure is encephalopathy which can be divided into 4 stages: grade I – confusion; grade II – drowsiness; grade III – severe confusion and drowsiness and grade IV – coma. Other features include bruising, GI bleeding, jaundice and oliguria.

Investigations and complications

Cerebral oedema: this may develop in patients with grade IV encephalopathy and is characterized by systemic hypertension, bradycardia, pupillary dilatation and opisthotonis.

Renal failure: this is common and can be divided into acute tubular necrosis with a high urinary sodium with low osmolality and functional renal failure with low urinary sodium and high osmolality.

Sepsis: this is also common and may develop without obvious signs other than deterioration in clinical condition.

Bleeding: due to coagulopathy secondary to impaired hepatic synthetic function and DIC. Bleeding may be subcutaneous, gastrointestinal, renal or intracerebral.

Cardiopulmonary disturbance: characterized by shock and ARDS.

Metabolic: derangement in metabolism is usual with hypoglycaemia, hyponatraemia, hyperkalaemia, metabolic acidosis and hypoxia being common.

Management and prevention Prophylactic measures which are appropriate in all patients include: skilled nursing with patients semirecumbant and head-up position, dextrose infusion, H_2-antagonist therapy and broad spectrum antibiotics. Where appropriate the following should be instituted: mechanical ventilation to correct hypoxia and treat cerebral oedema, haemodialysis and/or ultrafiltration to treat renal failure and volume overload, Swan-Ganz pressure monitoring to ensure adequate cardiac filling volumes to cardiac output, 10% mannitol administration 100 ml over 20 minutes to treat intracranial hypertension and the administration of FFP and platelets to correct coagulopathy associated with haemorrhage. Liver transplantation should be considered in patients who are deteriorating and in whom recovery is predicted as being unlikely.

Prognosis This is poor but is greatly influenced by skilled intensive care management. Overall the mortality for patients who develop grade IV encephalopathy is around 70%. However the cause is important with the mortality in such patients with paracetamol poisoning and hepatitis A and B being approximately 50% compared with a mortality of 90% in those due to non-A, non-B hepatitis or halothane hepatitis with grade IV encephalopathy. However it should be remembered that those patients who survive usually make a full and complete recovery.

OESOPHAGEAL VARICES

Portal hypertension develops as a consequence of increased splanchnic blood flow and increased hepatic vascular resistance in patients with liver disease. This leads to the opening up and dilatation of portosystemic anastomoses the most important of which are at the lower end of the oesophagus. Only 30% of patients with varices ever bleed and this is commonest in those with the largest varices. Other risk factors are poorly understood.

Clinical features   Brisk haematemesis is the commonest presentation although occasionally varices may bleed slowly with melaena or anaemia. In many stigmata of chronic liver disease are present.

Investigation   The diagnosis should be made at endoscopy which should be undertaken urgently in patients with known or presumed liver disease. Endoscopy allows identification of the bleeding site as well as a means of treatment.

Management

Acute bleeding: Resuscitation followed by injection sclerotherapy by a skilled operator. Where unavailable or unsuccessful iv vasopressin, 10 IU bolus followed by 0.4 IU/minute, with nitroglycerin infusion 200 µg/minute should be introduced. This latter drug reduces the toxicity of vasopressin and improves efficacy. If bleeding continues balloon tamponade with a Sengstaken tube is usually successful. Oesophageal transection should be considered in those who do not respond to such measures.

Rebleeding: this is common after all the above medical procedures and can be reduced by injection sclerotherapy to obliterate varices. Propranolol 160 mg LA/day also reduces the risk of rebleeding.

Prophylactic: many patients with varices never bleed and sclerotherapy for all patients with varices is not appropriate. Propranolol 160 mg LA/day reduces the risk of bleeding and should be used in those with large varices without contraindications to β-blockade.

ENCEPHALOPATHY

This is a neuropsychiatric syndrome in which changes in intellect and behaviour occur along with reduced conscious level in patients with acute or chronic liver disease. It occurs in the setting of fulminant hepatic failure where progression to coma, cerebral oedema and death is common and in those with portosystemic shunts usually as a consequence of chronic liver disease.

Aetiology It is believed that some substance derived from protein breakdown in the intestine is absorbed and reaches the brain either because of shunting around the liver or when the liver is incapable of removing it. The exact nature of this substance is unclear but false neurotransmitters derived from aromatic aminoacids or gamma aminobutyric acid (GABA) are currently believed the most likely.

Clinical features In acute liver failure progression from confusion (grade I), through drowsiness (grades II & III) to coma (grade IV) occurs. Foetor hepaticus, a flapping tremor (asterixis) and hyperreflexia are characteristic. The condition responds in parallel with the underlying liver function. In chronic liver disease encephalopathy usually develops along with some complication such as upper GI bleeding, infection, hypokalaemia, high protein intake, constipation or sedative drugs. In mild cases abnormalities can be detected by poor performance at joining sequences of scattered numbers (number connection tests) and constructional apraxia eg drawing a five-pointed star. Progression to coma is unusual.

Investigations Diagnosis is largely clinical but can be confirmed by EEG which shows a reduced α-rhythm, increased θ activity and large-voltage slow waves.

Management In acute liver failure treatment is directed to supporting the patient whilst liver recovery takes place. Hypoglycaemia may mimic encephalopathy in these patients and should be avoided by careful monitoring of the blood glucose concentration. In those with chronic liver disease identification and correction of the underlying complication such as sepsis, variceal haemorrhage or electrolyte imbalance is essential. Additional measures include reducing protein intake, reducing faecal content by lactulose (20 ml tid) and enemas. The use of branch chain aminoacids, vegetable protein diets and bromocriptine are still controversial and are not advocated in general clinical practice.

ASCITES

The presence of excess free fluid within the peritoneal cavity can occur in a large number of situations including cirrhosis, intra-abdominal malignancy, nephrotic syndrome,

Meig's syndrome, constrictive pericarditis, Budd-Chiari syndrome and tuberculous peritonitis. Abdominal swelling due to fluid should be differentiated from fat, flatus, faeces and fetus.

Ascites in cirrhosis

Aetiology Two theories exist: the overflow hypothesis in which excess fluid occurs secondary to renal salt retention and overflows into the peritoneal cavity, and the underfill hypothesis in which peripheral vasodilatation leads to a reduction in renal blood flow with secondary salt and water retention which then overflows into the peritoneal cavity because of portal hypertension. The latter is more popular and factors such as hypoalbuminaemia, secondary hyperaldosteronism and increased hepatic lymph flow exacerbate the problem.

Clinical features

Symptoms: Include abdominal swelling, rapid weight gain and often ankle swelling.

Signs: bilateral shifting flank dullness and a fluid thrill. Other stigmata of chronic liver disease may be present.

Investigations • US is especially useful in confirming the diagnosis and identifying other features such as splenomegaly • A diagnostic paracentesis of 20 ml should be carried out in all patients to identify the protein content, exclude malignant cells, bacteria and determine the WBC concentration. A WBC count >250/mm (predominantly polymorphs) is highly suggestive of spontaneous bacterial peritonitis, commonly due to coliforms. The presence of more than one type of organism should raise the possibility of bowel perforation.

Management Step-wise approach starting with bed-rest, reduced salt intake (no added salt) and spironolactone 50–100 mg daily. Aim for a weight loss of 0.5 kg per day. If no response increase spironolactone gradually to 300 mg before adding 20–40 mg frusemide. Care should be taken when introducing loop diuretics not to precipitate hepatorenal syndrome with rising creatinine, oliguria and hyponatraemia. Once the ascites has resolved maintenance doses of spironolactone of 50–200 mg are required along with dietary salt restriction. (Patients with malignant ascites may require large doses of frusemide 80–120 mg to control ascites). This approach fails in 10% in whom a therapeutic paracentesis of 5 l accompanied by iv salt-poor albumin (0.5–2 l) may start a diuresis. A low salt diet of 40–60 mol/day should be started. In refractory cases a Le Veen (peritoneo-venous) shunt may be the only way to control ascites.

In those in whom spontaneous bacterial peritonitis is suspected by a high WBC count in the ascitic fluid cefuroxime 500 mg qid with metronidazole 500 mg tid should be started and modified once the bacteriology is known.

LIVER TRANSPLANTATION

More than 2000 liver transplants have been undertaken since 1963. Two major types are recognized: ● auxillary homotransplantation where a liver is transplanted in an ectopic place leaving the existing liver in place and ● orthotopic transplantation where a new liver is inserted in place of the old. The latter is by far the most popular. Successful liver transplantation is a joint medical and surgical effort.

Indications

Children: biliary atresia, if corrective surgery is delayed beyond 2–3 months, inborn errors of metabolism eg α_1-antitrypsin deficiency, Wilson's disease, tyrosinaemia, glycogen storage disease, and primary hepatic malignancy.

Adults: subacute or fulminant hepatic failure eg due to hepatitis B, and end-stage cirrhosis due to PBC, CAH and cryptogenic and primary hepatic malignancy.

Selection ● Less than 65 years, patent portal vein and hepatic artery, satisfactory renal and cardiopulmonary function and receptive psychological attitude ● Correct timing: before the patient becomes too ill is important. Previous upper abdominal surgery makes the surgery more difficult ● HLA typing is not necessary ● Contraindications: ● metastatic disease ● sepsis ● recent variceal haemorrhage and ● active alcoholism.

Immunosuppression Prednisolone, azathioprine and cyclosporin. The former two can usually be withdrawn with time.

Complications

Early: acute rejection, vascular thrombosis, haemorrhage and sepsis.

Late: biliary infection, opportunistic infection, chronic rejection (vanishing bile duct syndrome) and disease recurrence eg malignancy.

Prognosis 1-year survival is between 60–70% for adults and 80% for children. Transplantation for malignancy has a poorer outlook than for benign disease because of disease recurrence. Transplantation for acute liver failure in those predicted unlikely to survive eg fulminant hepatic failure due to non-A, non-B hepatitis, halothane hepatitis or paracetamol poisoning accompanied by gross coagulopathy or a bilirubin >100 µmol/l, if performed before the development of cerebral oedema, has a good prognosis.

7

Nephrology

135

A thorough history and examination are fundamental to the investigation of patients with suspected renal disease and will identify those with a history of analgesic abuse or associated diseases such as hypertension, diabetes mellitus and connective tissue disorders.

Biochemistry Urea, creatinine, calcium, urate and glucose. Creatinine, especially in the elderly is insensitive and severe impairment of renal function may exist with only minimal increases in serum creatinine. Creatinine clearance is more sensitive but is subject to inaccuracies related to urine collection.

Urine examination Stick testing for protein, blood, glucose, ketones and pH. Microscopy for bacteria, WBCs and casts. Bacterial counts greater than 100 000/ml indicate significant infection in a proper MSU. Casts containing RBCs occur in conditions with glomerular inflammation; granular casts may indicate tubular damage whilst hyaline casts occur in chronic renal disease and in normal individuals after exercise. Pink urine occurs in haemoglobinuria, myoglobinuria, acute intermittent porphyria and ingestion of pigments and dyes eg beetroot, senna and phenolphthalein but only the first two give rise to positive tests for haemoglobin.

Ultrasound This will assess kidney size and any dilatation of the proximal renal tract or bladder.

Radiology The plain abdominal film may identify the size, shape and position of the kidneys as well as radio-opaque calculi and nephrocalcinosis. Intravenous urography assesses the size of the kidneys, obstruction and to some extent renal function but may be nephrotoxic in acute renal failure and myeloma. Retrograde pyelography is used to identify the site and degree of ureteric obstruction. The micturating cystogram is invaluable in assessing vesicoureteric reflux.

Radionuclide scan This is useful in assessing asymmetrical renal function. Dynamic computer analysis allows assessment of renal blood supply as well as the degree and rate of excretion. It is particularly useful in differentiating acute tubular necrosis from renal ischaemia in renal transplants.

Renal biopsy This is essential for establishing the diagnosis when this is unclear and when renal size is normal but carries a 1% risk of serious complications such as haemorrhage. Electron microscopy and immunohistochemistry has greatly increased its diagnostic sensitivity. Its value in those with bilateral small shrunken kidneys where management is unlikely to be influenced is limited.

ACUTE RENAL FAILURE (ARF)

> This condition characterized by oliguria (<15 ml urine/h) or anuria with a rising serum creatinine and potassium is common and frequently reversible with appropriate therapy.

Aetiology   Causes are traditionally divided into 3 groups:

Prerenal: due to volume depletion secondary to dehydration and haemorrhage or reduced cardiac output. It is characterized by oliguria and a high urinary specific gravity (>1.020) and low urinary sodium (<10 mmol/l). If the underlying insult is prolonged acute tubular necrosis (ATN) develops typified by oliguria of urine with low specific gravity (<1.010).

Intrinsic: due to renovascular disease, acute glomerulonephritis, malignant hypertension, myoglobinuria, toxins eg paracetamol, carbon tetrachloride.

Postrenal: due to outlet obstruction in the renal tract eg prostatic hypertrophy, ureteric stones, bladder or pelvic tumours.

Clinical features   Confusion, nausea, vomiting, dehydration, oliguria. In some volume overload is present with pulmonary and peripheral oedema and hyponatraemia.

Investigations   ● Serum urea, creatinine and potassium ● ECG looking for recent MI or tented T waves in hyperkalaemia ● urine excretion rate, specific gravity or osmolality and microscopy ● accurate fluid balance assessment ● blood culture and US ● An IVU is best avoided because of toxicity.

> **Management**   This is aimed at reversing life-threatening complications and identifying the underlying cause.
>
> *Hyperkalaemia* (>6 mmol/l):
>
> ● iv bicarbonate 1.26% infusion (200–500 ml)
>
> ● iv calcium gluconate 10% (10–20 ml slowly)
>
> ● Insulin/glucose infusion (15 units soluble insulin per 50 g glucose)
>
> ● Calcium resonium 15 g 3–4 times daily orally in water (not fruit juice) or by enema 30 g tid.
>
> ● Haemodialysis if hyperkalaemia is persistent and severe
>
> *Fluid balance:*   assess state of hydration; replace with CVP monitoring if depleted; iv frusemide 40–250 mg if overloaded. If persistently oliguric replace previous day's output plus 750 ml (more if vomiting, diarrhoea or blood loss).

Acid/base state: usually metabolic acidosis; if pH<7.0 give iv 1.26% bicarbonate to raise pH to >7.1 (usually 200–500 ml).

Dialysis: this is indicated for persistent hyperkalaemia or acidosis or to remove excess fluid eg pulmonary oedema.

POLYCYSTIC RENAL DISEASE

This inherited disorder may be associated with cystic disease of other organs eg liver and pancreas. Two main forms exist: ● the infantile autosomal recessive variety and ● the adult autosomal dominant form. Both kidneys are involved with cysts, primarily cortical, increasing in size with time.

Clinical features Renal angle pain, haemautria, hypertension and uraemia. Renal masses related to cysts or renal tumours may be palpable. Intracranial vascular malformation giving rise to bruit or CVA may be present.

Investigations ● U+Es ● creatinine ● creatinine clearance ● abdominal US, IVU and retrograde pyelography

Management Symptomatic with treatment of renal failure with dialysis or transplantation when indicated. Screening of relatives over the age of 25 years by renal US should be undertaken in association with genetic councelling.

Prognosis End-stage renal failure develops in middle age. Death may be from cardiac failure or stroke as well as uraemia.

RENAL TUBULAR ACIDOSIS

This results from failure of acid secretion in the distal tubule or proximal bicarbonate absorption. It may be inherited or secondary (→ Table 7.1, p 139).

RENAL CALCULI

Renal stones affect 1% of the population and occur when solutes come out of solution either because they are present in excessive quantities, the urine is over-concentrated or because of lack of inhibitors of crystallization. The majority are composed of calcium (75%), magnesium-phosphate mixtures (15%) or urate (5%).

Table 7.1
Types and causes of RTA

	Distal RTA	Proximal RTA
Type	I	II
Cause Primary	Autosomal dominant	Familial
Secondary Renal disease	Pyelonephritis Medullary sponge kidney Hydronephrosis Transplanted kidney	Nephrotic syndrome Transplanted kidney
Drugs	Lithium	Tetracycline
Metabolic	Hypercalcaemia Amyloidosis Hyperglobulinaemia Cryoglobulinaemia	Hypercalcaemia Cystinosis Tyrosinosis Amyloidosis
Miscellaneous	Connective tissue disease, eg PBC, SLE	Heavy metal poisoning

Clinical features

Symptoms: These may be asymptomatic especially if intra-renal. Loin pain, renal colic with pain radiating to groin, sweating, nausea and vomiting, strangury.

Signs: often few, haematuria, loin tenderness, pyrexia if associated infection.

Investigation To identify stone: ● plain abdominal X-ray (calcium and magnesium phosphate stones are radio-dense and urate stones radio-lucent) ● renal US ● IVU ● collect and sieve urine. To identify cause ● history of dehydration, excessive calcium intake, diuretic or vit D therapy, gout or bowel disease ● U+Es, plasma and urinary calcium, urinary pH and culture, plasma uric acid and bicarbonate ● Cystinuria is rare but a family history of stones should prompt exclusion by urinary cystine measurement ● IVU or US will identify causes such as medullary sponge kidney

Management Analgesia: this usually requires opiates eg pethidine 100 mg im although NSAID such as indomethacin 50 mg tid or diclofenac 50 mg bd/tid may also be useful. Antispasmodic agents such as probanthine 10 mg tid may be useful. High fluid intake eg 250–500 ml/hour. Most stones pass spontaneously but intervention is necessary in those in whom infection and/or obstruction is identified. In such cases the stone may be extracted cystoscopically with a Dormia basket if in the distal ureter, operatively if proximal or be fragmented by ultrasonic lithotripsy.

Prevention of recurrence Attention to high fluid intake and avoidance of dehydration. Where a precipitating factor such as excessive calcium intake is suspected dietary modification is advisable.

RENAL TRACT TUMOURS

RENAL ADENOCARCINOMA (HYPERNEPHROMA)

This arises from renal tubular epithelium and is commonest in males in the 5th decade. Risk factors include smoking, renal cysts in dialysis patients and von Hippel-Lindau disease.

Clinical features

Symptoms: Haematuria, loin pain, fever and fatigue.

Signs: include palpable mass, anaemia or polycythaemia.

Investigations • Urinalysis • biochemistry for hypercalcaemia • haematology for anaemia or polycythaemia • CXR for metastases • renal US, IVU • angiography and CT scanning.

Management Nephrectomy if no evidence of metastatic disease offers a 5-year survival of 70%. If spread is identified progesterone therapy may induce remission. Rarely resection of solitary metastases is indicated.

TRANSITIONAL CELL TUMOURS OF THE RENAL PELVIS

Risk factors include smoking and analgesic abuse. Presentation, diagnosis and treatment similar to hypernephroma.

BLADDER TRANSITIONAL CELL TUMOURS

These are commoner in males over 40 years. Risk factors include smoking, exposure to industrial chemicals, cyclophosphamide therapy and *Schistosoma haematobium* infection.

Clinical features   Painless haematuria or symptoms of urinary retention.

Investigation   • Urinary cytology and cystoscopy.

> *Management*   Superficial disease can be adequately treated by endoscopic resection with follow-up surveillance. Intravesical chemotherapy may be useful. Advanced disease requires surgery and chemotherapy.

PROSTATIC CANCER

The third commonest malignancy in males, this occurs in the elderly and may be very slow growing.

Clinical features   Urinary obstruction commonest although distant metastases eg to vertebrae may produce symptoms.

Investigations   • PR may reveal a craggy gland with obliteration of the median furrow • Serum acid phosphatase is commonly elevated • Transrectal prostatic biopsy.

> *Management*   Transurethral resection of prostate (TURP) relieves symptoms of prostatism. Stilboestrol 1 mg/day or buserelin nasal spray, which suppresses gonadotrophin release, reduce tumour growth as does orchidectomy. Radiotherapy in selected cases.

Prognosis   Very variable from months to many years.

URINARY TRACT INFECTION

> Infection within the urinary tract can be conveniently divided into that affecting the kidney (pyelonephritis) or the bladder (cystitis). They are not mutually exclusive. UTI is particularly common and 50% of women will experience symptoms of UTI sometime during life. Bacteria involved:
>
> *Enterobacteriaceae:* eg *Enterobacter* spp., *Escherichia coli*, *Klebsiella* spp., *Proteus* spp., *Serratia* spp.
>
> *Pseudomonadaceae:* eg *Pseudomonas aeruginosa*
>
> *Gram-positive cocci:* eg *Enterococci*, *Staph.* spp., *Strep.* Group B, D and G, *Strep. viridans,*
>
> *Other:* eg *Flavobacterium* spp.

Clinical features

Symptoms: There may be none. Commonly dysuria, frequency, urgency, fever, incontinence and retention.

Signs: include haematuria and tenderness suprapubically (cystitis) or over the renal angle (pyelonephritis) and features of uraemia. Features of cystitis without evidence of infection occur in the urethral syndrome.

Investigations ● Urine analysis, microscopy and culture. Microscopic haematuria and proteinuria are common. More than 100 000 organisms/ml on a fresh MSU indicates UTI despite any lack of symptoms and should be treated in the elderly, children and during pregnancy. Pyuria without obvious organisms occurs with renal TB and with analgesic abuse ● BP ● plasma electrolytes and creatinine should be checked and an ● IVU considered particularly if infection is recurrent or in childhood.

Management

Symptomatic: drink frequently eg 3–4 l/day, administration of sodium bicarbonate 2 g qid to alkalinize the urine and avoid sexual intercourse.

Antibiotics: ideally tailored according to sensitivity determined from urine culture. Most usually amoxycillin 250 mg tid or two 3-g sachets over 24 hours or trimethoprin 200 mg bd for 5 days.

Causes of failure to respond to treatment or relapse include: failure to complete course of antibiotics, re-infection from septic site eg renal calculi or bladder tumour, urinary retention eg neurogenic bladder, resistant organisms and postmenopausal urethral atrophy.

CHRONIC RENAL FAILURE

This refers to the gradual permanent loss of renal function leading to uraemia.

Aetiology Diabetes mellitus, GN, pyelonephritis, hypertension, renal stones, vesicoureteric reflux, bladder outlet obstruction, connective tissue diseases, polycystic kidneys, myeloma and hypercalcaemia.

Clinical features

Symptoms: Pruritus, nocturia, polyuria, anorexia, dyspnoea, confusion, neuropathy and vomiting.

Signs: pallor, pleural effusions, pericarditis, LVF, hypertension, bruising, ascites, peripheral oedema and increased pigmentation.

Investigations

Biochemistry: increased urea and creatinine, hyperkalaemia, hyponatraemia, hyperphosphataemia, hypocalcaemia and metabolic acidosis ● Urine: microscopy for casts, analysis for protein, specific gravity and creatinine clearance (this may be significantly reduced with a normal serum creatinine especially in the elderly)

Radiology: plain film. US to demonstrate renal size and possible obstruction. Retrograde pyelography if ureteric obstruction is suspected ● Renal biopsy only usually considered if renal size is normal.

Management Dialysis should be considered in those with symptoms and creatinine >500 μmol/l or bicarbonate <12mmol/l and in asymptomatic patients with a serum potassium >5 mmol/l; this may be either haemodialysis or chronic ambulatory peritoneal dialysis (CAPD). The choice of treatment must be tailored to the individual patient. Abdominal surgery or sepsis and poor patient motivation are contraindications to CAPD whilst coagulopathy, HBV carriage and poor venous access are factors against haemodialysis. For patients fit for surgery renal transplant must be considered to improve the quality of life.

Other measures: control of hypertension with metoprolol 50–100 mg/day and/or nifedipine 10–20 mg tid; reduction of hyperphosphataemia with calcium carbonate in doses titrated to reduce phosphate to normal; prevention of renal bone disease with 1 α vitamin D 0.25 μg/day; avoidance of nephrotoxic drugs eg tetracycline, aminoglycosides and potassium sparing diuretics eg spironolactone and amiloride. Low protein diets (40 g/d) and good BP control may delay the progression of renal failure. A restricted fluid intake is required in the majority both before and after dialysis. A low salt diet is indicated in some patients with hypertension. Erythropoietin to correct anaemia.

DIALYSIS AND RENAL TRANSPLANTATION

DIALYSIS

Treatment of acute and chronic renal failure is most commonly with dialysis in which the patient's blood is perfused across a semipermeable membrane against dialysis solution thereby removing salt, water and low molecular weight solutes such as urea. The membrane may be synthetic as in haemodialysis or natural as in peritoneal dialysis. As well as treating acute and chronic renal failure dialysis is indicated in the treatment of severe poisoning with lithium, aspirin and methanol.

Indications: ARF when complicated by water overload, hyperkalaemia, acidosis or uraemia. CRF when symptoms of uraemia develop.

Haemodialysis access This is usually via a radiocephalic arteriovenous (Cimino) fistula although short-term dialysis is possible via large central veins. Haemofiltration whereby large volumes of fluid can be removed is possible via more peripheral veins. Despite haemodialysis many of the manifestations of CRF such as anaemia and lethargy persist although erythropoietin therapy may be important in the future.

Complications: infection and thrombosis of vascular access, haemorrhage, hypotension, hypoxia, cramps, seizures, air embolism, haemolysis.

Peritoneal dialysis In ARF intermittent peritoneal dialysis is effective in removing fluid, solutes and balancing electrolytes. In CRF CAPD is an effective alternative to haemodialysis in cooperative patients. Its main advantages include freedom from the dialysis machine and lack of requirement for vascular access. The main disadvantage is infection.

TRANSPLANTATION

Now an accepted therapeutic alternative which allows the patient to return to near normal life. The donor kidney must be HLA and DR matched with the recipient to reduce the risk of rejection and this may be further reduced by pretransplant blood transfusions. The 5-year survival for an HLA identical kidney is approximately 75%. Immunosuppressive drugs, usually prednisolone, azathioprine and cyclosporin are necessary to prevent rejection. The transplanted kidney is usually sited in the right iliac fossa where subsequent biopsy is easy.

Complications: acute rejection, thrombosis, ATN, opportunistic infections, cyclosporin renal toxicity, chronic rejection, hypertension and increased risk of malignancy.

GLOMERULONEPHRITIS

Acute glomerulonephritis is characterized by haematuria, proteinuria, hypertension, oedema, uraemia and often oliguria. It is believed to be due to humoral immune mechanisms. Numerous causes are recognized and associated with different clinical features.

Poststreptococcal GN
This is less common now than formerly. It is commonest in

childhood developing 1–3 weeks after streptococcal laryngitis or skin infection. Diagnosis is by a positive skin or throat swab for Lancefield group b haemolytic streptococci, rising ASO titre, reduced plasma C3 and biopsy showing diffuse proliferative GN. Treatment is supportive, correcting fluid and electrolyte imbalance and hypertension, bed-rest initially, 40 g protein and 100 mmol sodium diet and penicillin if streptococcal infection still present. Haematuria and proteinuria may persist for 1–2 years but rarely progresses to CRF.

Postinfective GN
This is similar but often milder than poststreptococcal GN and often resolves after adequate treatment of the underlying infection.

Henoch-Schönlein purpura
This generalized vasculitis, commonest in children, is characterized by purpura, GN, abdominal pain and arthralgia. Serum IgA is increased in 50%. Treatment is supportive and the value of steroids is unproven.

Rapidly progressive GN
Characterized by a gradual onset of proteinuria, haematuria and renal failure over a period of weeks or months. The cause may be secondary to infection eg subacute bacterial endocarditis and hepatitis B, connective tissue disease eg SLE, Goodpasture's vasculitis, Wegener's granulomatosis, polyarteritis nodosa or idiopathic. Renal biopsy shows crescents of fibrosis in Bowman's capsule; linear IgG or immune complex deposits in the glomerular basement membrane may or may not be present. Treatment depends upon the underlying disease. In the idiopathic form plasmapheresis, steroids, anticoagulants and cytotoxic agents may be useful in some patients.

Membranous GN
This usually presents with proteinuria and often nephrotic syndrome (urinary protein >3 g/day with oedema and hypoalbuminaemia <30 g/l)(→ Table 7.2, p 146). Haematuria and hypertension are usually absent. Renal vein thrombosis is a common complication. Underlying conditions such as connective tissue disorders, neoplasia and drug reactions eg penicillamine may be present. Renal biopsy shows subepithelial IgG deposits with a thickened basement membrane. Steroids may reduce proteinuria but not the progression of disease which ends in uraemia in 30%.

Mesangiocapillary GN
This usually affects young patients presenting with haematuria, hypertension, reduced GFR and hypocomplementaemia and progressing to renal failure over some years. Renal biopsy identifies two variants: type 1 with large subepithelial deposits

and type 2 with deposition within the lamina densa of the basement membrane. Treatment with prednisolone in those with associated SLE and/or aspirin and dipyridamole may slow progression.

Minimal change GN

This is commonest in childhood causing 80% of cases of nephrotic syndrome. It is responsible for 30% of nephrotic syndrome in adults. Renal biopsy reveals normal glomeruli on light microscopy although electron microscopy shows fusion of podocytes. Immune-complex deposition is not seen. The proteinuria is selective and is steroid sensitive.

Focal glomerulosclerosis

This is a slowly progressive disease with hypertension, haematuria and reduced GFR. It may follow minimal change GN or be due to vesicoureteric reflux, iv drug abuse or HIV infection. Renal biopsy shows fibrosis of some of the juxtamedullary glomeruli. Approximately 50% respond to steroids.

Table 7.2
Causes of nephrotic syndrome

Primary glomerular disease 75%
Membranous GN
Minimal change GN
Focal glomerulosclerosis
Membranoproliferative
Mesangiocapillary

Infections
SBE, HBV infection, malaria (commonest world-wide), sickle cell disease, syphilis

Metabolic
Diabetes mellitus, amyloidosis

Drugs
Penicillamine, gold, NSAID, captopril, tolbutamide, iv drug abuse

Malignancy
Lymphoma, leukaemia, GI and breast tumours

Neurology

More than in any other system examination of the nervous system relies upon thorough clinical examination. Further investigations to a large part serve to confirm or refute clinical suspicions.

Lumbar puncture Indications include suspected meningitis or subarachnoid haemorrhage and to provide a route to administer antibiotics or contrast media. Once the subarachnoid space is entered the pressure should be measured and CSF taken for naked eye examination, biochemical, cytological and bacteriological analysis. Complications include headache, introduction of infection and cerebellar herniation (in those with raised intracranial pressure (ICP)). In those where raised ICP is suspected an LP should be avoided until excluded by CT.

CT scan This is essential in the accurate diagnosis of subdural and extradural haematoma, intracranial tumours, cerebral oedema and atrophy and hydrocephalus. Also valuable in differentiating cerebral haemorrhage from infarction. Contrast CT scanning may identify cerebral aneurysms and arteriovenous malformations.

Angiography Required for the accurate diagnosis of vascular occlusions, stenosis and aneurysms and to determine the vascular anatomy of tumours prior to surgery. Carotid Doppler may be useful in identifying abnormalities in blood flow.

Electroencephalography Primarily used in the diagnosis of epilepsy and monitoring metabolic brain disorders eg hepatic encephalopathy.

EEG Pattern in adults:

Normal:

- α 8–12 Hz in occipital and parietal regions
- β >12 Hz in frontal regions
- Slower wave patterns during sleep.

Abnormal:

- θ 4–7 Hz
- δ <4 Hz
- Paroxysmal sharp high-voltage waves in epilepsy (eg 3 Hz spike and wave pattern in petit mal).
- Absence of activity in normothermic patients not exposed to sedative drugs indicates brain death.

Nuclear magnetic resonance Principally used to identify spinal-cord lesions, abnormalities at the cranio-vertebral junction eg syringomyelia and areas of demyelination in multiple sclerosis.

Myelography Required for the visualization of the spinal canal and cord for the diagnosis of intervertebral disc herniation, and spinal tumours.

Evoked responses These measure electrical activity within the cortex from visual, auditory and tactile stimuli. Useful in detecting abnormalities within sensory pathways where structural lesions cannot be identified and for monitoring disease progression.

Electromyography Essential in distinguishing neuropathies from myopathies.

Perimetry, audiometry and labyrinthine function tests Used to confirm and quantitate sensory neurological deficit.

Brain biopsy This is indicated only infrequently such as in the diagnosis of herpes simplex encephalitis.

Tensilon test The administration of edrophonium (Tensilon) 10 mg iv improves power for 3–5 minutes in myasthenia gravis and is useful diagnostically.

CEREBROVASCULAR ACCIDENT

Cerebrovascular accident or stroke results from ischaemic infarction or haemorrhage within the brain. It affects 1–2/1000 per year and is the third commonest cause of death. Risk factors include hypertension, diabetes mellitus, smoking, hyperlipidaemia, the oral contraceptive pill and age.

Aetiology Thrombosis, embolism, haemorrhage and vasculitis.

Clinical features these depend upon the cause eg thrombosis or haemorrhage, and the vessel involved: thrombosis is commoner and symptoms develop over hours often during sleep whilst cerebral haemorrhage usually presents abruptly during waking hours often with a premonitory headache ● strokes can be divided into ● completed stroke (rapid onset with persistent deficit) ● stroke-in-evolution (gradual step-wise development) ● transient ischaemic attack (symptoms resolve completely within 24 hours) and ● progressive diffuse disease (no major incidents but gradual deterioration in cerebral function leading to multi-infarct dementia with bilateral pyramidal signs).

Vessel occluded: ● middle cerebral artery results in contralateral hemiplegia. Hemianaesthesia and hemianopia is also common. Dysphasia occurs when the dominant hemisphere is affected. Lesions within the carotid artery frequently present with similar features.

- Anterior cerebral artery results in hemiplegia affecting the lower more than the upper limb. Apraxia and expressive dysphasia are common.

- Posterior cerebral artery results in contralateral homonymous hemianopia with macular sparing and occasionally thalamic pain on the contralateral side.

- Brain-stem arteries result in vertigo, nystagmus, ataxia and diplopia often with involvement of an ipsilateral cranial nerve and contralateral pyramidal signs.

Investigations • BP noting that this is frequently increased temporarily after stroke • previous hypertension should be sought from the CXR, ECG and fundoscopy • FBC to exclude anaemia, thromboctyopaenia or polycythaemia • ESR and autoimmune screen to identify vasculitides such as cranial arteritis • glucose to exclude hypoglycaemia • ECG for AF and evidence of hypertension • Syphilis is now rare but should be excluded by serological studies • A carotid bruit in those with a TIA is an indication for carotid angiography and surgery if the event occurred in the same territory.

Management This is directed to reduce the risk of further CVA and promote rehabilitation. Controlling BP is important but overaggressive reduction in pressure should be avoided as it may result in extension of the stroke. Aspirin 300 mg daily may reduce the risk of further strokes and cigarette smoking must be discontinued. Physiotherapy is valuable in accelerating recovery although the long-term benefit is less clear. Treatment of the elderly presenting with a severe stroke is controversial although many would advocate iv fluids for 2–3 days followed by nasogastric feeding until self-feeding or death.

CEREBRAL TUMOURS

These account for 2% of deaths and although may be histologically malignant primary tumours rarely metastasize outwith the brain. 50% of brain tumours are metastases from other sites, 25% gliomas, 20% meningiomas and 5% neuromas, pituitary adenomas and craniopharyngiomas.

Clinical features These are due to local damage and/or raised intracranial pressure.

Symptoms: include headache, blurred vision, epilepsy, focal weakness, drowsiness, vertigo, vomiting and personality change.

Signs: bradycardia, papilloedema (if unilateral with optic atrophy in the other eye = Foster Kennedy syndrome), cranial nerve (often VI) palsy, nystagmus, grasp reflex.

Investigations • CXR and skull X-ray, CT and NMR scanning. If metastatic disease is suspected likely sources eg lung, breast and colon should be screened • CSF cytological examination provided there is no evidence of raised ICP • Stereotactic or open-brain biopsy.

Management *Medical:* only palliative to reduce symptoms related to cerebral oedema and raised intracranial pressure. Dexamethazone 4 mg qid may produce dramatic improvement in symptoms. Less often larger doses and intravenous mannitol 20% are required. Some pituitary adenomas may be reduced in size by such drugs as bromocryptine.

Surgery: represents the only hope of cure for most tumours. Meningiomas and neuromas are usually more accessible to surgery than gliomas. In some cases palliative surgery, removing the bulk but not all the tumour, is indicated.

Radiotherapy: may be used to reduce tumour size in some cases and such tumours such as medulloblastomas, microgliomas and lymphomas are markedly radiosensitive and potentially curable.

CENTRAL NERVOUS SYSTEM INFECTIONS

MENINGITIS

Inflammation of the meninges may be due to bacterial, viral, spirochaetal, protozoal or fungal infection. Viral infection is the commonest whilst syphilis and tuberculous infection are now rare.

Clinical features These may develop rapidly or in tuberculous infection over weeks and consist of features due to infection, meningism and raised intracranial pressure.

Symptoms: include lethargy, headache, neck pain, photophobia and fever.

Signs: neck stiffness (inability to bend the patient's head so that the chin touches the chest), Kernig's sign (inability to straighten the leg below the knee once the hip is flexed to 90°), drowsiness and rarely papilloedema. In meningococcal meningitis a purpuric skin rash may be obvious.

Investigations Lumbar puncture with examination of the CSF (→ Table 8.1).

Table 8.1
Causes of CNS infections and CSF finds

Cause	Microscopy	Biochemistry
Bacteria	Polymorphs and organisms eg Gram-negative diplococci	Low glucose High protein
Viral	Lymphocytes, no organisms	Normal glucose Mild protein ↑
TB	Lymphocytes and TB bacilli on Z-N stain	Low glucose High protein
Malignancy	Mixed inflammatory and malignant cells	Low glucose High protein

Management Specific antibiotic treatment for bacterial meningitis depends upon identification of the organism: meningococcus and pneumococcus: iv benzylpenicillin 1.2–2.4 g 4 hourly; *H influenzae:* chloramphenicol 3–5 g daily (or ampicillin); TB: rifampicin, isoniazid, ethambutol and pyrazinamide; cryptococcus: iv amphotericin and oral flucytosine. Treatment of presumed bacterial meningitis before microbiological confirmation is usually with penicillin in adults and chloramphenicol in children. Treatment of viral meningitis is generally symptomatic except for herpes simplex treated with acyclovir and CMV treated with ganciclovir.

Prognosis This depends upon the cause and in bacterial meningitis the delay before diagnosis and treatment.

ENCEPHALITIS

The majority of viruses which cause meningitis can cause encephalitis (infection of the brain tissue). The commonest cause in the UK is herpes simplex, although HIV infection is increasing. Other types include measles, mumps, varicella, poliomyelitis, measles, subacute sclerosing panencephalitis, encephalitis lethargica and progressive multifocal leucoencephalopathy.

Clinical features

Symptoms: These include headache, drowsiness and fits.

Signs: focal neurological deficit eg. aphasia, hemiplegia, cranial nerve lesions and pyrexia.

Investigations ● Differentiation from encephalopathy, cerebral abscess and CNS tumours ● Lumbar puncture after CT scanning, CSF pressure is usually increased with raised protein and lymphocytic pleocytosis ● EEG shows diffuse slowing with epileptiform discharges in herpetic encephalitis ● Increased temporal lobe isotope uptake on a brain scan may be a feature of herpetic disease. Since this condition is potentially treatable a brain biopsy is sometimes indicated ● Virological and immunological studies of the CSF and serum may be useful in confirming the diagnosis but the results are not usually available in the acute phase.

Management With the exception of herpes simplex encephalitis treatment is symptomatic. Acyclovir iv 5–10 mg/kg infusion tid with dexamethasone 4 mg tid is indicated if herpetic encephalitis is suspected. Vaccination against poliomyelitis has virtually eliminated polio-encephalomyelitis.

Prognosis This is good in most patients although neurological deficit may remain. The poorest outlook occurs in herpes simplex with a mortality rate of 15–20% and subacute sclerosing panencephalitis.

PARKINSONISM

A clinical syndrome characterized by hypokinesia, tremor, rigidity and postural instability. The underlying pathology is dopamine depletion within the basal ganglia the cause of which is usually idiopathic (Parkinson's disease). Less common causes include drugs, especially phenothiazines, cerebral tumours, Wilson's disease, repeated head trauma and following encephalitis lethargica.

Clinical features Usually in subjects over 40 years, presenting with hypokinesia or slowness and delay in movement typified by a slow shuffling gait. The tremor is slow and gives rise to the characteristic pill-rolling movement and is often made worse by stress and embarrassment. Other causes of tremor such as thyrotoxicosis, anxiety, alcoholism and cerebellar disease are usually easily differentiated. Dementia and hypothyroidism may mimic the slowness and paucity of movement. Atherosclerotic dementia with bilateral spasticity may mimic Parkinsonism. Rigidity on passive movement often 'cog-wheel' in nature due to the associated tremor. Power is well maintained. Fluctuations in symptoms is typical particularly in those on levodopa therapy for some years and is known as the 'on-off' effect.

Investigations the diagnosis is essentially clinical and the cause can usually be obtained from ● the history eg drug therapy and examination.

> *Management* Levodopa in combination with peripheral dopadecarboxylase inhibitors in preparations such as 'Sinemet' or 'Madopar' are the mainstay of treatment in most patients and these are effective in relieving particularly the hypokinesia. Adverse reactions such as nausea, vomiting and hypotension are well recognized. Other therapies used in combination or alone include anticholinergics eg benzhexol 5–15 mg/d, dopamine receptor agonists eg bromocryptine 30–60 mg/day and amantidine 200–300 mg/day. It has recently been demonstrated that the monoamine-oxidase-B inhibitor selegiline 5 mg bd reduces L-dopa requirement and reduces 'end-of-dose' akinesia. Stereotactic thalamotomy is rarely indicated for severe tremor. Transplant surgery to implant dopamine producing cells within the brain is entirely experimental.

Prognosis This is variable and although drug treatment improves symptoms it does not affect the natural history and may even accelerate progression. Mortality is three times greater than in the general population.

MULTIPLE SCLEROSIS

> This demyelinating disorder affects 1 in 1000 of the population. The aetiology is unknown but risk factors include habitation in temperate zones of both the northern and southern hemisphere, HLA A3, B7, Dw2/DR2 and a family history of the disease. Both autoimmune mechanisms and slow viral infection have been implicated.

Clinical features

Symptoms: These are very variable. Age of onset is usually 20–50 years, and commoner in women. Presentation is commonly with blurred vision or transient weakness or paraesthesia of one limb. Diplopia, vertigo and ataxia are common. Characteristically the symptoms appear suddenly before resolving partially or completely. A hot bath may markedly, though temporarily, exacerbate motor symptoms. A relapsing remitting course is typical.

Signs: include optic disc pallor, nystagmus, hyperreflexia, ataxia, scanning speech, spasticity and intention tremor.

Investigations ● History and clinical features are usually highly suggestive ● CSF oligoclonal bands of IgG are present in the majority ● CT scanning may identify disseminated lesions within the white matter but ● NMR scanning is even more sensitive identifying periventricular lesions in 95% of clinically definite cases. However this appearance is non-specific over the age of 45 yrs • Delayed auditory, visual and sensory evoked potentials are useful in detecting abnormalities when not clinically apparent.

Management   No cure is currently available. Steroid therapy often shortens the duration and severity of relapse but does not influence the natural history. Azathioprine or cyclophosphamide may reduce the relapse rate but are too toxic for general use. Treatment using baclofen 20–60 mg/day and low dose diazepam is helpful symptomatically in those with spasticity. Hyperbaric oxygen therapy is considered to be useful by some but proven value has not been supported by clinical trials. Clonazepam may benefit some patients with intention tremor.

DEMENTIA

This is defined as a global decline of cognitive function, the most obvious characteristic of which is an impairment in recent memory. This may affect up to 10% of the population over the age of 70 years but its severity and age of onset varies considerably.

Aetiology   Approximately 70% of cases are due to Alzheimer's disease, a condition of unknown cause. A minority of cases are due to strokes (often multiple), metabolic causes, including Korsakoff's psychosis, cerebral tumours, infections, normal pressure hydrocephalus, subdural haematoma, major or multiple minor head injury, HIV infection, Jakob-Creutzfeldt disease and Huntington's disease.

Clinical features

Symptoms: Memory loss, impaired judgement, changes in personality, dysphasia, apraxia, disorientation and impaired concentration. A simple series of questions regarding the date, patient's address, prime minister and recent significant news events usually suffice to confirm the diagnosis.

Signs: these are usually absent in Alzheimer's disease but in multi-infarct dementia, cerebral tumour and Wernicke-Korsakoff's disease features such as pseudobulbar palsy, long-tract signs, nystagmus and ataxia respectively may be obvious. Normal pressure hydrocephalus is said to present with the triad of dementia, urinary incontinence and gait disturbance.

Investigations   • Treatable causes of dementia such as cerebral tumours, subdural haematoma and normal pressure hydrocephalus should be excluded by CT scanning if indicated

● Rare causes such as myxoedema madness and pernicious anaemia are easily excluded by biochemical and haematological tests ● Syphilis requires exclusion by VDRL assay (and CSF examination if +ve) ● Cryptococcus can be excluded by CSF examination and HIV encephalopathy by serology ● EEG may demonstrate characteristic appearances of Jakob-Creutzfeldt disease in those with rapidly progressive dementia.

> **Management** Unfortunately Alzheimer's disease is untreatable and effort should be exerted in maximizing support services. For the minority of those discovered to have other causes such as normal pressure hydrocephalus, vitamin B_{12} deficiency or myxoedema appropriate medical or surgical treatment should be administered without delay.

EPILEPSY

> This is defined as a periodic disturbance in neurological function, often with changes in consciousness, due to abnormal excessive electrical discharge within the brain. Numerous classifications exist but the most commonly used is that where seizures are divided into ● generalized or ● partial attacks. The former may be tonic/clonic (grand mal), tonic or clonic in isolation, myoclonic or associated with absence (petit mal). The latter may be divided into simple partial (motor or sensory) with retained awareness or complex partial with impaired awareness and may progress into generalised or grand mal seizures.

Aetiology This varies with age.

• Infants: hypoxia, metabolic disorders, infection.

• Adolescents: trauma, alcohol/drugs, tumours.

• Elderly: tumours, CVA, metabolic.

Clinical features

Symptoms: Generalized seizures result in disturbance of consciousness the classical variety progressing through tonic, clonic and postictal phases. In absence or petit mal seizures cessation of mental activity occurs without prostration for less than 30 seconds. Partial seizures may present with physical, sensory, autonomic or psychic features without loss of consciousness. These may be primarily behavioural and difficult to diagnose in temporal lobe epilepsy.

Signs: these are often absent between attacks although the stigmata of cerebral tumours such as papilloedema may be present. Gum hyperplasia is characteristic of phenytoin therapy, port-wine naevi in Sturge-Weber syndrome, cafe-au-lait spots in neurofibromatosis and adenoma sebaceum in tuberous sclerosis. Evidence of previous CVAs with long-tract signs may also be obvious.

Investigation • Biochemical tests such as blood glucose, calcium, alcohol, urea and drug levels of anticonvulsant drugs are essential • CT and NMR scans may be necessary in those suspected of having focal neurological deficit • EEG may provide evidence of focal activity but a normal test does not exclude the diagnosis.

Management Generalized or tonic clonic seizures respond to phenytoin, carbamazepine or valproate therapy. Partial seizures require carbamazepine or phenytoin. Absence attacks require valproate and ethosuximide. Over or underdosage may result in increased epileptic attacks and drug levels should be monitored after administration of the initial doses (→ Table 8.2).

Table 8.2
Initial doses and therapeutic ranges

Phenytoin	100 mg bd	10–20 mg/l
Carbamazepine	100 mg bd	4–10 mg/l
Valproate	200 mg bd	Limited value
Ethosuximide	250 mg bd	40–80 mg/l

STATUS EPILEPTICUS

This is defined as repeated episodes without the patient having recovered consciousness from the previous attack. Repeated generalized seizures are readily apparent but epilepsia partialis continua may require EEG monitoring to diagnose. It is important that the patient is assessed at presentation for respiratory or cardiovascular insufficiency.

Management

- Intubate if required.
- Establish an iv line and administer 10% dextrose and 100 mg thiamine.
- iv diazepam 5–15 mg (repeat if required).
- Controlled infusion of chlormethiazole, closely monitoring respiration, or iv phenytoin 15–20 mg/kg followed by 30–50 mg/min infusion.
- If control is not achieved phenobarbitone 300 mg initially followed by 25–50 mg/minute infusion.
- Deep sedation and paralysis with thiopentone and suxamethonium with assisted ventilation is required in a minority.

NEUROPATHY

This can be divided into abnormalities which affect individual nerves (mononeuropathy) or several peripheral nerves either symmetrically (polyneuropathy) or asymmetrically (mononeuritis multiplex).

MONONEUROPATHY

Aetiology Single nerves: trauma, diabetes; numerous nerves: diabetes, sarcoidosis, polyarteritis nodosa, malignancy and amyloidosis.

Clinical features The commonest affected nerves involved in mononeuropathy, irrespective of the cause, include: median nerve (C5–T1), ulnar nerve (C8–T1), radial nerve (C5–T1), sciatic nerve (L4–S2), lateral popliteal nerve (L4–S2) and tibial nerves (S1–3). The clinical abnormality for each lesion is predictable from the nerve roots involved affecting both motor and sensory modalities. (→ Fig 8.1).

Investigation The cause of the underlying abnormality is usually apparent on clinical examination.

POLYNEUROPATHY

This is a more generalized disturbance in peripheral nerves, typically starting distally giving rise to the 'glove-and-stocking' distribution. A sensorimotor pattern is commonest but a pure motor, sensory or autonomic neuropathy may develop depending upon the cause (→ Table 8.3).

Table 8.3
Causes of polyneuropathy

Motor	Sensorimotor
Guillain-Barré	Alcohol abuse
Glandular fever	Thiamine or vit. B_{12} deficiency
Diphtheria	Carcinoma
Toxins eg thallium	Diabetes
Porphyria	Amyloidosis
	Drugs eg phenytoin, vincristine, isoniazid
	Toxins eg lead, arsenic
	Connective tissue disorders
	Hypothyroidism

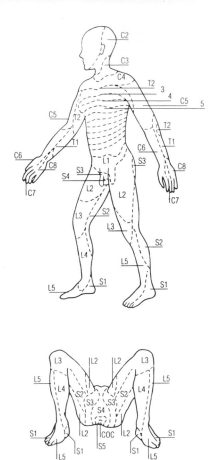

Fig. 8.1
Dermatomal anatomy.

Investigations ● FBC, glucose, ESR, creatinine, plasma vitamin B$_{12}$, thyroxine, CXR, porphyrins ● Neurophysiological studies and nerve biopsy are useful in selected cases.

MYOPATHY

Primary disorders of skeletal muscle are unusual and may have a wide range of causes.

**Table 8.4
Causes of myopathy**

Inherited	Metabolic	Toxic
Duchenne's	Glycogen storage	Alcohol
Becker's	disorders	Drugs eg
Myotonic dystrophy	Cushing's syndrome	cimetidine
Facioscapulo-humeral	Thyrotoxicosis	penicillamine
dystrophy	Hypercalcaemia	procainamide
Limb-girdle and	Hypokalaemia	azathioprine
distal dystrophy	Hypomagnesaemia	barbiturates
Central core disease	Diabetes mellitus	chloroquine
	Osteomalacia	

Aetiology ($\rightarrow$ Table 8.4) In a small number infectious causes can be implicated eg staphylococcal, streptococcal, cysticercosis and *Clostridium welchii* infection. Connective tissue disorders such as polymyalgia rheumatica and dermatomyositis should be excluded.

Clinical features

Symptoms: The most common are weakness, myalgia and cramps.

Signs: include proximal muscle wasting, tenderness and early fatigue provoked by exercise. In certain conditions characteristic associated features such as frontal baldness, ptosis, cataracts, sternomastoid muscle atrophy and testicular atrophy (in dystrophia myotonica) may be present. In Duchenne's dystrophy apparent hypertrophy of involved muscle is obvious.

Investigations ● An accurate family, drug and social history is essential ● Biochemistry; serum calcium, potassium and magnesium levels as well as serum thyroxine and cortisol concentrations. Elevated levels of serum creatine phosphokinase indicate active muscle damage ● The ESR is typically elevated in polymyalgia rheumatica ● An EMG and muscle biopsy may be essential in establishing the precise cause. These latter may however be normal in certain cases where obvious clinical disease exists.

Management For the inherited varieties no treatment exists and genetic counselling assumes high priority. In those acquired cases due to metabolic or toxic causes correction of the metabolic defect or removal of the drug or toxin may result in rapid clinical improvement. Corticosteroid treatment is highly effective in polymyalgia rheumatica.

9

Endocrinology

THYROTOXICOSIS

The commonest cause in the UK is autoimmune (Graves' disease) due to stimulating antibodies to the TSH receptor. Less often a toxic nodule or a thyroid adenoma may over-produce thyroxine and very rarely self-administered thyroxine may be the cause.

Clinical features Females outnumber males 5:1.

Symptoms: include sweating, heat intolerance, amenorrhoea, palpitations, weight loss, increased appetite and anxiety.

Signs: tachycardia, atrial fibrillation, exophthalmos, lid-lag, proximal myopathy, fine tremor and goitre (sometimes with a bruit). Pretibial myxoedema and acropachy are found in 5% of Graves' disease.

Investigations ● Serum T3, T4 and TSH. Undetectable TSH levels are virtually diagnostic and the TRH stimulation test is now seldom required ● TRH stimulation test is useful in bor-der-line cases ● An isotope iodine scan is useful in identifying toxic nodules and ● thyroid autoantibodies indicate an auto-immune aetiology.

Management Three forms exist.

Antithyroid drugs: eg carbimazole 15 mg tid initially reduc-ing to 5 mg tid for 12–18 months, with β-blockers: for symptomatic relief. Relapse occurs in approximately 70% within two years and is commoner with large goitres and severe disease. Adverse reactions such as rashes and neu-tropenia are relatively common.

Radio-iodine: is usually withheld in the UK in women of childbearing potential. Hypothyroidism is common after treatment, the frequency increasing with time after therapy, necessitating long-term surveillance. Some authorities ad-vocate administration of a large dose with early thyroxine replacement.

Surgery: this should only be undertaken once the thyro-toxic state has been controlled with propranolol and/or car-bimazole. Hypothyroidism is common and relapse of thy-rotoxicosis and hypoparathyroidism may occur. Damage to the recurrent laryngeal nerve is rare. Indications include medical failure in the young and large goitres causing stri-dor or dysphagia.

Extrathyroid complications Exophthalmos is best treated with high dose corticosteroids but may require tarsorrhaphy and/or orbital decompression. Cardiac arrhythmias espe-cially AF may respond poorly to digoxin and β-blockers are often required. Once the patient is euthyroid cardioversion should be considered. Thyrotoxic crisis, manifested by high-output cardiac failure, requires treatment with propranolol 80 mg qds, carbimazole 60–120 mg followed by potassium iodide 60 mg daily, dexamethasone 2 mg qds and fluid replacement.

HYPOTHYROIDISM

The commonest cause worldwide is iodine deficiency but in the UK autoimmune disease (Hashimoto's disease if associated with a goitre) is commonest, followed by post-operative and post ^{131}I therapy. Primary atrophic hypothyroidism, dyshormonogenesis, iodine excess and hypopituitarism are less common.

Clinical features

Symptoms: include weight gain, cold intolerance, depression, tiredness, menorrhagia, constipation and slowing in mental function.

Signs: slow relaxation of tendon reflexes, myxoedema (deposition of subcutaneous mucopolysaccharide), hair loss, hoarse voice, cold skin, bradycardia and slowness of movement.

Investigations • Low T4 with high TSH will identify the great majority. In hypopituitarism a low T4 is accompanied by a low TSH • Associated abnormalities include hypercholesterolaemia, anaemia and low voltage ECG complexes • Thyroid autoantibodies are present in the autoimmune variants.

Management Thyroxine replacement starting at a low dose such as 50 µg/day and increasing to 100 or 200 µg/day. The replacement dose should be judged against symptoms and restoring TSH levels to normal. In patients with angina replacement should be very slow and β-blockers may need to be introduced concomitantly.

THYROID CANCER

Thyroid cancer is rare but is important as some types have a good prognosis if treated early. The main types are:

Papillary (60%): all age groups, presents with a slow growing nodule and sometimes metastasizes to cervical lymph nodes.

Follicular (20%): middle age commonest, tends to metastasize via the blood stream to bones and lung.

Anaplastic (15%): old age, presents with a rapidly growing firm thyroid mass resulting in stridor, vocal-cord paralysis and weight loss.

Medullary (5%): presents as a solitary nodule often with spread to cervical nodes and the mediastinum. About 20% are associated with MEN. The tumours may secrete calcitonin, serotonin, ACTH and other peptides causing intractable diarrhoea and flushing. *Lymphoma (<1%):* rare.

Investigations Patients are usually euthyroid ● US shows a solid mass within the thyroid which is 'cold' on isotope scan ● Fine-needle aspiration is increasingly used for histological typing ● Calcitonin levels are high in medullary carcinoma.

> **Management** Papillary and follicular tumours are usually treated by total thyroidectomy followed by radiotherapy with long term thyroid replacement therapy and further radiotherapy for recurrences. Medullary carcinoma is not radiosensitive and is usually treated surgically. Anaplastic tumours have a poor prognosis irrespective of therapy.

DIABETES MELLITUS

> This exists when there is persistent hyperglycaemia due to deficiency or reduced effectiveness of endogenous insulin. A random blood glucose >14 mmol/l is diagnostic as is a fasting glucose >8 mmol/l. In equivocal cases a 75 g oral glucose tolerance test (OGTT) is indicated. A blood glucose >10 mmol/l 2 hours after the glucose load is diagnostic of diabetes mellitus (DM). Higher early glucoses which normalize (<7 mmol/l) at 2 hours (lag-storage curve) may result in glycosuria and occur in situations associated with rapid gastric emptying.

Classification Type I or insulin dependent DM which commonly presents in the young with ketoacidosis and type II or non-insulin dependent DM, more characteristic of the obese elderly subject. These clinical characteristics are by no means universal as some diabetic children do not require insulin while many elderly subjects do.

Aetiology Although the cause of diabetes remains unclear an autoimmune aetiology is likely in type I DM, perhaps triggered by viral infection whilst type II DM has a significant genetic component and is strongly related to obesity. Other factors which may induce or precipitate DM are drugs eg steroids, thiazides, pancreatic disease, stress eg trauma or surgery and endocrine disorders eg Cushing's disease and acromegaly.

Clinical features These vary in type I and II DM.

Type I: weight loss, dehydration, ketonuria, short duration of symptoms and hyperventilation.

Type II: obesity, weight gain and an insidious onset.

Common to both types: polyuria and polydipsia, lethargy, boils, pruritus vulvae and infections.

Investigations ● Random blood glucose is usually diagnostic and fasting and 2-hour post-prandial blood glucose will establish the diagnosis in the majority ● Glycosuria without hyperglycaemia occurs in those with a low renal glucose threshold and in those with a lag-storage curve ● Ketonuria occurs in type I DM and in fasting patients ● In those in whom ketoacidosis is considered blood glucose, U+Es, blood gas analysis, CXR, MSU and blood cultures are indicated ● Long-term monitoring of diabetic control as assessed by home blood glucose measurements and urinalysis supplemented by regular clinic measurements of blood glucose and $HbA1_C$ ● Screening for complications includes regular serum creatinine or creatinine clearance measurements as well as retinoscopy, attention to foot care, the peripheral circulation and detection of peripheral neuropathy.

Management

Type I: if ketoacidosis is present immediate and aggressive treatment with iv fluids and insulin is indicated ($\rightarrow$ p 311). In those without ketosis, hyperglycaemia associated with weight loss, rapid onset of symptoms and dehydration insulin therapy is also indicated. Many different regimens of insulin administration exist but the majority combine short and long-acting preparations usually twice daily eg Actrapid and Monotard. Approximately 1 unit of insulin per kg body weight is required per day. Many patients find greater flexibility and better control with a 'basal/bolus' regimen (long-acting insulin before bed with short-acting insulin before meals). Pumps delivering continuous insulin infusions have not gained popularity because of the rapid development of ketoacidosis due to pump failure. Dietary control and patient education are essential for good diabetic control and patient confidence.

Type II: many patients respond well to dietary treatment to reduce weight and restrict carbohydrate intake. In obese subjects who cannot or will not lose weight the addition of a biguanide drug eg metformin 500 mg tid often improves control. In others in whom dietary treatment alone does not provide adequate control sulphonylurea agents eg glipizide 5–10 mg tid or gliclazide 80–320 mg daily are useful.

Complications DM may result in damage to almost any organ. Poor diabetic control accelerates organ damage and good control reduces the risk. CNS damage may also accrue from frequent episodes of hypoglycaemia which may accompany overzealous attempts at normoglycaemia.

Kidneys: the earliest manifestation of damage is microalbuminuria which indicates risk of development of frank proteinuria due to diffuse glomerulosclerosis, chronic pyelonephritis or papillary necrosis.

Eyes: microvascular damage results in microaneurysms (dots), haemorrhage (blots), infarction (cotton wool spots), exudates and neovascularization. Vitreous haemorrhage, rubreosis (new vessel formation on the iris) and cataracts are other complications.

Heart: IHD is more common, and there is a specific diabetic cardiomyopathy.

Circulation: large vessel disease due to atheroma may result in intermittent claudication or stroke. Small vessel disease may produce distal gangrene in the presence of good peripheral pulses.

Skin: abnormalities may develop at the site of insulin injection including abscess formation, fat necrosis and fat hypertrophy. Repeated injection in the latter results in highly variable blood glucoses.

Nervous system: peripheral neuropathy in a glove-and-stocking distribution is common. Mononeuropathy eg VI nerve palsy is well recognized as is autonomic neuropathy which may manifest as diarrhoea, vomiting, impotence, postural hypotension and cardiac arrhythmias.

Prognosis The standard mortality rate of DM is greater than the general population, the excess mortality in type I being due to renal disease and in type II due to cardiovascular and cerebrovascular disease. Evidence exists that good diabetic control reduces the rate of development of complications.

PITUITARY DISEASE

The pituitary gland: the anterior pituitary gland secretes the gonadotrophins FSH and LH, growth hormone, prolactin, ACTH and TSH. The posterior pituitary secretes anti-diuretic hormone (ADH) and oxytocin.

HYPOPITUITARISM

This is complete or partial deficiency of anterior or posterior pituitary hormones.

Aetiology Most commonly due to anterior pituitary tumours, other causes include craniopharyngioma, metastatic tumour, autoimmune, granulomatous disorders eg sarcoidosis, and postpartum haemorrhage (Sheehan's syndrome). Surgery and radiotherapy for pituitary tumours may result in hypopituitarism.

Clinical features

Symptoms: Apathy, reduced libido, infertility, amenorrhoea, myxoedema, depression.

Signs: hypotension, small testes, reduced body hair, fine wrinkled skin, bitemporal hemianopia.

Investigations • Skull X-ray • CT scan • T4 and TSH levels, prolactin, gonadotrophins, testosterone and cortisol • Absence of the normal increases in gonadotrophins, TSH and cortisol after GnRH, TRH and insulin induced hypoglycaemia. This test should only be undertaken under medical supervision and with iv glucose available to reverse hypoglycaemia. It should be avoided in those with IHD or epilepsy.

Management Replacement therapy with deficient hormones, hydrocortisone 20 mg mane and 10 mg nocte, thyroxine 0.2 mg/day, testosterone 250 mg im 3-weekly in men and the combined oral contraceptive pill for premenopausal women.

DIABETES INSIPIDUS

Inability to produce concentrated urine due to complete or partial deficiency of ADH (central DI) or renal resistance to the antidiuretic action of ADH (renal DI).

Aetiology

Central DI: idiopathic (50%) and head injury commonest. Also posthypophysectomy, craniopharyngioma, sarcoidosis, post-meningitis and inherited.

Renal DI: drugs (lithium commonest), hypokalaemia, hypercalcaemia, renal disease and glycosuria.

Clinical features Polyuria, nocturia and polydipsia. If deprived of water, dehydration and confusion develop.

Investigations • 24-hour urine output to confirm polyuria • Exclude DM and renal failure • Water deprivation test; if after 12 hours of fluid deprivation the urine osmolality is >800 DI is excluded; if below administer desmopressin 20 µg intranasally – if urine osmolality increases to >800 = central DI, if not = nephrogenic DI. • In difficult cases plasma ADH levels can be measured during hypertonic saline infusion.

> **Management**
>
> *Central DI:* treatment of the underlying cause may cure the DI; if not administer desmopressin 10–20 µg bd intranasally.
>
> *Nephrogenic DI:* treat the underlying cause. In refractory cases thiazide diuretics 5–10 mg/day may be beneficial.

PITUITARY TUMOURS

These are usually adenomas and can be divided into those which secrete hormones; eg acidophilic adenomas which secrete growth hormone or prolactin and basophilic adenomas which secrete ACTH; and non-functional tumours usually chromophobic adenomas.

Clinical features These may be due to local pressure effects eg bitemporal quadrantic or hemianopia, cranial nerve palsy, optic atrophy and hypothalamic disturbance eg sleep and eating disturbance. Other effects may be due to hormone secretion which results in:

Acromegaly: characterized by insidious onset with headaches, coarsening of features, enlargement of extremities, prognathia, enlarged tongue, sweating, hypertension, cardiac failure and glucose intolerance.

Hyperprolactinaemia: characterized by amenorrhoea, infertility, galactorrhoea and impotence.

Cushing's disease: with proximal myopathy, central distribution of fat, abdominal striae, 'moon face', proximal myopathy, hirsutism, osteoporosis, bruising, hypertension and oedema.

Features of hypopituitarism may develop due to pituitary compression.

Investigations ● Skull X-ray, CT scan, visual-field assessment ● Acromegaly is diagnosed by high GH levels which do not suppress during a 75 g OGTT ● Prolactin levels >1000 mU/l (normal <400 mU/l) which do not rise in response to iv TRH or metoclopramide suggest a prolactinoma ● For diagnosis of Cushing's disease → p 170 ● It is important to measure gonadotrophins, sex hormones, T4, TSH and to perform a short synacthen test to screen for associated hormone deficiency.

> **Management** Deficient hormones must be replaced prior to surgery, which should be covered with iv hydrocortisone. Acromegaly should be treated with hypophysectomy followed by pituitary irradiation; post-operatively DI and hypopituitarism may develop. Somatostatin therapy can also

be used. Prolactinomas can be successfully treated with bromocryptine 2.5–30 mg/day, although radiotherapy and surgery may be indicated. Non-secreting tumours are best treated by hypophysectomy to relieve local pressure effects on the optic chiasma and cavernous sinus.

ADRENAL INSUFFICIENCY

Adrenal insufficiency may be primary (Addison's disease), when adrenal disease occurs following autoimmune destruction (80%), tuberculosis, metastatic disease or intra-adrenal haemorrhage or secondary due to pituitary, hypothalamic disease or withdrawal of chronic corticosteroid therapy.

Clinical features

Symptoms: Acute adrenal insufficiency, usually due to sudden cessation of steroid therapy or failure to increase dosage during stress, results in shock, nausea, abdominal pain and bowel disturbance. Chronic adrenal insufficiency presents with lethargy, weakness, weight loss, postural dizziness, anorexia, nausea, constipation and amenorrhoea.

Signs: include hypotension, vitiligo, hyperpigmentation of mucous membranes and those areas exposed to light or pressure.

Investigations • Careful history eg of steroid therapy • BP • U+Es usually revealing hyperkalaemia, hyponatraemia, elevated urea and hypoglycaemia • CXR and abdominal film to identify evidence of TB • Serum cortisol levels are low and do not increase following parenteral synacthen • ACTH levels are high in Addison's disease and low in secondary adrenal failure • Adrenal antibodies may be positive.

Management If this follows withdrawal of corticosteroids immediate replacement therapy is essential although gradual withdrawal over weeks may allow endogenous corticosteroid synthesis to resume. In other cases corticosteroid therapy is required indefinitely. Therapy of choice is hydrocortisone: 20 mg mane and 10 mg nocte is the usual dose. Serum cortisol levels before and after oral administration should be checked. Cortisol therapy should be increased at times of stress eg surgery and during acute illness. The majority of patients with Addison's disease also require mineralocorticoid replacement with fludrocortisone 0.05–0.15 mg/day. Mineralocorticoid therapy is not usually required in secondary adrenal insufficiency.

Treatment of acute adrenal insufficiency This is characterized by profound hypotension, abdominal pain and hyperkalaemia. IV fluid replacement as well as parenteral hydrocortisone (100 mg qid) administration is required. Clinical improvement is usually dramatic and steroid therapy should never be withheld in those in whom the diagnosis has been considered whilst the results of tests are awaited.

CUSHING'S SYNDROME

Prolonged exposure to abnormally high serum cortisol levels causes Cushing's syndrome. Causes other than iatrogenic can be divided into: ACTH dependent eg pituitary dependent disease (Cushing's disease 60%), ectopic ACTH from tumours eg small cell bronchial carcinoma (20%); and non-ACTH dependent eg adrenal adenoma (10%), adrenal carcinoma (5%) and alcohol-induced psuedo-Cushing's (5%).

Clinical features   Same as for Cushing's disease p 168. Additional features may be present due to associated pathology eg bronchial carcinoma. Pigmentation is prominent in ectopic ACTH syndromes but absent in non-ACTH dependent causes.

Investigations   ● U+Es may show hypokalaemia, glucose intolerance may be present as may hypertension ● CXR to exclude bronchial carcinoma ● Failure to suppress 09:00 hour serum cortisol to <170 nmol/l after overnight (23:00 h) dexamethasone 2 mg, elevation of 24-hour urinary free cortisol and loss of diurnal variation in serum cortisol levels are useful screening tests ● ACTH levels are high in pituitary disease, very high in ectopic ACTH syndromes and low in adrenal disease ● A high-dose dexamethasone suppression test 2 mg qid and the metyrapone test (750 mg 4 hourly for 24 h) may help differentiate ACTH dependent from adrenal disease ● CT scan of the pituitary and adrenals may identify a tumour and inferior petrosal sinus sampling for ACTH may localize pituitary tumours.

Management   Surgery is indicated for most pituitary and adrenal tumours and may be appropriate for some cases of ectopic ACTH syndrome, although pituitary radiotherapy is also used for Cushing's disease. The use of metyrapone and aminoglutethimide which inhibit cortisol production, are necessary preoperatively, and may produce benefit in cases not amenable to surgery. Iatrogenic Cushing's syndrome responds to reduction in steroid dosage when possible. Drugs such as azathioprine may be used in conjunction with steroids to enable lower doses to be used to control the underlying disease.

PHAEOCHROMOCYTOMA

This is a rare catecholamine secreting benign (90%) tumour usually arising in the adrenal medulla. Other sites include chromaffin tissues of the sympathetic nervous system eg para-aortic ganglia.

Clinical features   These depend upon the relative amounts of adrenaline and noradrenaline. Features may be episodic and include weight loss, hypertension, tachycardia, pallor, sweating, headache, anxiety and nausea. Hyperglycaemia may exist.

Investigations   • 24-hour urine for total metadrenalines • Location of the tumour by CT scanning and venous sampling for noradrenaline if necessary.

Management   Surgical excision under α and β-blockade using phenoxybenzamine and propranolol. These should be given for at least three days preoperatively. Special care necessary during surgery because of blockage of sympathetic nervous system.

HYPERALDOSTERONISM

Primary hyperaldosteronism
This is a condition where high aldosterone levels exist independent of the renin-angiotensin system, is rare and due in most cases to an adrenocortical adenoma; Conn's syndrome.

Clinical features   These are often asymptomatic. Hypertension, lethargy and muscular weakness due to hypokalaemia.

Investigations   • Hypokalaemia (<3.5 mmol/l) in patients not taking diuretics, steroids, laxatives, potassium • Plasma renin, angiotensin and aldosterone levels taken in the early morning before the patient moves from the supine position • CT scan may identify an adrenal mass.

Management   Surgery to remove the adenoma in Conn's syndrome after 4–6 weeks spironolactone 300 mg/day. If due to adrenal hyperplasia spironolactone therapy alone is usually sufficient.

Secondary hyperaldosteronism
This is said to exist when high aldosterone levels are present due to activation of the renin-angiotensin system. Causes include renal artery stenosis, decompensated liver disease, accelerated hypertension, cardiac failure and nephrotic syndrome.

> *Management* Remove the underlying cause if possible.

PARATHYROID DISEASE

PRIMARY HYPERPARATHYROIDISM

> High levels of PTH occur in primary hyperparathyroidism, usually due to a ● parathyroid adenoma, less commonly ● hyperplasia and rarely ● carcinoma. Hyperparathyroidism is the commonest component of the multiple endocrine neoplasia syndromes.

Clinical features These may be absent and many cases are detected by identifying hypercalcaemia on routine blood screening. Hypercalcaemia may cause anorexia, weakness, constipation, vomiting and confusion. Renal colic, backache, hypertension, nephrolithiasis, nephrogenic DI and pseudogout are also well recognized. Corneal calcification is rare.

Investigations ● Ionised calcium if available, otherwise serum calcium avoiding the use of a tourniquet and correcting for hypoalbuminaemia ● Other causes of hypercalcaemia eg malignancy, sarcoidosis, myeloma and vitamin D excess require exclusion ● The serum phosphate is usually low as is plasma bicarbonate and high plasma chloride in primary hyperparathyroidism ● X-rays of the hands and skull may reveal subperiosteal erosions of the phalanges or a 'pepper-pot' skull in primary hyperparathyroidism whilst an abdominal film may reveal nephrocalcinosis ● US of the neck may identify a parathyroid adenoma as may a radioactive thallium technetium extraction scan ● New 2-site radioimmunoassays for PTH can reliably differentiate primary hyperparathyroidism (high PTH) from the hypercalcaemia of malignancy (low PTH).

> *Management* Surgery to remove a parathyroid adenoma is highly successful although in elderly asymptomatic patients conservative therapy may be indicated. In those with parathyroid hyperplasia resection of all four glands with subsequent transplantation of parathyroid tissue to the forearm is also successful. Treatment of severe hypercalcaemia requires adequate rehydration with iv saline along with oral phosphate sodium cellulose phosphate or disodium etidronate. Steroid therapy and the use of calcitonin are seldom required for the hypercalcaemia due to hyperparathyroidism in comparison to that associated with malignancy.

SECONDARY HYPERPARATHYROIDISM

This occurs following prolonged hypocalcaemia eg associated with renal failure or malabsorption, which stimulates PTH secretion in order to correct the hypocalcaemia. Occasional PTH secretion may become autonomous in these circumstances leading to hypercalcaemia (tertiary hyperparathyroidism).

> **Management**   Correct the underlying cause.

HYPOPARATHYROIDISM

This may be either primary (autoimmune, associated with hypothyroidism and Addison's disease) or secondary, usually after thyroid surgery.

Clinical features   If acute this may give rise to tetany, perioral and peripheral paraesthesia, cramps and fits. Occult tetany may be revealed by Trousseau's and Chvostek's tests. If chronic it is associated with abnormalities of nails, teeth and hair. Cutaneous moniliasis is more common in the autoimmune variant. Less often cataracts and rarely papilloedema are found.

Investigations   • Low serum calcium, increased phosphate and normal alkaline phosphatase • Skull X-ray may reveal basal ganglia calcification • Plasma PTH levels low • Decreased urinary execretion of AMP which rises following PTH infusion.

> **Management**   In acute cases of hypocalcaemia give 10–20 ml 10% calcium gluconate iv. If hypomagnesaemia exists iv magnesium chloride should be given. Long-term management requires therapy with 1 α vit D$_3$. Calcium supplements are not usually required to maintain normal serum calcium levels.

PSEUDOHYPOPARATHYROIDISM

This is a rare inherited disorder with resistance to PTH. Similar biochemical features to hypoparathyroidism are found in association with short stature, mental retardation, short 4th and 5th metacarpals, a 'moon' face, cerebral calcification and hypothyroidism.

OSTEOMALACIA / RICKETS

> Failure of organic bone matrix (osteoid) to mineralise normally produces rickets during bone growth and osteomalacia following epiphyseal closure.

Aetiology:

Low dietary vit D_2

Lack of sunlight – reduced level of vit D_3

Malabsorption/impaired absorption of vit D_2/vit D_3
– coeliac disease, bowel resection, biliary cirrhosis, phytates,
   excessive aluminium hydroxide

Impaired activation vit D_3 – renal failure

Resistance to vit D_3

Drugs – phenytoin

Clinical features

Symptoms: skeletal pain, proximal muscular weakness, lethargy

Signs: bony tenderness, swelling of distal ends of radius and
ulna, rickety rosary (costochondral swelling), delayed dentition, waddling gait, tetany, spontaneous fractures, knock-knees,
bow legs.

Investigations: • hypocalcaemia, hypophosphataemia, raised
alkaline phosphatase, low vitamin D • bone biopsy shows in
complete mineralisation • radiology (pseudo-fractures in pubic
rami, scapula, upper ends humerus and femur, cupped and
ragged metaphyseal surfaces in rickets).

> ***Management*** Replace deficient vitamin D (dose depends
> on aetiology). Treat any underlying condition. Monitor
> calcium level.

MULTIPLE ENDOCRINE NEOPLASIA

May occur spontaneously or familially (autosomal dominant).

MEN I (Wermer's Syndrome)
  Pancreatic endocrine tumour (insulinoma, gastrinoma,
    vipoma, glucagonoma)
  Parathyroid adenoma
  Pituitary adenoma (eg prolactinoma)

MEN IIa (Sipple's Syndrome)
  Parathyroid adenoma
  Medullary carcinoma of the thyroid
  Phaeochromacytoma

MEN IIb
  Medullary carcinoma of the thyroid
  Phaeochromocytoma
  Mucosal neuromas
  Marsanoid habitus

10

Haematology

INVESTIGATIONS

Full blood count: RBC, WBC and platelet counts; RBC morphology; WBC differential.

Blood film: RBC, WBC and platelet morphology.

Erythrocyte sedimentation rate ($\rightarrow$ Table 10.18, p 189).
Normal range   1–5 cm in adult males
                     1–8 cm in adult females.

Bone marrow/aspiration/trephine/culture

Serum protein estimation: protein electrophoresis, immunoglobulins, plasma viscosity, haptoglobins, haemopexin.

Bence Jones protein: free immunoglobulin light chains in the urine.

Surface marker studies: rosetting techniques, immunofluorescence.

Haemoglobin studies: sickle cell screening, haemoglobin electrophoresis, oxygen dissociation curves, methaemoglobin detection, 2, 3 DPG quantification, G-6-P dehydrogenase assay.

Isotope studies: red cell mass, plasma volume, red cell survival, iron absorption.

DEFINITIONS

Microcytosis: reduction in average volume of RBCs MCV <78 fl.

Macrocytosis: increase in average volume of RBCs MCV >98 fl.

Hypochromia: red cells contain less than the normal amount of haemoglobin, MCHC <30 g/dl.

Poikilocytosis: irregularity of red blood-cell shape.

Anisocytosis: variation in size in red blood cells.

Elliptocytosis: elliptical red blood cells.

Ovalocytosis: oval red blood cells.'

Spherocytosis: spherical RBCs, loss of central pallor eg congenital or aggressive haemolysis.

Dimorphic: dual population of RBCs in the peripheral circulation eg sideroblastic anaemia.

Reticulocytosis: the presence of immature red blood cells in the peripheral blood.

Polychromasia: blue tinge to red blood cells in the blood film due to the presence of immature red blood cells.

Nucleated RBC: indicates overactive erythropoiesis eg leukaemia, marrow infiltration.

Blast cells: nucleated precursor cells eg leukaemia.

Schistocytes: red cell fragments secondary to mechanical trauma eg prosthetic heart valves, DIC.

Punctate basophilia: indicates damaged RBCs eg severe anaemia, lead poisoning, β-thalassaemia.

Leucocytosis: increase in total circulating WBCs (>11.0 × 10^9/1) eg pyogenic infection.

Leucopenia: decrease in total circulating WBCs (<4.0 × 10^9/1) eg TB, overwhelming infection

Eosinophilia: increase in total circulating eosinophils eg parasitic infection, lymphoma, worms and drug reactions.

Monocytosis: increase in circulating monocytes eg TB and malaria.

Leucoerythroblastic: blood film containing immature RBCs and WBCs, usually in association with tumour infiltration of the bone marrow.

Thrombocytopenia: decrease in circulating platelets eg marrow suppression or drug reaction (<150 × 10^9/1).

Thrombocytosis: increase in circulating platelet count (>350× 10^9/1).

Extramedullary erythropoiesis: production of RBCs outside the bone marrow eg liver, spleen.

Burr cells: irregularly shaped RBCs seen in uraemia.

Howell-Jolly bodies: nuclear remnants seen in the RBCs in post-splenectomy cases, leukaemia, megaloblastic anaemia.

Target cells: RBCs with central staining surrounded by a ring of pallor and an outer ring of staining eg thalassaemia, severe liver disease.

Heinz bodies: denatured haemoglobin in RBCs.

Haemolysis: excessively rapid red cell breakdown.

Left shift: increase in immature white cells eg infection.

Right shift: hypersegmented polymorphs eg uraemia, liver disease and megaloblastic anaemia.

ANAEMIA

Anaemia exists if the haemoglobin level is less than that which is expected when both age and sex are taken into account. The haemoglobin level at birth is high (20 g/dl), but falls during the first three months of life to a nadir (10 g/dl) before rising again to the adult value (>12 g/dl in females and >13 g/dl in males).

Aetiology (→ Table 10.1).

Table 10.1 Aetiology of anaemia	
Loss of blood	Acute or chronic
Impaired RBC formation	Congenital: marrow aplasia, red cell aplasia Nutritional deficiencies: iron, B_{12}, folate, vitamin C, protein (kwashiorkor) Immune dysfunction: SLE, RA Infection: viral – EBV, HIV, TB Bone marrow invasion: leukaemia, carcinoma, fibrosis Endocrine abnormalities: hypothyroidism, hypoadrenalism, hypopituitarism, hypogonadism Drugs/toxins: antibiotics – sulphonamides, chloramphenicol antimalarials – pyrimethamine anti-inflammatory – gold salts, indomethacin, phenylbutazone antithyroid – carbimazole anticonvulsants – phenytoin antidepressants – chlorpromazine cytotoxics – dose dependant ionising radiation solvents – benzene Thalassaemia Sideroblastosis Porphyria: erythropoietic Hepatic failure Renal failure
Haemolysis	Congenital red cell defects: membrane defects – spherocytosis; enzyme defects – G6PD; defects in Hb structure – sickle cell anaemia Acquired: B_{12}/folate deficiency infections: malaria trauma: prosthetic valve chemicals: drugs antibodies: autoimmune, isoimmune toxins tumours

Clinical features These depend on the degree of anaemia present and on the speed of its development.

Symptoms: are lethargy, malaise, headache, increasing breathlessness, palpitations, dizziness, syncope, and angina.

Signs: include pallor of the conjunctivae, mucous membranes and skin, tachycardia, systolic flow murmurs and peripheral oedema. Hypotension may be present. Splenomegaly, pigmented gallstones and jaundice may be present in haemolytic anaemia. Leg ulceration in hereditary haemolysis.

Investigations • FBC: red cell indices often give a pointer to the underlying aetiology.

Microcytic anaemia (MCV <76 fl, MCH <27 pg, MCHC <30 g/dl): iron deficiency ($\rightarrow$ Table 10.2), inherited sideroblastic anaemia, thalassaemia, chronic disease.

Normocytic anaemia: haemolytic conditions, following haemorrhage, aplastic anaemia, combined deficiencies eg iron and folate, chronic disease eg RA, uraemia, infection, malignancy, aplastic anaemia.

Macrocytic anaemia (MCV >96 fl): megaloblastic erythropoiesis ($\rightarrow$ Table 10.3, p 182): B_{12} deficiency, folate deficiency; normoblastic erythropoiesis: reticulocytosis, marrow infiltration/suppression, aplastic anaemia, hypothyroidism, hypopituitarism, alcoholism, liver disease.

• Peripheral blood film • ESR • BM examination • iron binding capacity • ferritin • vitamin B_{12} and folate levels • Schilling test, and • reticulocyte count • Tests for haemolysis include increased bilirubin, increased urinary urobilinogen, reduced or absent serum haptoglobin, haemoglobinuria, reticulocytosis, haemosiderinuria, methaemalbuminaemia, RBC morphology – spherocytes, elliptocytes, fragmentation, target cells • Reduced RBC survival can be assessed using labelled ^{51}Cr, and antibodies against RBC by direct antiglobulin test (Coombs' test).

Management Treat the underlying cause. Remove any provoking drugs. Blood transfusion may be required. Replace vitamin or mineral deficiencies eg oral ferrous sulphate 200 mg 3 × daily, parenteral iron is only rarely needed, vitamin B_{12} as im hydroxycobalamin 1 mg 2 × during the first week followed by 1 mg weekly until the blood count is normal. B_{12} injections may be needed three monthly for life. Folate 5 mg daily. Never give folate alone in pernicious anaemia as subacute combined degeneration of the spinal cord may be provoked. Steroids (40–60 mg/d initially) or splenectomy may be needed in haemolytic anaemia.

Table 10.2
Causes of iron deficiency anaemia

Inadequate diet
Malabsorption Coeliac disease
Blood loss GI malignancy, ulceration, varices, gastritis,
menorrhagia, haematuria, hookworm,
inflammatory bowel disease, diverticulitis,
haemorrhoids
Achlorhydria
Previous gastric surgery
Increased physiological demand Pregnancy, growth
Intravascular haemolysis Paroxysmal nocturnal
haemoglobinuria, RBC
fragmentation due to prosthetic
valves
Delayed weaning from the breast
Bleeding diathesis

PERNICIOUS ANAEMIA

Disorder characterized by megaloblastic change in the bone
marrow and anaemia, often with neurological abnormalities. It
is due to a failure of secretion of gastric intrinsic factor and has
an autoimmune basis. F>M, usually presents between 45–65
years. Higher incidence in people with blood group A. Achlorhydria and atrophic gastritis are present. Bone marrow morphology reflects failure of DNA synthesis with maturation arrest of
RBC, granulocyte and platelet precursors. Haemolysis occurs.

Clinical features Insidious onset and a profound degree of
anaemia may be present at the time of diagnosis. Weight loss
and diarrhoea are common, mild pyrexia, jaundice due to
haemolysis and pallor give the skin a lemon-yellow tinge. The
tongue is smooth, atrophic and may be tender. Splenomegaly
is common. Degenerative changes in the posterior and lateral
tracts of the spinal cord may cause subacute combined degeneration which presents with 'glove-and-stocking' impairment
of superficial sensation with loss of both proprioception and
vibration sense. The tendon reflexes may be brisk but the ankle
jerks are often lost. The plantar reflex is extensor. Ataxia and
a toxic confusional state may be present. If no treatment is
given dementia follows.

Differential diagnosis Any cause of megaloblastic anaemia
(→ Table 10.3). Exclude any other coexisting autoimmune
diseases eg vitiligo, DM, hypothyroidism, ovarian failure,
myasthenia gravis.

Table 10.3
Causes of megaloblastic anaemia

Vitamin B$_{12}$ deficiency:	Inadequate diet <1–2 μg/day
	Alcohol abuse
	Malabsorption:
	intrinsic factor deficiency
	– pernicious anaemia, previous gastric surgery, congenital absence, atrophic gastritis, Zollinger-Ellison Syndrome
	Terminal ileal disease:
	– ileal resections, Crohn's disease, ulcerative colitis, tropical sprue
	Infection:
	– blind loop syndrome, fish tapeworm
	Pancreatic insufficiency
	Drug induced:
	– neomycin, colchicine, metformin
	Increased requirements:
	– pregnancy, hyperthyroidism, increased erythropoiesis transcobalamin II deficiency
Folate deficiency:	Inadequate diet
	Malabsorption:
	— coeliac disease, jejunal resection, tropical sprue, Crohn's disease, Whipple's disease, GI lymphoma
	Increased requirements:
	— pregnancy, lactation, puberty, prematurity, dialysis, increased erythropoiesis, psoriasis, severe dermatitis
	Defective utilization:
	— drugs eg alcohol, methotrexate, trimethoprim, isoniazid, OCP
	Congenital enzyme deficiency:
	— dihydrofolate reductase
Pyridoxine deficiency	
Thiamine deficiency	
Preleukaemic leukaemia	
Lesch-Nyhan Syndrome	

Investigations ● FBC shows macrocytic anaemia ● Aniso-cytosis, poikilocytosis and RBC fragmentation may be present. Low reticulocyte count. Leucopenia and hypersegmentation of neutrophils are common. Platelet count is usually normal ● BM aspiration confirms a megaloblastic picture ● Serum vit B_{12} level is low (<160 ng/l), serum folate is not reduced ● Schilling test shows lack of B_{12} absorption ● Autoantibodies may be detected eg intrinsic factor (50%) or parietal cell (80%) ● Pentagastrin-fast achlorhydria ● Atrophic gastritis.

> ***Management*** im Hydroxycobalamin as for any case of B_{12} deficiency ($\rightarrow$ p 180). Reticulocytosis may be >50% by the tenth day. Iron (ferrous sulphate 200 mg 8-hourly) and po-tassium (KCl 1.2 g 8-hourly) supplements may be needed. Blood transfusion if the degree of anaemia is critical but should be given slowly with diuretic cover to avoid precipi-tating cardiac failure.

AUTOIMMUNE HAEMOLYTIC ANAEMIA

Antibodies are formed against RBC antigens leading to prema-ture destruction of the cells (normal life span 120 days). Two types of antibody exist based on thermal characteristics: 'warm' IgG (occasionally IgA or IgM) antibodies are most active at 37°C, 'cold' IgM antibodies at 4°C.

Aetiology ($\rightarrow$ Table 10.4).

Table 10.4
Causes of autoimmune haemolytic anaemia

'Warm' antibody type	Idiopathic, SLE, lymphoma, chronic lymphatic leukaemia, ovarian teratoma, Evan's Syndrome, drugs eg methyldopa
'Cold' antibody type	Cold haemagglutinin disease, paroxysmal cold haemoglobinuria (PCH) mycoplasma pneumonia, lymphoma, infectious mononucleosis, SLE, viral infections, chronic lymphatic leukaemia
Drug related	Drug absorbed onto RBC surface: penicillin, cephalosporins Immune complex mediated: sulphonamides, quinidine
Immune disease of the newborn	
Secondary to blood transfusion	

Clinical features

Warm' type: insidious onset, lethargy, jaundice, splenomegaly, purpura, fever and rarely renal failure. F>M.

'Cold' type: anaemia precipitated by cold conditions, Raynaud's phenomenon, cyanosis, acrocyanosis and non-specific symptoms of any anaemia.

Investigations ● FBC shows macrocytic anaemia ● demonstrate evidence of antibody attack against RBC by direct antiglobulin test (Coombs' test) at various temperatures to classify the responsible antigen ● Reticulocytosis ● Evidence of excessive RBC destruction (rise in unconjugated bilirubin and LDH, fall in concentration of haemoglobin scavenger levels – haptoglobin and haemopexin, free haemoglobin may bind to albumin-methaemalbumin, or spill over into the urine with haemoglobinuria or haemosiderinuria) ● Donath-Landsteiner IgG antibody is present in PCH. Look for underlying cause.

Management

'Warm' type: prednisolone 40–60 mg/day initially reducing slowly after 4 weeks. If this fails splenectomy or other immunosuppressive agents may be needed eg azathioprine (50–100 mg/d). Transfuse if necessary. Folate supplements if required, thymectomy may be useful occasionally in infants. '

'Cold' type: keep extremities warm, avoid transfusions if possible (always pre-warm), steroids and splenectomy are less successful.

APLASTIC ANAEMIA

Decrease in haemopoietic bone marrow with resultant pancytopenia.

Aetiology   (→ Table 10.5)

Clinical features M>F, peak incidence around 30 years. Insidious onset, symptoms are due to the deficiency of RBCs, WBCs and platelets with anaemia, bleeding and increased susceptibility to infection. Purpura, epistaxis, GI bleeding and haematuria are common. Skin and mucous membrane ulceration and infection.

Investigation   ● FBC: anaemia (normoblastic or macrocytic), reduced reticulocyte count, granulocytopenia, monocytopenia, lymphopenia, thrombocytopenia ● BM is hypocellular (multiple site biopsies) ● Elevated erythropoietin ● Radioactive iron studies show reduced clearance from the blood with poor marrow uptake.

Table 10.5
Causes of aplastic anaemia

Congenital	Fanconi's (autosomal recessive)	
Acute	Drugs:	cytotoxics
		chloramphenicol
		chlorpromazine
		oral anticoagulants
		indomethacin
		thiazide diuretics
		barbiturates
	Infections:	viral
		bacterial
		fungal
Chronic acquired	Idiopathic	
	Drugs (as above)	
	Chemicals: benzene	
	Radiation	
	Viral Infection: non A, non B hepatitis	
	PNH	
	Pregnancy	

Management Remove any identifiable cause eg drugs. Support with replacement therapy: RBC, granulocyte and platelet transfusions. Treat infections: antibiotics, antiviral agents and antifungal agents as required. Folate supplements as needed. Stimulate haemopoiesis: androgenic steroids (testosterone, oxymetholone, nandrolone deconate or fluoxymesterone), glucocorticoids (methylprednisolone), BMT may be needed. Immunosuppressive agents (cyclophosphamide, chlorambucil, azathioprine and antilymphocyte globulin) as the disease may have an immune basis in some cases but this is not without risk.

Prognosis Only 50% one-year survival.

HAEMOGLOBINOPATHIES

The haemoglobinopathies are a group of conditions in which the structure/production of haemoglobin has been altered in some way (→ Table 10.6, p 186).

SICKLE CELL ANAEMIA

Widespread disease in equatorial Africa in which an inherited

Table 10.6
Classification of haemoglobinopathies

Structural haemoglobin variants
HbS : the sickle cell syndromes
Methaemoglobins

Defective haemoglobin synthesis
Thalassaemias

Persistence of foetal haemoglobin

mutation in the gene sequence leads to an abnormal amino acid structure in the β-globin chain of haemoglobin. The normal glutamine amino acid at position six is replaced by valine. When the sickle cell haemoglobin molecule (haemoglobin S – HbS) is deoxygenated aggregations of fibrils are produced which distort the RBC into a characteristic 'sickle' shape. This polymerisation is initially reversible when reoxygenation occurs but the distortion of the RBC membranes may become permanent if excessive hypoxia or acidosis is present. This condition is inherited in an autosomal fashion, the homozygote having sickle cell disease and the heterozygote sickle cell trait which is usually asymptomatic and seems to be confer resistance to *falciparum* malaria. The coexisting presence of other haemoglobinopathies eg HbA or HbF reduces the concentration of HbS and makes sickling less likely.

Clinical features The two major problems are haemolytic anaemia due to reduced RBC survival and vascular occlusions by sickled cells. Symptoms begin during the second six months of life when HbF levels are falling and HbS levels rising. Severe anaemia occurs, with lethargy, growth retardation, delayed puberty, increased susceptibility to infection, leg ulceration and hyperplasia of the bone marrow leading to bossing of the skull. The anaemia is due to marrow hypoplasia, haemolysis, splenic sequestration and folate deficiency. Vaso-occlusive crises produce pain because of infarction in bones, fingers (dactylitis), lungs, spleen, kidneys, bowel, liver and retina. They are precipitated by dehydration, infection or cooling but may appear spontaneously and are characterized by fever, malaise, pain and prostration.

Investigation ● FBC, blood film shows sickle shaped cells (not in sickle cell trait) ● Affected cells will sickle within 20 minutes when mixed on a slide with 2% sodium metabisulphate, haemoglobin electrophoresis.

Management Avoid precipitating factors eg treat infections, prevent cold, hypotension, acidosis, hypoxia and dehydration. Folate supplements if indicated. Treat crisis by hydration, warmth, antibiotics, antimalarials, non-narcotic analgesia, transfuse if necessary and fresh frozen plasma.

Prognosis Without treatment few children survive into adulthood.

THALASSAEMIAS

Inherited disorders in which the rate of synthesis of one or more globin chains is reduced or absent producing haemolysis, ineffective erythropoiesis and anaemia. β-chain production is most commonly affected. Both heterozygote and homozygote states exist. Commonly found in Africa, Orient, Middle East, Asia and Mediterranean.

β-thalassaemia

This is due to failure to synthesize β chains. Heterozygote form (minor) is mild and may be asymptomatic. Homozygotes (major) are unable to synthesize normal amounts of adult haemoglobin A and retain production of the much less effective haemoglobin F.

Clinical features There are symptoms of severe anaemia after the first two months of life, anorexia, failure to thrive, developmental delay and early death. Marrow hyperplasia leads to head bossing and mongoloid appearance. Hepatosplenomegaly and leg ulceration occur.

Investigation

Minor: ● mild iron deficiency anaemia resistant to iron therapy ● haemoglobin electrophoresis shows increased HbA2 to 4–6% (normal 1.5–3%) and slight, if any, elevation of HbF levels (2–5%).

Major: ● profound hypochromic anaemia with RBC dysplasia, erythroblastosis, absent HbA and raised HbF levels ● radiology shows expanded marrow cavity eg skull and phalanges and 'hair-on-end' appearance to skull vault.

Management Transfuse to maintain Hb >10 g/dl. This may lead to gross iron overload and subsequent haemochromatosis with cardiac failure despite treatment with the iron chelating agent desferrioxamine. This should be administered to all patients receiving regular transfusions. Treat folate deficiency with supplements. Splenectomy may be needed for hypersplenism.

These are characterized by uncontrolled proliferation of malignant cells derived from one of the haemopoietic precursor cells with resulting replacement of the normal bone marrow. There is often systemic involvement. They are usually progressive and ultimately fatal due to overwhelming infection, haemorrhage or anaemia. Aetiology is usually unknown but may be related to ionising radiation, cytotoxic drugs, viral infection, chromosome changes or chemical exposure eg benzene.

There are many different forms of this disease, each arising from a separate stem cell component. In acute leukaemia the disease tends to be aggressive with a short life expectancy and many primitive blast cells are seen in the blood film. The presence of Auer rods in the cytoplasm of blast cells indicates a non lymphoblastic type. Acute lymphoblastic anaemia (ALL) has a dual dermographic distribution with peaks in children and the elderly while acute myeloid leukaemia (AML) is commonest in the young and middle aged (→ Table 10.7).

Table 10.7
Classification of acute leukaemia

Lymphoblastic: (ALL)		T-Cell B-Cell Receptor silent Undifferentiated
Myeloid: (AML)	M0:	Undifferentiated
	M1:	Poorly differentiated
	M2:	Myeloblastic
	M3:	Promyelocytic
	M4:	Myelomonoblastic
	M5a:	Monoblastic
	M5b:	Monocytic
	M6:	Erythroleukaemia
	M7:	Megakaryoblastic

Clinical features This often appears as a flu-like illness with fatigue, fever, malaise, rapidly progressing anaemia, persistent bacterial, viral or fungal sepsis (mouth, throat, anorectal or tongue ulceration) in the absence of pus formation. Purpura, bruising, bleeding from the gums, nose and GI tract. DIC may be present. Lymphadenopathy and hepatosplenomegaly are present in ALL. Gum hypertrophy and diffuse skin involvement are features of the monocytic type of acute myeloid leukaemia. CNS involvement with cranial nerve palsies may occur. Muscle and joint pain are common.

ACUTE MYELOID LEUKAEMIA

This is a group of aggressive neoplastic diseases involving myeloid stem cells ($\rightarrow$ Table 10.7). They can arise de-novo or following myelodysplastic syndromes. The various subtypes are classified on the basis of peripheral blood and bone marrow morphology, cytochemical staining, immunophenotyping and cytogenetic studies.

Management Aggressive combination chemotherapy involving a series of 3–4 individual pulses of treatment at monthly intervals allowing marrow recovery between. Allogenic bone marrow transplant in first remission (<45 years) from an HLA matched sibling donor is the treatment of choice. The adverse reactions of chemotherapy are numerous and include anaemia, total alopecia, gastrointestinal mucocitis with diarrhoea and infections secondary to immunosuppression. The patient requires intensive red cell support, reverse barrier nursing with iv antibiotics, platelet support and nutritional support for several weeks after each pulse of treatment. Long-term consequences of treatment are less well defined: rashes are common and the risk of secondary neoplasia is increased.

Prognosis Chemotherapy achieves an initial remission rate of 80% though long-term cure is probably only around 30% with chemotherapy alone. Allogenic BMT improves long-term remission to 50%.

ACUTE LYMPHOBLASTIC LEUKAEMIA

Presentation is usually with bone marrow failure although generalized lymphadenopathy and splenomegaly are common.

Table 10.8
Good prognostic indices in ALL

WBC: <10 × 10⁹/l
Age: 2–10 years
Sex: Female
Cell markers: common ALL Ag
Remission: early (within 4 weeks)

Management Involves intensive combination chemotherapy with inductive, early and late consolidative and maintenance phases. CNS relapse is a significant problem and prophylactic cranial radiotherapy and intrathecal chemotherapy are given. An allogenic transplant may be performed in first remission in adults.

Prognosis 70% 5-year survival in children with good prognostic indices (→ Table 10.8, p 189).

MYELODYSPLASTIC SYNDROMES

The myelodysplastic syndromes comprise a spectrum of disorders including those that used to be regarded as 'preleukaemic states' (→ Table 10.9). There is progressive marrow failure leading to anaemia, leukopenia and thrombocytopenia. Approximately 30% of patients develop an acute leukaemia. An allogenic BMT should be considered in young patients. No other specific treatment is available other than supportive measures.

Table 10.9
Classification of the myelodysplastic syndromes

Refractory anaemia
Refractory anaemia with ring sideroblasts
Refractory anaemia with 'excess blasts'
Chronic myelomonoblastic leukaemia

MYELOPROLIFERATIVE DISORDERS

Neoplastic diseases involving a proliferation of the myeloid stem cell or its derivatives (→ Table 10.10). A degree of overlap exists between these various disorders. Patients are often diagnosed following a routine FBC although some present with symptoms of marrow failure or hyperviscosity (retinal haemorrhages, infarcts, papilloedema, renal failure, TIAs, cerebral infarction or intermittent claudication).

CHRONIC MYELOID LEUKAEMIA

A less aggressive neoplastic disorder than AML involving more differentiated myeloid cell lines.

Table 10.10
Classification of myeloproliferative disorders

Chronic myeloid leukaemia
Polycythaemia rubra vera
Essential thrombocythaemia
Myelofibrosis/Myeloid metaplasia

Clinical features Insidious onset, lassitude, weight loss, arthralgia, myalgia, epistaxis, priapism, gout, sweating, recurrent infections. Lymphadenopathy is not a prominent feature. Massive splenomegaly is characteristic.

Investigations ● Elevation of the WBC count with a predominance of mature neutrophils but a spectrum of less mature cells is often present in the peripheral blood ● BM aspiration and trephine biopsy with chromosome analysis demonstrates the Philadelphia chromosome in 90% of cases (translocation of the long arm of chromosome 22 to another site, usually chromosome 9) ● Monoclonal immunoglobulin bands may be present ● Serum urate may be elevated.

Management Control of the elevated WBC using hydroxyurea or busulphan. Interferon may be used. The disease can often be controlled for some time before some patients develop related myeloproliferative disorders eg myelofibrosis or an elevated platelet count. Inevitably the disease transforms to an acute leukaemia with a poor prognosis. Allogenic BMT is the only available treatment and is offered to patients <45 years of age. GVH may complicate the transplant and is due to the cytotoxic effect of donor lymphocytes which become sensitized to the tissues of the recipient which they regard as foreign. Acute GVH disease may occur and is characterized by mucositis, diarrhoea, hepatitis and dermatitis. It may respond to corticosteroids, cyclosporin or anti-thymocyte globulin. Chronic GVH disease mimics diffuse connective disease and may respond to corticosteroids and azathioprine.

POLYCYTHAEMIA RUBRA VERA

Excessive production of red cells occurs despite the presence of low levels of erythropoietin. The disease often terminates in acute leukaemia or myelofibrosis.

Polycythaemia indicates an increase in red cell concentration in the peripheral blood. Apparent polycythaemia is caused by a reduction in plasma volume, true polycythaemia reflects a real increase in red cell mass (→ Table 10.11, p 192).

Table 10.11
Causes of polycythaemia

Polycythemia rubra vera		
Secondary (physiological)	Hypoxia:	cardiac disease, pulmonary disease, altitude, obesity, sleep apnoea, methaemoglobinaemia, sulphaemoglobinaemia
	Increased erythropoietin:	smoking, tumours (kidney, cerebellum, uterus, adrenal, liver)
Hypertransfusion		
Benign familial		
Spurious		'Stress' (Gaisbock syndrome), dehydration

Clinical features M>F and usually occurs in middle age. Dizziness, lethargy, headache, visual disturbance, pruritus, poor concentration, blackouts, dyspepsia, thrombosis and gout. Patients are plethoric, hypertensive, have engorged retinal veins and hepatosplenomegaly.

Investigations • FBC: Hb >18 g/dl in males and 16 g/dl in females, RBC $8–12 \times 10/l$, raised PCV, WBC is usually raised, thrombocytosis in 50%, secondary iron deficiency anaemia may occur • ESR usually low • BM usually hypercellular • Isotope studies provide a measure of red cell mass, plasma volume and total blood volume. Red cell mass is increased and plasma volume normal • Whole blood viscosity raised. • Neutrophil alkaline phosphatase (NAP) score elevated • Urate often high • Serum vitamin B_{12} often raised, folate normal • Exclude secondary causes (CXR, ABG, Hb electrophoresis, IVU).

Management Repeated venesection. Iron supplements are withheld to curb erythropoiesis. Radioactive phosphorus and busulphan.

Prognosis Average survival exceeds 10 years.

MYELOID METAPLASIA AND MYELOFIBROSIS

Both are myeloproliferative disorders ($\rightarrow$ Table 10.10, p 191). Myeloid metaplasia is the appearance of marrow stem cells in abnormal sites eg liver and spleen. The BM contains increased amounts of fibrous tissue (myelofibrosis). Unknown aetiology.

Clinical features Fatigue, malaise, weight loss, heat intolerance and night sweats. Gross splenomegaly is present. Bone pain and dyspepsia are common.

Investigations • Blood film is leukoerythroblastic and characteristic 'tear-drop' poikilocytes are present • Thrombocytosis occurs • NAP score is elevated as is the serum urate level. • BM aspiration often produces a 'dry' tap due to the extensive fibrosis but the trephine biopsy is helpful.

Management Supportive with transfusions, steroids for thrombocytopenia, allopurinol for gout and folate if required. Splenectomy may be needed. Radiotherapy for bone pain or for hypersplenism. Chemotherapy is rarely useful.

Prognosis Usually progressive disease with a mean survival of 5 years. Death is usually due to acute leukaemia or marrow failure.

LYMPHOPROLIFERATIVE DISORDERS

Table 10.12
Classification of lymphoproliferative disorders

Chronic lymphatic leukaemia
Hodgkin's lymphoma
Non Hodgkin's lymphoma

CHRONIC LYMPHATIC LEUKAEMIA

CLL is a chronic lymphoproliferative disorder in which the predominant early feature is that of peripheral blood lymphocytosis though features of BM failure, generalized lymphadenopathy and splenomegaly develop in more advanced disease. An associated autoimmune haemolytic anaemia and thrombocytopenia may occur.

Table 10.13
Staging of CLL

Stage	Features
0	Peripheral blood lymphocytosis
1	Generalized lymphadenopathy
2	Splenomegaly
3	Anaemia
4	Thrombocytopenia

Management The peripheral blood count can usually be controlled using a combination of chlorambucil and prednisolone. Death usually occurs due to BM failure or intercurrent infection. Transformation to acute leukaemia does not usually occur.

HODGKIN'S LYMPHOMA

Usually arises in a group of lymph nodes and spreads to other adjacent nodes before metastasizing to non-lymphoid tissues. Uncommon before puberty but reaches a peak incidence 20–40 years and peaks again in the elderly. M>F. Unknown aetiology but viral infection may be important. The malignant cell is the Reed-Sternberg giant cell with paired mirror imaged nuclei and prominent nucleoli ('owl's eyes appearance'). A classification is given in Table 10.14.

Table 10.14
Histological classification of Hodgkin's lymphoma (Rye)

		Prognosis
Nodular sclerosing		Good
Non sclerosing:	Lymphocyte predominant	Good
	Mixed cellularity	Good
	Lymphocyte depleted	Poor

Clinical features Non-tender, rubbery discrete lymphadenopathy (commonly cervical initially) which extends to involve other nodes. The enlarged nodes compress adjacent structures producing dysphagia, dyspnoea, stridor, SVC obstruction, paraplegia, nerve root compression or jaundice. Splenomegaly may occur. Alcohol induced lymph node pain can occur. General features include intermittent pyrexia (Pel-Ebstein fever), pruritus, weight loss, night sweats and lethargy.

Investigations ● FBC: normochromic, normocytic anaemia, eosinophilia, autoimmune haemolysis, thrombocytopenia, increasing lymphocyte depletion is a poor prognostic sign ● BM involvement is uncommon initially ● Lymph node biopsy is diagnostic ● Staging includes inspection of Waldeyer's ring, CXR, liver and spleen isotope scan, CT scan of thorax and abdomen, bone scan, Gallium scan, IVU, and lymphangiogram (→ Table 10.15) ● A staging laparotomy (largely superceded by high resolution CT scanning) may be undertaken and includes splenectomy, liver biopsy and multiple node biopsies.

Differential diagnosis Infectious lymphadenopathy (TB, chronic bacterial infection, infectious mononucleosis, syphilis,

Table 10.15
Staging of Hodgkin's lymphoma (Ann-Arbor)

Stage I:	Single lymph node region/extra-lymphatic site
Stage II:	Two or more node regions on one side of the diaphragm/one node region plus one extra-lymphatic site on the same side of the diaphragm
Stage III:	Node regions on both sides of the diaphragm +/– extra-lymphatic or splenic involvement
Stage IV:	Disseminated involvement of one or more extra-lymphatic tissues

Each stage can be divided into separate categories (A or B) according to the presence or absence of systemic symptoms. The poorer 'B' group have: weight loss >10% in 6 months, fever >38°C, night sweats. Pruritus does not merit a 'B' category.

HIV infection), leukaemia, Non-Hodgkin's lymphoma, sarcoidosis, connective tissue diseases and secondary malignancy.

Management Depends on the stage of the disease.

Radiotherapy: stages I–IIIA, using a 'mantle' field supra-diaphragmatically and an 'inverted Y' field subdiaphragmatically.

Chemotherapy: stages IIIB–IV and cases relapsing after radiotherapy. Combinations of mustine, vincristine, procarbazine and prednisolone (MOPP) are used monthly and achieve remission in 80%. Adverse reactions are common: vomiting, alopecia, lethargy, marrow suppression with haemorrhage, anaemia and increased susceptibility to infection, peripheral neuropathy and constipation.

Prognosis Good prognostic factors: category A disease, nodular sclerosing and lymphocyte predominant histologies and normal Hb level. 5-year survival for stage IA exceeds 90% but for stage IIIB is 50%.

NON HODGKIN'S LYMPHOMA

Malignant proliferation of lymphoid cells (usually B cells). M>F, pre-adolescent peak followed by a nadir in incidence with a gradual rise thereafter. Unknown aetiology but certain predisposing factors may exist (→ Table 10.16, p 196).

Table 10.16
Possible predisposing factors to NHL

Viruses: Epstein-Barr
Radiation
Chemicals
Immunodeficiency: post transplant, SLE, HIV injection
                   primary immunodeficiency states
Chromosomal abnormalities: translocation of Ch. 8

Many different classification systems exist but the most important distinction is whether or not the nodular (follicular) structure of the lymph node is preserved. The nodular forms have a better prognosis than the more aggressive diffuse forms ($\rightarrow$ Table 10.17).

Table 10.17
Classification of NHL

		Prognosis
Low grade:	small lymphocytic	Good
	follicular types	Good
Intermediate grade:	diffuse types	Poor
High grade:	large cell	Poor
	lymphoblastic	Poor
Miscellaneous:	mycosis fungoides	Poor
	Burkitt's lymphoma	Good

Clinical features Painless lymphadenopathy, lassitude, weight loss, fever, sweating and anorexia. Spread occurs both via lymphatic channels and the blood stream thus the disease may be widely disseminated at the time of diagnosis. Hepatosplenomegaly may occur.

Investigations ● Lymph node biopsy is essential ● FBC shows anaemia, neutropenia and thrombocytopenia secondary to marrow involvement or hypersplenism ● Autoimmune haemolytic anaemia may be present ● Hypoalbuminaemia and hypergammaglobulinaemia are common ● BM aspiration and trephine to define marrow involvement ● Cell membrane receptor studies help to classify the disease ● Staging investigations as for Hodgkin's lymphoma can be performed but most patients are in stages III or IV at diagnosis ● HIV serology.

Management Depends on the grade of the disease. Low grade may be simply observed unless symptomatic as treatment at an early stage probably has little effect on survival. Intermediate or high-grade disease should be treated immediately as they are rapidly fatal. Combination chemotherapy is employed eg cyclophosphamide, doxorubicin, vincristine, bleomycin and prednisolone in pulses but the disease is often difficult to control. Radiotherapy can also be used and often produces good local control.

Prognosis Mean survival of follicular forms is about eight years but the diffuse forms only have a mean survival of two years.

MULTIPLE MYELOMA

A disease characterized by neoplastic B lymphocyte proliferation within the BM. The predominant cell type is the plasma cell and monoclonal immunoglobulins are secreted with an associated immunoparesis. In some cases only the light chains are produced and appear in the urine as Bence Jones proteins. IgG paraprotein is produced in >50%, IgA and Bence Jones in 20% each and IgD, IgE and IgM in the remainder. M>F, peak incidence between 60–70 years. There is usually progressive replacement of the BM by abnormal plasma cells. Rarely a solitary plasmacytoma may occur in either soft tissue or bone.

Clinical features Bone involvement: pain due to osteoporosis, erosion and stress fractures, nerve root compression. Hypercalcaemia leads to thirst, polyuria, constipation, abdominal pain and confusion. Haemopoietic dysfunction produces anaemia, leucopenia (increased infection rate) and thrombocytopenia (bleeding). Hyperviscosity causes lethargy, dizziness, headaches, gangrene, fundal haemorrhages. Renal failure may occur.

Investigation • Elevated ESR with rouleaux formation (→ Table 10.18, p 198) • BM shows a plasmacytosis >10% • Skeletal radiographs show osteoporosis, crush fractures and lytic lesions ('pepper-pot' skull) • Hypoalbuminaemia and hypergammaglobulinaemia are present • Plasma protein electrophoresis shows a monoclonal band (usually >10 g/l) • Bence Jones protein may be present • Urea, creatinine clearance, calcium, phosphate, alkaline phosphatase and urate • The combination of BM plasmacytosis, monoclonal band of plasma electrophoresis and lytic lesions on X-ray are diagnostic of myeloma • Occasionally plasma cells spill over into the peripheral blood producing plasma cell leukaemia.

Management Radiotherapy for skeletal problems. Chemotherapy (melphalan alone or in combination with cyclo-

phosphamide, vincristine and prednisolone). Hypercalcaemia is treated with rehydration, frusemide, corticosteroids
and disodium etidronate or mithramycin ($\rightarrow$ p 304). Plasmaphoresis for hyperviscosity. RBC transfusion if needed.
Solitary plasmacytomas can be treated by surgery or irra-
diation.

Table 10.18
Causes of abnormal ESR

Increased	
	Pregnancy
	Elderly
	Infection
	Multiple myeloma
	Collagen diseases
	Malignancy
	Cold agglutinin disease
	Injury
	Anaemia
Decreased	
	Polycythaemia
	Reduced plasma volume
	Newborn
	Sickle cell disease
	Clotted blood
	Cryoglobulinaemia

Prognosis   Mean survival is about two years and may be due
to AML. Poor prognostic factors are urea >10 mmol/l, Hb <7.5
g/dl and reduced activity.

WALDENSTRÖM'S MACROGLOBULINAEMIA

Rare B cell malignancy with monoclonal IgM production
and hyperviscosity. M>F, usually in the elderly.

Clinical features   Lethargy, haemorrhage, headaches, dizziness,
vertigo, confusion, increased susceptibility to infection,
Raynaud's phenomenon, thromboses, weight loss, lymphadenopathy and cardiac failure.

Investigations • FBC: normocytic anaemia, normal WBC
and platelet counts • elevated ESR • BM shows infiltration
with lymphocytes and plasma cells • IgM monoclonal band on
protein electrophoresis.

Management Plasmaphoresis, chlorambucil, cyclophosphamide and corticosteroids.

Prognosis Mean survival is five years.

AMYLOIDOSIS

Group of disorders characterized by tissue infiltration by
eosinophilic material which demonstrates emerald green
birefringence with Congo red stain. The classification is
given in Table 10.19.

**Table 10.19
Classification of amyloidosis**

Type	Associated disease	Nature of deposit
Immunocytic:	myeloma, Waldenström's	AL amyloid fibrils similar to monoclonal light chains
Reactive systemic	RA infections, hypernephroma, lymphoma	AA amyloid fibrils, formed from serum precursor SAA (induced by interleukin 1)
Hereditary:	familial Mediterranean fever, other familial types	AA amyloid fibrils AF amyloid fibrils (similar to prealbumin)
Senile	Senile cardiac amyloid	As amyloid fibrils
Endocrine tumours:	MEN II	Hormones eg calcitonin (AEmct fibril)

Clinical features Protean depending on the tissue involved
eg peripheral neuropathy, carpal tunnel syndrome, macroglos-
sia, malabsorption, arthropathy, cardiomyopathy, haemorrhage,
nephrotic syndrome, hepatosplenomegaly and confusion.

Investigations ● Tissue biopsy (usually rectum, kidney or
liver) ● monoclonal gammopathy ● search for underlying condition.

Management Supportive eg cardiac or renal failure and
treat the underlying condition. Colchicine in familial
Mediterranean fever.

BLEEDING DISORDERS

Normal haemostasis involves a complex series of steps including spasm of small vessels in response to injury, formation of platelet plugs on the damaged endothelial surface and finally the triggering of the coagulation cascade mechanism ($\rightarrow$ p 202) to arrest the haemorrhage. There are thus many ways in which haemostasis can be adversely affected with resultant haemorrhage. The site of bleeding varies with different abnormalities.

Cutaneous/mucosal bleeding: vessel/platelet disorder.

Skin ecchymoses/haemarthroses: coagulation disorder. The classification is given in Table 10.20.

Table 10.20
Classification of bleeding disorders

Blood vessel defect:	vascular purpuras
	– drugs: aspirin, NSAID, frusemide
	– infections: meningococcus, typhoid, SBE
	– anaphylactoid: Henoch-Schönlein
	– metabolic: uraemia, liver failure
	– scurvy
	hereditary haemorrhagic telangectasia
Platelet defect:	thrombocytopenia
	– idiopathic, secondary
	thrombocythaemia
	thrombobasthaenia
Coagulation cascade defect:	hereditary
	– haemophilia A, haemophilia B, von Willebrand's disease
	acquired
	– oral anticoagulants, liver disease, vitamin K deficiency, malabsorption, DIC

General Investigation ● FBC, blood film, bone marrow and trephine, template bleeding time (2–7 min) ● platelet studies (count, adhesion and aggregation) ● coagulation studies: extrinsic system and intrinsic system ($\rightarrow$ p 202) ● Assay of specific coagulation factors (eg VIII). Fibrinogen level and FDPs are measured if DIC is suspected. Inhibitors of haemostasis (antithrombin III) can also be estimated.

THROMBOCYTOPENIA

Thrombocytopaenia can occur for a number of different reasons (→ Table 10.21).

Table 10.21
Causes of thrombocytopenia

Decreased marrow production:	Fanconi's syndrome, marrow infiltration, lymphoproliferative disorders, alcoholism, uraemia, viral infection
Decreased platelet survival:	ITP, SLE, drugs – thiazides, NSAID, rifampicin, sulphonamides; post incompatible transfusion
Increased platelet consumption:	DIC, haemolytic uraemic syndrome, drugs – heparin; infections – meningococcus, SBE
Platelet sequestration:	hypothermia, hypersplenism
Platelet loss:	massive haemorrhage

Idiopathic thrombocytopenic purpura

This follows a viral infection and is characterized by a severe reduction in the number of circulating platelets. Probably due to IgG antibody attack. Acute form M=F, peak incidence in childhood. Chronic form F>M: 3:1, usually occurs in adults. The normal platelet count is $150–350 \times 10^9/l$, if the count falls below $50 \times 10^9/l$ the patient will have a bleeding diathesis and if the count falls below $20 \times 10^9/l$ there is a high risk of spontaneous intracranial haemorrhage.

Clinical features Skin bleeding (purpura, ecchymoses), epistaxis, GI and intracranial bleeding and haematuria. Headache and dizziness. The spleen is often enlarged but not usually palpable.

Investigations ● BM; thrombocytopenia with normal or increased numbers of megakaryocytes ● Normal Hb and WBC levels ● Platelet antibodies can be demonstrated.

Management Usually self limiting in childhood and seldom needs active treatment. In adults prednisolone 60 mg/day initially. Splenectomy may be needed. Post-splenec-

COAGULATION CASCADE

Consolidation of the platelet plug is achieved through the formation of cross-linked fibrin polymers ($\rightarrow$ Fig. 10.1). The coagulation protein precursors (zymogens) are converted into active proteases by the action of their predecessors in the cascade system. This produces rapid amplification of the clotting process producing a stable fibrin mesh. The system is held in check by inhibitory factors which neutralize the activated factors rapidly (eg antithrombin III, C_1 esterase inhibitor, proteins C and S and α_1-antitrypsin). The fibrin polymer is destroyed by the fibrinolytic system ($\rightarrow$ Fig. 10.2).

The extrinsic system requires tissue thromboplastin for activa-

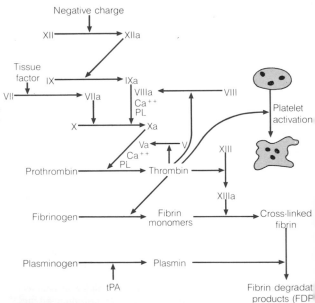

Fig. 10.1
Coagulation cascade.

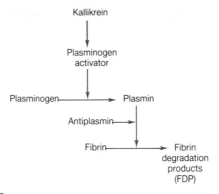

Fig. 10.2
Fibrinolytic system.

tion which is released by damaged tissues. The extrinsic and common pathways are reflected in the INR and are affected by warfarin (decreases hepatic synthesis of factors II, VII, IX and X). The intrinsic system requires factor XII activation through contact with subendothelial tissues or enzymes such as kallikrein. The intrinsic and common pathways are reflected in the Partial thromboplastin time with kaolin (PTTK). Heparin acts by augmenting the effect of antithrombin III and control is best measured by PTTK or Activated partial thromboplastin time (APPT). Warfarin overdosage can be reversed in the short term by FFP. IV vitamin K will reverse the bleeding diathesis within 24–48 hours but makes the patient refractory to further warfarinization for 1–2 weeks. Heparin overdosage can be reversed by protamine.

HAEMOPHILIAS

The haemophilias are a group of genetic disorders giving rise to deficiency of one of the coagulation pathway factors.

Haemophilia A
X-linked recessive disorder affecting males and carried by females and characterized by a deficiency of one subunit of factor VIII (factor VIII C). Factor VIII RAG and factor VIII RiCoF levels are normal. If >5% of the factor is present the disease is mild, 1–5% moderate and <1% severe. Occasionally no genetic link can be established and the disease is then thought to arise by mutation.

Clinical features Excessive bruising and haemarthroses from the time of crawling. Pain, swelling, heat and eventually deformity occur in the affected joints. Bleeding into muscles often occurs. Intra-abdominal, retroperitoneal and intracranial bleeding may all occur. Hepatitis B, and C and HIV infection can complicate this disease following transfusion of blood products.

Investigations ● Clinical history ● factor VIII assay.

Management Early treatment eg at home is vital. Factor VIII levels can be elevated by the administration of cryoprecipitate or freeze dried factor VIII concentrate. Repeated administration is needed as the half life of factor VIII is only 8 hours. Oral antifibrinolytics eg tranexamic acid or desmopressin can reduce the need for factor VIII administration. Factor VIII inhibitors can develop and large doses of factor VIII or plasmaphoresis may be needed to overcome them. Early mobilization helps prevent contractures. Antenatal diagnosis is now possible.

Haemophilia B: Christmas disease

X-linked deficiency of factor IX. Ten times less common than haemophilia A. Clinical features are identical to haemophilia A. Treatment is by factor IX replacement (contained in FFP).

Von Willebrand's disease

Autosomal dominant inheritance, M=F. Variable deficiency of both factor VIII RAG and factor VIII RiCoF subunits with relatively normal factor VIII C level. Factor VIII RAG is important for the normal adherance of platelets to endothelium thus this disease is characterized by an abnormally long bleeding time.

Clinical features Skin/mucous membrane bleeding eg after tooth extraction. Haemarthroses are uncommon.

Investigations ● Family history ● prolonged bleeding time ● normal platelet count but abnormal function (● poor aggregation by ristocetin and impaired adherance to glass beads) ● reduced factor VIII RAG and factor VIII RiCoF assay levels.

Management FFP, cryoprecipitate, factor VIII concentrate or DDAVP.

DISSEMINATED INTRAVASCULAR COAGULATION

The process in which coagulation and fibrinolysis occur simultaneously in the circulation.

Aetiology ($\rightarrow$ Table 10.22).

Table 10.22
Causes of DIC

Bacterial toxins	Septicaemia – meningococcal, Gram negative
Parasitaemia	Malaria
Viral infection	Yellow fever
Acute pancreatitis	
Shock	Hypovolaemic, anaphylactic, burns
Major surgery	
Heart-lung bypass	
Incompatible blood transfusion	
Pulmonary embolism	
Fat embolism	
Obstetric	Amniotic embolism, placental abruption intrauterine death, eclampsia
Malignancy	Leukaemia, hepatoma, renal, breast, lung, GI tract, prostate
Diabetic ketoacidosis	
Aortic aneurysm	
Snake venom	
Vasculitis	

Clinical features Extensive bruising, oozing from venepuncture sites, mucosal bleeding. Patient is usually gravely ill (hypotensive, hypoxaemic, pyrexial, confused).

Investigations ● Thrombocytopenia ● red cell fragmentation on blood film ● prolongation of PTR, PTTK and thrombin time ● reduced fibrinogen level ● raised FDPs.

Management Identify and treat the underlying cause, supportive measures eg oxygen, antibiotics, fluid expansion. Replace coagulation factors to stem haemorrhage (fresh blood, cryoprecipitate, platelets). Heparin can be used to try to 'switch off' coagulation. Rarely antifibrinolytic agents eg tranexamic acid are employed.

BLOOD PRODUCTS AND THEIR USAGE

450 ml of blood is usually collected from donors at each donation. The collection pack consists of two or three separate bags so that fractionization can be undertaken with minimal external interference thus reducing the risk of introducing infection (Fig. 10.3, p 206).

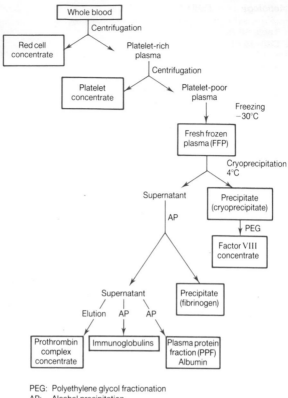

Fig. 10.3
Blood fractionation

PEG: Polyethylene glycol fractionation
AP: Alcohol precipitation

☐ : Available blood products

AVAILABLE BLOOD PRODUCTS

Whole blood

Only occasionally used for the rapid restoration of red cells following massive haemorrhage. The viability of whole blood declines rapidly with storage: after 4–5 days the platelet and coagulation factor components have deteriorated.

Red cell concentrate

The preparation of choice for the management of active bleeding and for the elective correction of chronic anaemia. A single unit of RCC contains approximately 300 ml of fluid with a haematocrit of 70%. The red cells are stored in an optimal additive solution to release the plasma for other uses.

Platelet concentrate

Prepared by centrifugation of platelet-rich plasma. Each unit contains approximately 50×10^9 platelets, 5 units are usually given at each transfusion. Some individuals develop antibodies to platelet derived HLA antigens, and should be provided with single donor platelets.

White cell concentrate

Only used rarely as it is difficult to give sufficient quantities of leucocytes to combat infection (t1/2 is only 8 hours). Neutrophils express HLA and leucocyte specific antigens very strongly and development of antibodies with non-haemolytic transfusion reactions are very common. Most patients with sepsis and leucopenia respond to broad spectrum antibiotics.

Plasma products

Do not contain cells and do not require cross-matching but blood grouping is required.

Fresh frozen plasma: platelet poor plasma can be stored at $-30°C$ with a shelf-life of 3–6 months. FFP contains all the components of normal plasma and is particularly useful in situations where replacement of several factors is required as in DIC, massive red cell transfusion or replacement of coagulation factor deficiencies due to liver failure or warfarin overdosage.

Cryoprecipitate: prepared from FFP by allowing it to thaw slowly at $+4°C$. A precipitate is formed which is rich in factor VIII, VWF, fibrinogen and factor XII. The precipitate can be refrozen and stored for 3–6 months.

Factor VIII concentrates: prepared by further fractionation of cryoprecipitate and is specifically indicated for haemophilia A. Plasma from a large number of donors is pooled in the preparation and in the past suboptimal sterilization techniques have lead to a high viral infection rate in haemophiliacs, especially with hepatitis B and C and HIV. Current sterilization techniques involve heat treatment of the lyophilized product.

Prothrombin complex concentrate: contains factors II, VII, IX and X and is indicated in haemophilia B.

Human immunoglobulin: non specific immunoglobulin is used in congenital and acquired immunodeficiencies and in the treatment of severe ITP. Specific immunoglobulins are used after exposure to certain serious viral infections by a non-immune patient eg hepatitis B, rubella (in pregnant women), herpes zoster, rabies, tetanus and measles (in the immunosuppressed).

Albumin containing solutions: a number of products are available with various degrees of albumin purity eg PPS, human albumin solution. These are useful in two clinical situations – as plasma expanders in a patient with acute haemorrhage whilst awaiting blood and to maintain plasma albumin levels in patients with severe malnutrition or a protein losing state. Salt poor albumin is expensive and usually only used in liver failure.

BLOOD TRANSFUSION

There are many potential hazards present whenever any blood product is transfused. Unfortunately all of these donated products have the potential to contain unwanted infectious material eg HIV virus, hepatitis B and C despite extensive screening precautions and they must thus be used wisely. The complications are listed in Table 10.23.

Table 10.23
Complications of blood transfusion

Incompatible blood transfusion	
Circulatory overload	
Febrile reactions	Allergy due to sensitisation by previous transfusions
Infections	Hepatitis B and C, CMV, HIV, infectious mononucleousis, syphilis
Potassium/citrate toxicity	
Thrombophlebitis	
Transfusion siderosis	
Massive transfusion	DIC, acidosis, hyperkalaemia, thrombocytopenia

INCOMPATIBLE BLOOD TRANSFUSION

May be due to: clerical errors, careless ABO blood typing or incompatible subgroup typing eg rhesus. Always administer blood transfusions slowly and monitor pulse rate, BP, urinary output and temperature closely.

Clinical features Begin within minutes of the transfusion beginning. Restlessness, rigors, urticarial rash, bronchospasm, itching, nausea, vomiting, chest pain, loin pain, hypotension, poor peripheral circulation, pyrexia, jaundice and oliguric renal failure in severe cases.

Investigations ● Double check the identity of the patient, blood group of the patient and the donor ● FBC, haemolysis screen, full clotting screen.

> **Management** Stop the transfusion immediately and return the blood product to BTS. IV hydrocortisone 100–200 mg and iv chlorpheniramine 10 mg. Mannitol may be needed to induce a diuresis. ARF and shock are dealt with in the standard fashion.

TISSUE TYPING

RBC membranes contain a number of surface antigens including ABO, rhesus, Lewis, P and Ii which are autosomally inherited. The function of these antigens is unknown but they may help to maintain the integrity of the membranes. Red cell antibodies are present in the serum and are produced in response to stimulation by the appropriate antigen on the RBC membrane but may also be present in bacteria and in certain foodstuffs. For prevalence of various blood groups (→ Table 10.24). Blood group O are universal donors and AB universal recipients.

Table 10.24
Occurrence of ABO blood groups and serum antibodies in the UK

Blood group	Serum antibody	UK frequency (%)
A	Anti-B	42
B	Anti-A	8
AB	None	3
O	Anti-A/anti-B	47

Approximately 85% of the European population contain the D antigen on the RBC surface and are known as rhesus (Rh) positive.

HLA SYSTEM

Human leucocyte antigens are important in producing the immune response which rejects foreign tissues including tissue allografts. They are genetically determined and coded for by an area on chromosome 6 known as the MHC. HLAs are found on cells in most tissues and can be divided into types: HLA-A, HLA-B, HLA-C, HLA-D, HLA-DR and HLA-DW. Certain genotypes are associated with disease (→ Table 10.25, p 210).

Table 10.25
Association of HLA and disease

Rheumatoid arthritis	: DR4
Addison's disease	: B8, DW3
Seronegative arthritis	: B27
Thyrotoxicosis	: B8, DR3
IDDM	: B8, B15, DR3, DR4
Myasthenia gravis	: B8
Haemochromatosis	: A3, B14
Multiple sclerosis	: DRW2
Coeliac disease	: B8

HLA tissue typing is performed before organ transplantation (except liver) as matched tissue has the best chance of survival.

11

Rheumatology

RHEUMATOID ARTHRITIS

> A chronic inflammatory, destructive and deforming poly-
> arthritis associated with systemic disturbance, many extra-
> articular lesions and the presence of circulating antiglob-
> ulin antibodies (rheumatoid factors).

Aetiology and pathogenesis Unknown aetiology, adult prevalence approximately 3%, commonly commences in early adult
life and associated with a significant increase in HLA-D4 and
HLA-DR4. There is also an increase in urban dwellers sug-
gesting that environmental factors may be important. F>M:3:1.
Evidence points to persistent immune overactivity, autoimmu-
nity and the presence of immune complexes at sites of articular
and extra-articular lesions. Circulating IgG, IgM and IgA
antiglobulins (rheumatoid factors) are produced in response to
some unknown antigen and the immune system is triggered
with resulting inflammation and tissue destruction. The joint
synovial membrane becomes swollen and congested with lymphocytes, neutrophils, plasma cells and macrophages. It has
the histological appearance of granulation tissue and is known
as 'pannus'. This pannus destroys the articular cartilage and
subchondral bone producing bony erosions. Fibrosis and bony
ankylosis are produced, joint effusions occur and adjacent
muscles atrophy. Subcutaneous nodules contain fragmented
collagen fibres, cellular debris and exudate and are surrounded
by pallisades of mononuclear cells. There is no evidence as yet
to suggest that any one particular bacteria or virus is the
triggering antigen.

Disease remission often occurs during pregnancy and relapse
may occur following the menopause.

Clinical features Insidious onset of symmetrical joint pain,
stiffness and swelling which is most marked in the mornings
and usually affects the hands, feet and wrists first. Swelling of
the proximal (PIP), but not the distal, (DIP) interphalangeal
joints gives the fingers a 'spindled' appearance and swelling of
the metatarsophalangeal joints (MTP) produces 'broadening'
of the forefoot. As the disease progresses other joints become
involved including the elbows, shoulders, knees, ankles, tarsal
joints, cervical spine and temperomandibular joints. The hips
are usually spared. Systemic features including fever, malaise,
night sweats and weight loss may also be present. Popliteal
cysts (Baker's cysts) may be produced and mimic DVT. Joint
destruction occurs causing increasing joint instability, subluxation, ankylosis and decreasing mobility.

Characteristic deformities are produced and include ulnar
deviation of the fingers due to subluxation at the metacarpo-
phalangeal joints, loss of finger function due to hyperextension
of the PIP joints with fixed flexion of the DIP joints 'swan

necking' or fixed flexion of the PIP joints with hyperextension of the DIP joints 'boutonnaire' or Z deformity of the thumb. Rupture of the extensor tendons of the hand can occur secondary to either tenosynovitis or stretching over a prominent ulnar styloid process. Foot involvement leads to clawing of the toes and a painful sensation of 'walking on pebbles' due to exposure of the metatarsal heads. Severe cervical pain may be present and the potentially fatal complication of atlantoaxial subluxation may occur. For other manifestations (→ Table 11.1).

Table 11.1
Extra-articular manifestations of RA

Anorexia
Weight loss
Malaise
Lethargy
Myalgia

Rheumatoid	*nodules* over bony prominences eg elbows, occiput, scapulae, Achilles tendon, flexor tendons of the fingers (cause 'triggering')
Vasculitic lesions	eg nail bed or finger pulp infarcts, skin necrosis, pyoderma gangrenosum
Raynaud's phenomenon	
Lymphadenopathy	
Osteoporosis	
Eye signs	eg keratoconjunctivitis sicca, episcleritis, scleromalacia, nodular scleritis, scleromalacia perforans
Cardiac	eg pericarditis, myocarditis, conduction defects, endocarditis, aortic regurgitation, cardiomyopathy
Pulmonary	eg pleural effusions, interstitial fibrosis, pneumothorax, bronchitis, nodules, pleurisy, stridor due to cricoarytenoid arthritis, obliterative bronchiolitis, pulmonary vasculitis, rheumatoid pneumoconiosis (Caplan's)
Neurological	eg mononeuritis multiplex, entrapment neuropathy, distal sensory neuropathy cervical myelopathy
Haematological	eg anaemia – normochromic, normocytic, iron deficiency due to GI blood loss or defective utilisation, Coomb's +ve haemolytic, Felty's syndrome, macrocytic (folate deficiency), hyperviscosity, thrombocytosis
Renal	eg proteinuria, amyloid, glomerulonephritis
Tenosynovitis	
Bursitis	

Investigations ● FBC, ESR ● C-reactive protein, low albumin level, hypergammaglobulinaemia, increased fibrinogen level, circulating complement levels are usually normal (synovial fluid levels low) urinalysis for protein ● arthroscopy and synovial biopsy ● rheumatoid factor titre eg Rose Waaler for protein. Rheumatoid factor may however be negative during the early stages of the disease and indeed may remain negative in up to 30% cases. False positive values also occur (→ Table 11.2). Radiological features are listed in Table 11.3.

**Table 11.2
Causes of a false positive rheumatoid factor**

Scleroderma
SLE
SBE
Chronic active hepatitis
TB
Leprosy
Syphilis
Sarcoidosis
Paraproteinaemia eg multiple myeloma
Sjogren's syndrome
Mixed connective tissue disease
Chronic juvenile arthritis
Malaria

**Table 11.3
Radiological features of RA**

Early:	soft tissue swelling
	periarticular osteoporosis
	periostitis
	erosions – periarticular
	subarticular cysts
Late:	narrowed joint spaces
	articular surface irregularity
	osteoporosis
	subluxation
	ankylosis
	secondary osteoarthritis

Differential diagnosis Gout, SLE, polyarteritis nodosa, rheumatic fever, dermatomyositis, mixed connective tissue disease, infective arthritis eg TB, bacterial or viral, Reiter's syndrome, hypertrophic osteoarthropathy, sarcoidosis, osteoarthritis, psoriatic arthropathy, arthritis due to inflammatory bowel disease, polymyalgia rheumatica, seronegative arthritides.

Management Bed-rest, joint splinting, physiotherapy, occupational therapy, NSAID eg aspirin, mefenamic acid, flurbiprofen, diclofenac, indomethacin or naproxen +/– simple analgesic eg paracetamol or coproxamol. All NSAID may cause GI bleeding and skin rashes. Intra-articular injections of corticosteroids eg methylprednisolone acetate or triamcinolone may be extremely useful on a limited basis. Rarely systemic corticosteroids may be needed. Some drugs may have a disease modifying role and actually slow down disease progression (such drugs include gold, penicillamine, sulphasalazine and chloroquine derivatives but they all have potentially serious adverse reactions (→ Table 11.4). Immunosuppressive agents can also be used both as 'disease modifying' agents and also in a steroid sparing capacity but they are reserved for very severe cases eg cyclophosphamide, azathioprine and chlorambucil. Surgical intervention may also be needed eg arthroplasty, arthrodesis, synovectomy, tendon transplants, cervical spine stabilization and spinal-cord decompression.

Table 11.4
Adverse reactions of disease modifying rheumatoid drugs

Penicillamine	Rashes, loss of taste, fever, nausea vomiting, glomerulonephritis, Goodpasture's syndrome, SLE-like syndrome, myasthenic syndrome, thrombocytopenia, pancytopenia, mouth ulcers
Gold	Mouth ulcers, nephrotic syndrome, pruritic rash, entercolitis, aplastic anaemia, glomerulonephritis
Sulphasalazine	Bone marrow suppression, rashes, nausea
Chloroquine	Diarrhoea, ocular toxicity – reversible corneal deposits on drug withdrawal, permanent retinopathy, haemolytic anaemia

Prognosis Most patients follow a chronic course with remissions and relapses. After 10 years 25% will have complete remission, 40% moderate impairment, 25% severe impairment and 10% will be crippled by their disease. Poor prognostic factors include progressive disease without periods of remission, high titres of rheumatoid factor, rheumatoid nodules, and the development of extra-articular manifestations.

SERONEGATIVE SPONDARTHRITIDES

A group of conditions characterized by inflammatory asymmetrical oligoarthritis, sacroiliitis, anterior uveitis, high incidence of HLA-B27 but negative rheumatoid factor tests.

Types:
- Ankylosing spondylitis
- Psoriatic arthritis
- Bechet's syndrome
- Reiter's syndrome
- Reactive arthritis
- Whipple's disease
- Enteropathic arthritis
- Juvenile chronic arthritis.

ANKYLOSING SPONDYLITIS

A disease of young men M>F 9:1, teenage peak age of onset. Unknown aetiology but strong link with HLA-B27.

Clinical features Initially low back pain, especially in the mornings, bilateral sacroiliitis, progressing to thoracic backache, pleuritic chest pain, rigid spine with increasing kyphosis. Failure to obliterate lumbar lordosis on forward flexion. Achilles tendinitis and pain over iliac crest. Anterior uveitis, aortic regurgitation, apical pulmonary fibrosis, osteoporosis, myopathy, amyloidosis, atlanto-axial subluxation.

Investigations • FBC (leucocytosis), high ESR • C-reactive protein, hypergammaglobulinaemia • negative rheumatoid factor • HLA-B27 • radiology (sacroiliitis, 'bamboo spine', erosions, sclerosis and ankylosis)

Management Maintain mobility, physiotherapy, hydrotherapy, NSAID, rarely radiotherapy or surgery.

PSORIATIC ARTHRITIS

This affects 7% psoriatic sufferers. Various types exist: DIP joint involvement with nail changes, seronegative RA, arthritis mutilans with digit destruction, ankylosing spondylitis and asymmetrical disease affecting the hands and feet.

Clinical features Think of the diagnosis when psoriasis coexists with arthritis. Nail pitting common in DIP joint disease.

Investigations ● As for ankylosing spondylitis ● Radiology shows asymmetrical disease, DIP joint involvement and little peri-articular osteoporosis.

Management NSAID, gold in severe disease but avoid chloroquine derivatives. Sulphasalazine may be useful.

BECHET'S SYNDROME

An association of arthritis, iritis and recurrent oral and genital ulceration. Commoner in Eastern Mediterranean and Japan. M>F. Associated with HLA-B5. Unknown aetiology.

Clinical features As above. Vasculitis eg erythema nodosum, thrombophlebitis, synovitis, meningitis, encephalitis, pericarditis, and sacroiliitis may also be present.

Investigations As for ankylosing spondylitis.

Diagnosis Usually clinical.

Management Symptomatic to oral and genital ulcers eg local anaesthetic cream, NSAID, systemic corticosteroids and immunosuppressives for severe disease especially if the eyes are involved. Azathioprine and cyclosporin may have a role in the future.

REITER'S SYNDROME

A triad of conjunctivitis, urethritis and seronegative lower limb oligo-arthritis. Two forms exist.

The genital form: occurs after genital infection.

The intestinal type: follows enteric infection with *Shigella, Salmonella, Yersinia* or *Campylobacter* in genetically predisposed individuals. M>F 20:1 (but urethritis is often asymptomatic in females).

Clinical features As above, usually affects the knees 1–4 weeks after exposure, may be recurrent although the urethritis may not always be recurrent. Backache, heel pain (due to calcaneal spur enthesopathy), tender fingers. Skin lesions are common eg circinate balanitis, keratoderma blenorrhagica, macules, papules, pustules, nail dystrophy and scales. Rarely pleurisy and pericarditis.

Investigations As for anklosing spondylitis, the diagnosis is suggested by the classical presentation.

REACTIVE ARTHRITIS

This is similar to Reiter's disease but follows enteric infection.

WHIPPLE'S DISEASE (intestinal lipodystrophy)

A rare disease, M>F, unknown aetiology.

Clinical features Malabsorption, weight loss, lymphadenopathy, abdominal pain, migratory polyarthritis (usually knee or ankle), sacroiliitis, pyrexia and increased skin pigmentation.

Investigations ● Negative rheumatoid factor ● small intestinal biopsy shows PAS positive staining macrophages.

> **Management** NSAID, tetracycline 1 g daily for at least a year.

ENTEROPATHIC ARTHRITIS

This is the association of a seronegative arthritis with either infection or inflammatory bowel disease eg ulcerative colitis or Crohn's disease or with intestinal bypass operations performed for obesity.

Clinical features Acute and often migratory oligo-arthritis of weight bearing joints or sacroiliitis which classically follows exacerbations of bowel disease. Aphthous ulceration, erythema nodosum or uveitis may be present.

Investigations As for ankylosing spondylitis ● bowel investigations as indicated eg barium studies, endoscopy.

> **Management** NSAID, physiotherapy, treat the underlying bowel disease eg corticosteroids or sulphasalazine.

JUVENILE CHRONIC ARTHRITIS

Disease onset before 16 years. Various types: Still's disease (systemic juvenile chronic arthritis), polyaricular juvenile chronic arthritis, seropositive polyarticular disease and pauci-articular juvenile chronic arthritis.

Clinical features   These depend on the type but may include fever, malaise, lymphadenopathy, myalgia, arthralgia, pleurisy, pericarditis, weight loss, growth retardation and polyarthritis which may affect large or small joints and the spine. The eyes may be affected.

Investigations   As for any seronegative arthritis.

Management   Bed-rest during acute exacerbations, continue education, physiotherapy, hydrotherapy, NSAID, try to avoid corticosteroids because of growth retardation secondary to adrenal suppression. Intra-articular corticosteroids may be useful. Disease modifying drugs eg gold, penicillamine or chloroquine derivatives can be used as long as the patient is closely monitored for possible adverse reactions. Surgery may be needed in severe cases.

OSTEOARTHROSIS

A disorder which is the end result of a variety of conditions which produce joint destruction. It is characterized by destruction of articular cartilage, and proliferation of new bone, cartilage and fibrous supporting tissue. Extremely common condition affecting in excess of 80% of people older than 65 years although not all of these cases are symptomatic. Primary is commoner in females. Damp environmental conditions are associated with increased symptoms.

Aetiology and pathogenesis   (→ Table 11.5, p 220) This is unknown but two main theories exist. The first considers that the initial feature is fatigue fracture of the collagen support network underlying the articular cartilage. This leads to an increased level of hydration of the cartilage with subsequent unravelling of the proteoglycans. The alternative hypothesis suggests that the initiating event in joint destruction is the development of microfractures in the subchondral bone whose healing produces increased stress on the overlying cartilage with subsequent fracture of its surface exposing the underlying bone. The joint is eventually destroyed with loss of normal function.

Clinical features   These may be asymptomatic. Pain which is usually worse on activity and eased by rest, joint swelling, stiffness, limitation of movement and muscle wasting. Crepitus may be elicited. Deformity due to articular cartilage damage

Table 11.5
Aetiology of osteoarthrosis

Primary	Unknown cause	
Secondary	Traumatic:	malaligned fractures excessive wear and tear
	Metabolic:	haemochromatosis, chondrocalcinosis,
	Endrocrine:	acromegaly, hypothyroidism
	Inflammatory:	gout, alkaptonuria
	Aseptic necrosis:	corticosteroids, sickle cell disease
	Paget's disease	
	Developmental:	slipped femoral epiphysis, Perthes' disease
	Neuropathic:	Charcot's joint, diabetes mellitus
	Haemophilic arthritis	

and bony remodelling may be present. Heberden's nodes are gelatinous cysts or bony outgrowths on the dorsal aspects of the TIP of the hands and are characteristic of primary OA. Bouchard's nodes are similar but occur at the proximal interphalangeal joints. The joints which are characteristically involved are weight bearing eg hips, knees and spine, MTP joint of the great toe, TIP joints in the hands, carpometacarpal of the thumb, temporomandibular and sternoclavicular joints.

Investigations • Radiology: joint space narrowing, subchondral sclerosis, osteophytes, cysts, erosions, chondrocalcinosis • FBC and ESR are both normal • RF is negative unless the initiating condition is RA • Synovial fluid aspiration/microscopy • serum uric acid if gout is considered.

Management Symptomatic only eg rest, reduce weight, NSAID, physiotherapy, heat or US treatment. Treat the underlying condition. Surgical replacement of the affected joint may be required.

CRYSTAL DEPOSITION DISEASES

GOUT

Metabolic disorder of purine metabolism characterized by hyperuricaemia and recurring attacks of arthritis. In the later stages of the disease chronic arthritis, tophi and renal failure may develop. Commonest in middle age and may be inherited in an autosomal dominant manner in some cases. Predisposing factors are listed in Table 11.6

Table 11.6
Factors predisposing to hyperuricaemia and gout

1: Impaired excretion of uric acid (75%)
Undefined genetic defect
Drugs – low dose salicyclates, thiazides,
          alcohol, sulphonamides, pyrazinamide
Chronic renal failure
Lactic acidosis – alcohol, exercise, starvation,
                toxaemia of pregnancy
Hypothyroidism
Down's syndrome
Hyperparathyroidism
Lead poisoning
Cystinuria
Type 1 glycogen storage disease

2. Increased production of uric acid (25%)
Myeloproliferative disorders – chronic lymphatic
                      leukaemia,
                      polycythaemia vera
Psoriasis
Enzyme deficiencies – HGPRT, Glucose-6-phosphatase

Clinical features

Acute attack: classically a monoarthritis with sudden onset of severe pain in the MTP joint of the great toe. May also affect the ankle, knee, small joints of the feet and hands, wrist or elbow. Joint is hot, tender, and swollen with shiny overlying skin. Fever, nausea and mood swings may be present. Attacks last 2–10 days and resolution may be accompanied by pruritus and local desquamation. The attack can be precipitated by dietary excess, alcohol, trauma, uricosuric drugs or during initiation of allopurinol therapy.

Chronic gout: produces progressive joint destruction with deformity. Tophi may be produced in the cartilage of the ear, bursae and tendon sheaths. They are composed of monosodium urate, cholesterol, calcium and oxalate. Urate urolithiasis occurs in 10% and rarely chronic urate nephropathy with renal failure.

Differential diagnosis Septic arthritis, RA, trauma, cellulitis, bunion, chondrocalcinosis, seronegative arthritis.

Investigations ● serum urate (serum uric acid level >0.42 mmol/l in adult males or >0.36 mmol/l in adult females) is usually raised but may be normal ● aspiration and polarized light examination of synovial fluid (negative birefringence of needle shaped particles) ● radiology shows osteoporosis, 'punched out' erosions, secondary osteoarthritic changes ● leucocytosis and raised ESR during an acute attack.

Management NSAID should be used as early as possible during an acute attack eg naproxen 250 mg 6–hourly. Alternatively colchicine 1 mg stat followed by 0.5 mg 2-hourly may be used but it may be poorly tolerated due to vomiting and diarrhoea. Once the acute attack is controlled long-term prophylaxis can be undertaken using allopurinol 300–900 mg daily to reduce the serum urate level. Lower doses of allopurinol should be used in renal impairment. Allopurinol should not be started until several weeks after the last acute attack. Avoid precipitating factors eg alcoholic binges and reduce weight if obese. Uricosuric drugs can also be used as prophylaxis eg probenecid 0.5–1.0 mg bd together with colchicine 0.5 mg bd but must be avoided in renal failure, urate urolithiasis and in gross uricosuria. If urate calculi are present push fluids and alkalinize the urine to pH >6.

PYROPHOSPHATE ARTHROPATHY

Calcium pyrophosphate dihydrate crystals are deposited in cartilage (chondrocalcinosis) where they are associated with degenerative changes. Shedding of the crystals into the joint space produces acute synovitis and a clinical picture which resembles acute gout. It is associated with a number of underlying conditions eg metabolic diseases (hyperparathyroidism, hypothyroidism, haemochromatosis, Wilson's disease, oxalosis, gout. OA, dialysis and long-term steroid use). M=F incidence.

Clinical features Various forms exist.

Pseudogout: mimics an acute attack of gout.

Polyarticular attacks: multiple joint involvement with subacute attacks.

Chronic arthropathy: osteoarthritic like.

Chronic destructive arthropathy: produces a neuropathic joint.

Polymyalgic type: generalized muscle aches.

Asyptomatic form: noticed on X-ray.

Investigations ● Radiology shows linear opacification of articular cartilage ● synovial fluid examination under polarized light reveals positively birefringent crystals ● arthroscopy shows 'microtophi' on the synovial membrane ● Identify possible underlying conditions.

> **Management** NSAID, joint aspiration and injection of
> steroids, colchicine, rarely intra-articular yttrium-90.

CONNECTIVE TISSUE DISEASE

SYSTEMIC LUPUS ERYTHEMATOSUS

Systemic disease of unknown aetiology characterized by the
presence of non-organ specific autoantibodies. F>M 9:1, occasionally familial, associated with HLA-A1, B8 and DR3, and
much commoner in the Black population. May be precipitated
by a variety of drugs eg phenytoin, isoniazid, OCP, hydralazine
and penicillamine. Commonest during childbearing years and
exacerbations can occur during pregnancy and also during
menstruation. There may be a past history of spontaneous
abortion and thrombosis (antiphospholipid antibody syndrome).

Clinical features   ($\rightarrow$ Table 11.7)

Table 11.7 Clinical features of SLE	
General	Fever, malaise, lethargy
Locomotor	Arthralgia, arthritis, tenosynovitis, myalgia
Skin	'Butterfly rash'. erythematous or maculopapular rash, vasculitis, purpura, Raynaud's phenomenon, alopecia, livido reticularis, chillblains, oral ulceration
Cardiovascular	Pericarditis, myocarditis, endocarditis (Libman-Sacks), lupus anticoagulant with recurrent venous or arterial thrombosis, thrombophlebitis
Pulmonary	Pleurisy, pleural effusions, atelectasis, breathlessness due to pulmonary fibrosis, 'shrinking lung syndrome'
Renal	Nephrotic syndrome, nephritis
Nervous system	Peripheral neuropathy, transverse myelitis, hemiparesis, seizures, psychosis, meningitis, cranial nerve palsies, dementia
Gastrointestinal	Ulceration, protein-losing enteropathy, abdominal pain, pancreatitis
Haematological	Haemolytic anaemia
Ophthalmic	Cystic bodies in retina, episcleritis, soft exudates
Hepatic	Jaundice, abnormal LFTs
Lymphadenopathy	
Splenomegaly	

Investigation • FBC (normochromic normocytic anaemia, leukopenia, thrombocytopenia, haemolytic anaemia, prolongation of INR in the presence of lupus anticoagulant) • elevated ESR • C-reactive protein (usually normal in the absence of infection), cold agglutinins, hypergammaglobulinaemia, low albumin, raised fibrinogen, cryoglobulins • low serum complement, raised immune complexes • antinuclear antibodies (ANF, anti-double stranded DNA, anti-histone, anti-extractable nuclear antibodies: anti-RNP, anti-Sm, anti-SSA, anti-SSB) • false positive RF • false positive tests for syphilis (VDRL or TPHA) • Renal function tests (urea, electrolytes, creatinine clearance, 24-hour urinary protein, urinary casts or RBCs) • synovial fluid examination (absence of crystals and infection) • Radiology may show changes indistinguishable from RA • Biopsy of skin or renal tissue.

Differential diagnosis Systemic sclerosis, polyarteritis, RA or mixed connective tissue disease, SBE, infective arthritis.

Management Mild cases need rest, NSAID and removal of any precipitating causes eg drugs or sunlight. Severe cases need systemic corticosteroid therapy eg 40–60 mg prednisolone daily initially, or 'pulse' therapy using methyl-prednisolone 1 g daily for 3 days to gain control of the disease. As the disease comes under control the dose of steroids can be gradually reduced to an alternate day regime if possible. Antimalarials eg chloroquine derivatives are useful in skin and joint disease. Immunosuppressive agents (eg azathioprine) or plasmaphoresis are reserved for those cases which cannot be controlled with steroids alone. Dialysis may be needed in renal failure. Anticoagulants are used when the lupus anticoagulant is present.

Prognosis Poor prognosis is indicated by childhood onset of disease, high urea, persistent proteinuria, evidence of arteritis, CNS and cardiopulmonary involvement and requirement for long-term corticosteroids. The overall 5-year survival for this disease is now in excess of 90%.

PROGRESSIVE SYSTEMIC SCLEROSIS

Generalized connective tissue disorder characterized by fibrosis. The skin is the predominant organ to be affected but the gut, heart, lungs and kidneys may also be involved. Unknown aetiology, associated with HLA-A1, B8 and DR3 haplotypes. F>M by a ratio of 4:1, and an increased incidence is present amongst miners.

Clinical features (→ Table 11.8)

Investigations • FBC (normochromic, normocytic anaemia)

Table 11.8
Clinical features of systemic sclerosis

Skin	Severe Raynaud's phenomenon, non-pitting shiny digital oedema, 'sausage shaped' fingers, atrophy and ulceration of finger tips, subcutaneous calcinosis, loss of hair follicles and sweat glands, sclerodactyly, puckering around mouth, 'pinched' nose, telangectasia localized morphoea
Musculoskeletal	Arthralgia, myositis, non-erosive arthritis
Gastrointestinal	Reflux oesophagitis, dysphagia, bowel dilatation causing abdominal pain, diarrhoea, malabsorption
Pulmonary	Lung fibrosis, cor pulmonale, alveolar cell carcinoma
Renal	Hypertension, renal failure
Cardiac	Pericarditis, myocarditis, cardiomyopathy

● raised ESR ● positive ANF in 50% (nucleolar or speckled staining pattern), antibodies to single stranded RNA are more specific: RF may be falsely positive ● Complement levels are normal ● Radiology reveals soft tissue calcification, resorption of the tufts of the terminal phalanges, pulmonary fibrosis and barium studies may show an hiatus hernia, oesophageal stricture or dysmotility.

Differential diagnosis CREST syndrome (calcinosis, Raynaud's phenomenon, oesophageal involvement, sclerodactyly and telangectasia), morphoea, eosinophilic fasciitis, amyloid, acromegaly, myxoedema.

Management None arrests the disease. Keep the hands and feet warm, treat infections, hypertension and dysphagia. Penicillamine and colchicine may be helpful. Corticosteroids may improve pulmonary fibrosis. NSAID for joint symptoms. 5-year survival is approximately 70%.

DERMATOMYOSITIS AND POLYMYOSITIS

Inflammatory conditions of unknown aetiology affecting the skin and striated muscle. Linked with HLA-B8 and DR3. Five categories exist:

● Primary (idiopathic) polymyositis

● Primary (idiopathic) dermatomyositis

● Dermatomyositis associated with malignancy

• Dermatomyositis associated with collagen disease

• Childhood dermatomyositis.

Clinical features The adult forms typically affect middle aged females and present with difficulty rising from the seated position. Examination reveals limb girdle weakness. The pharyngeal, laryngeal and respiratory muscles may also be involved leading to dysphagia, dysphonia and respiratory failure. Arthralgia, myalgia, Raynaud's phenomenon, swelling of the fingers, purple discolouration on the face and knuckles ('heliotrope rash'), and subcutaneous calcinosis may all occur. An underlying tumour of the breast, lung, ovary, prostate, GU tract or GI tract may be present in 3% of cases of polymyositis and 15% of dermatomyositis. In children the presenting features are usually muscle weakness, calcification, contractures and the heliotrope rash.

Investigations • FBC (normochromic, normocytic anaemia, leucocytosis) • raised ESR • raised serum muscle enzymes (CPK, aldolase) • autoantibodies are often positive (ANF, RF and extractable nuclear antigen PM-1) • EMG • muscle biopsy.

Management Prednisolone 40–60 mg/day initially to produce remission, reducing slowly to a maintenance dose of 5–15 mg/day. Immunosuppressive agents eg azathioprine can be used as a steroid sparing agent. Splinting and physiotherapy are important. Treatment directed at any underlying tumour can produce some improvement in the condition.

MIXED CONNECTIVE TISSUE DISEASE

Combines the features of two or more connective tissue disorders eg SLE, scleroderma or dermatomyositis. High incidence of Raynaud's phenomenon, arthralgia, erosive arthritis, myositis, oesophageal motility problems and hypergammaglobulinaemia. Low titres against DNA but high titer against an extractable nuclear antigen (ENA – ribonuclear protein). There is characteristically a good response to steroids.

INFECTIVE ARTHRITIS

Relatively rare in normal joints except when the joint space is breached by a foreign body eg nail, splinter or rose thorn.

Aetiology (→ Tables 11.9 & 11.10)

**Table 11.9
Causes of infective arthritis**

Bacterial	Staphylococci
	Streptococci
	Gonococcal
	Syphilis
	Tuberculosis
	Meningococcai
	Enteric fever
	Brucellosis
	Leprosy
	Lyme disease
	Chlamydia
Viral	Rubella
	Mumps
	Hepatitis A, B
	CMV
	Coxsackie B
	Parvovirus
	Arbovirus
	Varicella
	HIV infection
Fungal	Histoplasmosis
	Coccidioidomycosis
	Blastomycosis
	Spirotrichosis
	Aspergillosis
	Actinomycosis

**Table 11.10
Predisposing factors to joint infection**

Septicaemic spread from infective focus elsewhere
Abscess, bronchiectasis, enteric fever
Previous joint damage OA, RA
Immunosuppression Leukaemia, lymphoma, steroids,
cytotoxics
General debility Elderly, neonates, malignancy, diabetes,
alcohol
Sickle cell disease
iv drug abuse
Operations Orthopaedic procedures eg arthroplasty
Trauma
Neuropathic joint Diabetes, syphilis

Clinical features Pyrexia, lethargy, rigors. Affected joint is painful, swollen, hot and stiff with limitation of movement. Spinal infection may present as backache. The physical signs may be extremely subtle if the patient is immunosuppressed.

Investigations ● Multiple blood cultures before initiating antibiotic therapy ● FBC shows leucocytosis with a 'left shift' ● ESR ● C-reactive protein ● synovial fluid aspiration (culture, microscopy, Gram stain, examination for crystals and rheumatoid factor) ● ASO titre ● radiology shows soft tissue swelling acutely and in the chronic state some peri-articular osteoporosis and loss of cartilage may be present ● If tuberculosis is suspected a tuberculin test eg Mantoux, CXR, and specific culture for AAFB should be undertaken.

Differential diagnosis Trauma, haemarthrosis, monoarticular arthritis (RA, gout, seronegative arthritis), osteomyelitis or battered baby syndrome.

> *Management* Rest, analgesia, joint splintage and prompt iv antibiotic therapy following multiple blood cultures and joint aspiration. Surgical drainage may be needed (→ Table 11.11).

DISEASES OF BONE

OSTEOMYELITIS

Denotes infection of bone and is usually bacterial in origin. Organisms reach the bone to produce infection by one of three routes: ● haematogenous spread ● direct extension from a contiguous source of infection or ● direct introduction of organisms by trauma (including operations). Most common in children. The organisms most commonly involved are staphylococci, streptococci, salmonellae and *Mycobacterium tuberculosis*.

Clinical features Fever, malaise, nausea, vomiting, severe pain at the site of infection. An effusion may occur if the infection is close to a joint. The affected area is hot and tender.

Investigations ● FBC ● ESR ● multiple blood cultures ● glucose ● radiology shows bony destruction with radiolucent areas, radio-opaque sequestrae and involucrum formation but changes do not occur for some days or weeks ● Radioisotopic bone scans are useful.

> *Management* Early appropriate antibiotic therapy (as for infective arthritis → Table 11.11). Surgical decompression may be needed.

Table 11.11
Management of infective arthritis

Organism producing joint infection	Antibiotic
Staphylococcus	Flucloxacillin 500 mg 6 hourly
	Fusidic acid 500 mg 8-hourly
Streptococcus	Ampicillin 500 mg 6-hourly
	Benzylpenicillin 0.6 g 6-hourly
Haemophilus influenzae	Ampicillin
Pseudomonas, E. coli	Aminoglycoside
	eg Gentamicin (dose depends on weight, age and renal function)
	Cephalosporin
	eg Ceftazidime 1 g 8-hourly
	Cefuroxime 750 mg 8-hourly
Neisseria gonorrhoeae	Ampicillin
	Benzylpenicillin
Neisseria meningitides	Ampicillin
	Benzylpenicillin
Salmonellae	Ampicillin
	Cotrimoxazole 960 mg 12-hourly
Mycobacterium tuberculosis	Rifampicin +
	Isoniazid +
	Ethambutol +/−
	Pyrazinamide
Viral	Symptomatic
Fungal	Amphoteracin

PAGET'S DISEASE

Bone disorder of unknown aetiology characterized by increased osteoclastic bone absorption followed by disorderly, excessive osteoblastic new bone formation. This leads to softening, painful enlargement and bowing of the affected bones. The disease affects certain bones preferentially: skull, vertebrae, pelvis and long bones. It may be asymptomatic. Affects approximately 3–4% of the population over 50 years old rising to 10% in the 85+ age group. M>F.

Clinical features Bone pain (often at night), tenderness, compressive symptoms eg deafness, blindness, nerve entrapment, slowly progressive paraparesis), pathological fractures, high output cardiac failure and rarely the development of osteogenic sarcoma.

Investigations ● Normal FBC ● ESR may also be normal ● Serum calcium and phosphorus levels are usually normal unless the patient is immobilized when the calcium level can rise

• Alkaline phosphatase (bony isoenzyme) is raised and reflects increased osteoblastic activity • urinary hydroxyproline is also elevated and reflects increased osteoclastic activity • Acid phosphatase is normal • Hyperuricaemia may be present • Radiology reveals osteolytic lesions (cortical resorption), areas of osteosclerosis and bony distortion, stress fractures, and osteoporosis circumscripta in the skull (osteolytic but no osteosclerotic lesions) • Bone scan is positive at an early stage of the disease.

> **Management** None is necessary in asymptomatic cases. Calcitonin: peptide hormone secreted by the thyroid gland which inhibits osteoclastic activity. Human or salmon varieties 50–100 units sc or im daily for at least 6 months. Allergic reactions may occur. Adverse reactions include nausea, vomiting, flushing, sweating and diarrhoea. The drug is very expensive. Diphosphonates eg disodium etidronate and amino-hydroxy propylidene diphosphonate disodium (APD): synthetic analogs of pyrophosphate which act by stabilizing the bony matrix hydroxyapatite crystals thus impeding bony turnover. Active orally but slower acting than calcitonin. Dose 5 mg/kg/day. Main adverse reaction is the development of osteomalacia. Mithramycin: effective but requires iv administration and can produce marrow suppression. Dose 10–20 μg/kg/day for 7–10 days. NSAID for analgesia and physiotherapy are useful. Surgery is occasionally needed. Radiotherapy is rarely used.

OSTEOPOROSIS

Reduction in bone mass per unit volume. Histologically there is loss of bone matrix with secondary loss of bone mineral. The resultant bone is weak and apt to fracture. This loss of bone occurs with age and is linked to androgen/oestrogen deficiency, dietary lack of vitamin D and poor absorption of calcium. This is greatest in post-menopausal women. Clinically significant osteoporosis is rare in men.

Aetiology (→ Table 11.12)

Clinical features Bone pain, backache, crush vertebral fractures, kyphosis, fractures with minimal trauma (distal radius and neck of femur). Bones are not particularly tender.

Investigations • Serum biochemistry is normal (calcium, phosphate and alkaline phosphatase), unless a fracture is present or osteomalacia coexists • Radiology may reveal reduced bone density, fractures and vertebral wedge collapse • Assessment of bone density (CT scan, neutron activation analysis or photon densitometry) • A bone biopsy may be needed to confirm the diagnosis.

**Table 11.12
Causes of osteoporosis**

Ageing	Post-menopausal
Endocrine	Thyrotoxicosis
	hypogonadism
	Cushing's syndrome
	hyperparathyroidism
Nutritional	Calcium deficiency
	avitaminosis C or D
Hereditary	Marfan's syndrome,
	osteogenesis imperfecta
Inflammatory arthritis	RA
Bone marrow replacement	Lymphoma, leukaemia, myeloma,
	glycogen storage disease
Chronic renal disease	
Malabsorption	
Post-gastrectomy	
Chronic liver disease	
Immobility	

Management Correct underlying cause. Analgesia and physiotherapy. Cyclical oestrogen helps prevent postmeno-pausal osteoporosis but is linked with a small risk of endometrial carcinoma. Calcium and vitamin D if the diet is deficient. Fluoride supplements may be useful.

Infectious diseases

No attempt has been made to cover tropical diseases in any detail in this chapter.

History: This is vital and should include detailed questions about exposure to possible infection (occupation, travel, immunization ($\rightarrow$ Table 12.1), date of onset, place of onset, animal contact and recent operations. The cause of fever may be unknown (PUO) ($\rightarrow$ Table 12.2, p 236).

Examination: must be complete and include eyes, ears, mouth, nose, sinuses, lymph glands, skin, anus, vagina and external genitalia.

INVESTIGATIONS

These will be guided by the above and include ● FBC ● ESR ● C-reactive protein ● LFTs ● immunoglobulins and ● protein electrophoresis ● multiple blood cultures before starting antibiotics ● sputum Gram stain and culture ● MSU ● autoantibody profile (RF, ANF) ● Mantoux test ● CXR ● plain abdominal X-ray ● serology (paired acute and convalescent samples) ● CT scans ● US ● bone scans and ● Indium labelled WBC scans may be useful in localizing the site of sepsis.

SEPTICAEMIA

Bacteraemia is the spread of infection into the bloodstream and if organisms multiply there it is known as septicaemia. The

Table 12.1
UK Immunization schedule

Age	Visits	Vaccine
3–12 months	3 (at intervals of 6–8 weeks and 4–6 months)	'Triple' DTP + oral polio on each visit
12–24 months	1	Measles
First school year	1	Booster DT + oral polio
10–13 years	1	BCG (tuberculin negative) + Rubella (girls)
15–19 years	1	TT + oral polio

DTP Diphtheria, tetanus, pertussis
DT Diphtheria, tetanus, TT Tetanus toxoid

Table 12.2
Causes of pyrexia of unknown origin (PUO)

Infections	Tuberculosis, infective endocarditis, localised abscesses, brucellosis, HIV, relapsing fever, EBV, CMV, cholangitis, enteric fever
Malignancy	Hypernephroma, lymphoma, hepatoma, myxoma, leukaemia
Connective tissue diseases	RA, SLE, temporal arteritis
Drugs	Virtually any drug
Endocrine	Hypothalamic lesions, thyrotoxicosis, phaeochromocytoma
Myocardial infarction	
Pulmonary embolism	
Familial mediterranean fever	
Munchausen's syndrome	

primary site of infection is often unknown but is commonly the gall bladder, bowel, lungs, meninges or urinary tract. Dissemination may result in the formation of abscesses in multiple organs. A number of predisposing factors often exist including multiple trauma, surgery, diabetes, alcoholism, immunosuppression host or malignancy. Any infective organism can produce septicaemia but the commonest cause is the Gram negative group of bacteria.

Clinical features The classical features of septic shock are fever, hypotension, vasodilatation, tachycardia and tachypnoea. Multiple organ failure may result eg kidneys, heart, lungs (ARDS), DIC, pancreas, bowel, liver and brain.

Investigations • FBC • clotting screen, fibrinogen level, fibrin degredation products • urea and electrolytes, creatinine • LFTs • urinary electrolytes • creatinine clearance • glucose • ABG • ECG • CXR • multiple blood cultures (aerobic and anaerobic culture) • MSU • CSF • drain fluid • sputum Gram stain and culture.

Management Reverse hypotension, hypoxaemia, treat infection and improve tissue perfusion. Ensure adequate oxygenation (supplemental oxygen by face mask or nasal cannulae or endotracheal intubation and artificial ventilation if necessary). Establish intravenous access. Monitor pulse, BP, temperature and urine output hourly. Neurological observations may be needed. Central venous or pulmonary artery wedge pressure measurements are helpful. Blood pressure should be maintained with crystalloids, colloids or a combination of both. Dopamine, dobutamine or noradrenaline may be needed to maintain adequate cardiac and urinary outputs. Surgical drainage of any suspected areas of sepsis should be undertaken. Antimicrobial therapy should be commenced immediately (after blood cultures have been taken), and should be effective against a wide variety of organisms. The combination of a broad spectrum penicillin/cephalosporin, an aminoglycoside and an anti-anaerobic agent is often used eg azlocillin/cefotaxime and gentamicin/tobramycin and metronidazole. This regime can be altered once culture results become available. The role of corticosteroids (30 mg/kg methylprednisolone) is controversial. Individual types of organ failure are treated conventionally.

Prognosis Approximately 50% survival.

BACTERIAL INFECTIONS

STAPHYLOCOCCAL

Staph. aureus produces a variety of suppurative conditions including wound infections, boils, carbuncles, abscesses, bone and joint infections, cavitating pneumonia and endocarditis. The toxic shock syndrome is commonly due to toxins released following *Staph. aureas* infection of the female genital tract in association with tampon use. Multi-system involvement is common in this condition and includes vomiting, diarrhoea, renal failure, hepatitis, thrombocytopenia, DIC, rash and encephalopathy.

Management Flucloxacillin (500 mg 6-hourly oral or iv), if penicillin allergy: erythromycin (500 mg 6-hourly oral or iv and/or fusidic acid (500 mg 8-hourly oral or iv).

STREPTOCOCCAL

Streptococci produce a number of toxins and can rapidly produce septicaemia and disseminated infection (→ Table 12.3, p 238).

Scarlet fever
Strep. pyogenes infection involving the throat, tonsils and skin. Incubation period 2–4 days.

Clinical features Sudden onset fever, sore throat, headache, vomiting, cervical lymphadenopathy, yellow friable tonsillar exudate, erythematous rash affecting the arms, legs and behind

Table 12.3
Streptococci and disease

Variety	Disease
Group A (pyogenes)	Scarlet fever, impetigo, erysipelas, tonsillitis, cellulitis
Group B	Neonatal infection
Pneumoniae	Pneumococcal pneumonia
Faecalis	Pyelonephritis, endocarditis
Viridans	Endocarditis
Anaerobic	Abscesses

the ears and furred tongue (white or red "strawberry" tongue). Rarely rheumatic fever and nephritis.

Investigations Throat swab, antistreptolysin O titre (ASO).

Management Ampicillin (500 mg 6-hourly orally or iv), amoxycillin (500 mg 8-hourly orally or iv or erythromycin (500 mg 6-hourly orally or iv if penicillin allergy).

Pneumococcal pneumonia ($\rightarrow$ p 69).

Erysipelas ($\rightarrow$ p 289).

Impetigo ($\rightarrow$ p 289).

Cellulitis ($\rightarrow$ p 289).

Endocarditis ($\rightarrow$ p 46).

ANAEROBIC

Anaerobic bacteria are responsible for many different infections due to both tissue invasion and because of their ability to produce a variety of toxins ($\rightarrow$ Table 12.4).

Clinical features Anaerobic organisms produce putrid smelling pus at the site of sepsis eg gingivitis, dental abscess, mastoiditis, sinusitis, cellulitis, intra-abdominal infection, peritonitis, bone and joint infection, bites and diabetic foot ulcers. There is often synergistic infection with aerobic organisms.

Investigations • Gram stain and culture of pus in a medium containing 10% carbon dioxide.

Management Surgical exision of necrotic material. Metronidazole (500 mg 8-hourly iv, 1 g 8-hourly PR, 400 mg 8-hourly orally).

Table 12.4
Anaerobes and disease

Variety	Disease
Clostridium perfringens	Gas gangrene, foot ulcers necrotising enterocolitis food poisoning, abscesses endocarditis, intra-abdominal infection
Clostridium difficile	Pseudomembranous colitis
Clostridium botulinum	Food poisoning
Clostridium tetani	Tetanus
Actinomyces	Actinomycosis
Borrelia vincenti	Acute necrotising gingivitis

TETANUS

Infection due to *Clostridium tetani* which exists as a gut commensal as well as in the soil. The Gram positive bacilli remain localized at the portal of entry but they produce an exotoxin which acts on the CNS. Not transmissible. Incubation period 1–15 days.

Clinical features Fever, trismus ('lockjaw') due to masseter muscle spasm, myalgia, apprehension, alert, hypertonia, rigidity of face, neck and trunk muscles ('risus sardonicus' and opithotonos). Muscle spasm may occur in response to noxious stimuli (unexpected noise or touch) and can produce asphyxia. Autonomic instability occurs with cardiac arrhythmias, sweating and swings in BP. Umbilical sepsis is an important source in the Third World.

Investigations • Usually a clinical diagnosis. Isolation of the organism is rare.

Differential diagnosis Hysteria and phenothiazine dystonia.

Management Prevent the disease if possible: active immunization (→ Table 12.1, p 235) and adequate wound toilet following injury. Treat as soon as the disease is suspected: prevent further toxin absorption by wound toilet, iv/im human tetanus anti-toxin, iv benzylpenicillin 600 mg 6-hourly or erythromycin 500 mg 6-hourly orally or iv for 1 week, nurse in a quiet room and prevent muscle spasms with diazepam, or paralyse the patient if necessary with d-tubocurarine or pancuronium following intubation and artificial ventilation. Ensure adequate nutrition and hydration.

DIPHTHERIA

Acute epidemic notifiable disease caused by *Corynebacterium diphtheriae* spread by droplets. It is preventable by active immunization. Rare in the UK nowadays but still important in underdeveloped countries. Incubation period 2–4 days. Organisms remain localized in the throat but produce an exotoxin which damages the heart and brain.

Clinical features Sore throat with classical tonsillar appearance: oedematous yellow/haemorrhagic membrane with a well-defined edge which may extend onto the faucial pillars and the palate. In severe cases the neck may become swollen 'bull-neck diphtheria'. Marked tachycardia, mild pyrexia, husky voice and nasal discharge. Rarely solitary skin ulcers in tropical climates. In severe cases laryngeal obstruction, stridor, circulatory collapse and death may occur.

Investigations ● Clinical diagnosis confirmed by culture of throat swab.

Management Give diphtheria anti-toxin im immediately on clinical suspicion (anaphylaxis may occur as horse serum is used so adrenaline, chlorpheniramine, salbutamol and hydrocortisone should be available). Penicillin or erythromycin should be given for 1 week to eliminate *C. diphtheriae* from the throat. The disease should be prevented by active immunization of children aged 3–12 months (→ Table 12.1, p 235). Carriers should be identified in any outbreak and treated with a week of penicillin or erythromycin and kept in isolation until 6 daily throat swabs are negative.

Complications Neurological involvement includes palatal paralysis, extrinsic eye muscle paralysis, peripheral neuropathy and diaphragmatic weakness. Myocarditis with resultant arrhythmias and cardiac failure may occur.

PERTUSSIS (WHOOPING COUGH)

Gram-negative bacillus *Bordetella pertussis,* spread by droplets. Highly infectious. Usually affects pre-school children. Incubation period 7–14 days.

Clinical features

Catarrhal stage: rhinitis, conjunctivitis, unproductive cough.

Spasmodic stage: staccato coughing bouts, vomiting, exhaustion. Bronchial hyperactivity may remain for many months.

Investigations • Clinical diagnosis confirmed by culture of nasal swabs and serological examination.

> *Management* Prevent by active immunization of pre-school children (→ Table 12.1, p 235). The risk of vaccination induced brain damage is small and can be minimized if the vaccine is not given to babies with a history of birth injury, CNS damage, previous convulsions or a family history of such or a previous reaction to the vaccine. The established disease is treated with erythromycin during the catarrhal stage. Cough suppressants are useful. Adequate hydration and nutrition must be maintained. Ventilation may be required. Babies who have not been vaccinated can be given prophylactic erythromycin if they develop a cough for 24 hours.

Complications Secondary bacterial bronchopneumonia, bronchiectasis, asphyxia, cerebral anoxia, convulsions and death. Subconjunctival haemorrhages can be produced by paroxysms of coughing.

TYPHOID FEVER (ENTERIC FEVER)

Due to Gram-negative bacilli *Salmonella typhi*. Paratyphoid fever is due to *S. paratyphi*. Spread by human to human transfer especially under conditions of poor hygiene. Occurs sporadically or in epidemics. Following ingestion the organisms penetrate the mucosa of the GI tract to be taken up by reticuloendothelial cells where they multiply. Incubation period up to 18 days. Septicaemic spread then occurs throughout the body. The gall bladder may act as a reservoir for ongoing infection in carriers.

Clinical features Nonspecific headache, cough, lethargy, constipation, pyrexia, confusion, splenomegaly, macular rose spots and relative bradycardia during the first week. If untreated the patient deteriorates with dehydration, doughy abdomen, GI bleeding and possible perforation.

Investigation • Neutropenia • Blood, urine, rose spot and stool culture • Serological tests (Widal) to both the O and H antigens of the organism.

> *Management* Barrier nursing, rehydration, chloramphenicol 500 mg 4-hourly, amoxycillin 500 mg 6-hourly or cotrimoxazole 960 mg 12-hourly for 2 weeks (iv initially). Carriers can be treated with ciprofloxacin 500 mg bd but may need cholecystectomy.

TUBERCULOSIS

Chronic infectious disease caused by *Mycobacterium tuberculosis* or rarely by *M. bovis*. The disease is a major cause of both morbidity and mortality in Third World countries and although it is now less of a problem in the developed world it still occurs in some sections of society eg alcoholics, undernourished, ethnic communities and HIV population. *M tuberculosis* is a non-motile bacillus which is not discoloured by acid-alcohol when stained with carbolfuchsin and is therefore 'acid fast'. It is slow to grow and it may take six weeks for the culture result to become available. The BACTEC system allows identification of mycobacterial metabolites within two weeks but is not yet widely available.

Aetiology and pathogenesis The organisms enter the body via the skin, respiratory tract or alimentary tract. Clinical illness does not always occur and may depend on the degree of natural immunity existing, state of nourishment, age, coexisting disease (diabetes mellitus, malignancy), immunosuppression or even standard of living conditions of the affected individual. The primary infection usually occurs in the lung and a 'primary complex' is produced which is the combination of the primary focus (Ghon focus) of infection in the lung parenchyma plus caseous involvement of the regional lymph nodes (usually mediastinal). If the initial site of infection is the tonsil or the ileum the affected nodes will be the cervical or mesenteric respectively. In the vast majority of cases the primary complex then heals and calcifies and the person remains entirely asymptomatic but becomes sensitized to tuberculoprotein. In a few cases healing may not be entirely complete and progressive pulmonary tuberculosis results. Rarely haematogenous spread may occur to produce miliary tuberculosis with widespread involvement of lungs, bone marrow, kidneys, liver, brain, bones, joints and heart. Reactivation of a partially healed primary complex can occur many years later or the person may be reinfected from an outside source with resultant postprimary tuberculosis. Blood-borne dissemination is uncommon at this stage.

Clinical features

Systemic: lassitude, weight loss, night sweats, malaise, fever and anorexia. The disease may be asymptomatic and found incidentally.

Local: • Lungs: cough, sputum, haemoptysis, breathlessness, hoarseness, lobar collapse, bronchopneumonia.

• Pleura: pain, breathlessness, effusion.

- Pericardium/heart: pain, arrhythymias, constrictive pericarditis, cardiac failure.

- Intestine: diarrhoea, malabsorption, obstruction.

- Genitourinary tract: renal failure, haematuria, epididymitis, salpingitis, infertility.

- Skin: lupus vulgaris, erythema nodosum.

- Eyes: choroiditis, iritis, phlyctenular keratoconjunctivitis.

- Bones/joints: osteomyelitis, arthritis.

- Lymphatics: cold abscesses, lymphadenopathy, sinuses.

- Brain: meningitis, tuberculoma.

- Adrenal glands: Addison's disease.

Investigations • CXR: primary focus, lymphadenopathy, cavitation, pneumothorax, areas of calcification, pleural effusion/empyema, segmental/lobar collapse, miliary disease or secondary aspergilloma formation. Always compare with previous X-rays if possible • chest tomography • IVU • CT scanning • Tuberculin test: Mantoux test is an intradermal injection of purified protein derivative (PPD) usually injected into the flexor aspect of the forearm and read 48–72 hours later. A positive result is an area of induration at least 5 mm in diameter with surrounding erythema. 0.1 ml of 1 in 10 000 dilution should be used initially progressing to more concentrated solutions if the result is negative. Alternative tuberculin tests are available and useful for large-scale screening (Heaf and Tine tests) but they are not as accurate as the Mantoux test • Bacteriological examination: staining (Ziehl-Neelsen, fluorescent Auramine), culture and BACTEC analysis of sputum, pleural aspirate/biopsy, early morning urine samples (EMUs), laryngeal swabs, gastric aspirate, CSF, liver biopsy or BM aspirate.

Management Prevent the disease if possible by BCG vaccination, better living standards, adequate nutrition, notification of index cases and subsequent case finding. Isolation of infected cases is rarely needed but young children should be isolated from the index case until adequate chemotherapy has had a chance to be effective. Surgery is now rarely needed. The mainstay of treatment is antibacterial chemotherapy and various drug regimens are now employed. Five drugs are commonly used in the developed world: rifampicin, isoniazid, ethambutol, pyrazinamide and streptomycin. If these drugs are used in the correct combinations for an adequate period of time they are virtually 100% effective in curing tuberculosis (→ Table 12.5, p 244)

Table 12.5
Drug regimens in tuberculosis*

9 months duration	Initial phase (2 months): rifampicin + isoniazid + ethambutol/streptomycin Continuation phase (7 months): rifampicin + isoniazid
6 months duration	Initial phase (2 months): rifampicin + isoniazid + pyrazinamide + ethambutol/streptomycin Continuation phase (4 months): rifampicin + isoniazid

* Drug therapy can be modified according to bacterial sensitivity test results.

In developing countries less expensive drug regimens have to be used eg streptomycin + isoniazid twice weekly for 12 months but standard respiratory medicine textbooks should be consulted for details on suitable treatment regimes.

Rifampicin: 10 mg/kg (400–600 mg/d) best absorbed from an empty stomach. May cause a transient rise in LFTs which can be ignored but the drug must be discontinued if jaundice occurs. Produces reddish discolouration of body fluids eg urine, sweat and tears and may irreversibly stain contact lenses. Induces liver enzymes thus making OCP less effective and alternative forms of contraception must be used. May produce fever, vasculitis, influenza-like illness, nausea and vomiting.

Isoniazid: 200–300 mg/day in adults. Can produce a hypersensitivity reaction (erythematous skin rash and pyrexia) and occasionally polyneuropathy (especially in slow acetylators – minimized by concurrent treatment with pyridoxime 10 mg/d). Hepatotoxity is well recognized.

Ethambutol: 15 mg/kg/day in adults. May cause optic neuritis. Document visual acuity before starting treatment and at regular intervals thereafter and stop the drug if visual problems occur.

Pyrazinamide: 35 mg/kg/day up to a maximum of 2.5 g/day. May produce gout, hepatitis, arthralgia and hypersensitivity.

Streptomycin: 0.75–1.00 g/day. Dose depends on serum level. May cause vestibular disturbance, deafness and hypersensitivity.

All the drugs should be given together once daily to ensure adequate peak serum bactericidal levels. Corticosteroids may be needed in fulminating infection, secondary Addison's disease, tuberculous pleural and pericardial effusions, lymphadenopathy, genitourinary or meningeal involvement.

MALARIA

Infection due to *Plasmodium falciparum, P. ovale, P. vivax* or *P. malariae*. Spread by the bite of the female anopheline mosquito and rarely by blood transfusion or transplacentally. Endemic in many tropical and sub-tropical countries where drug resistance is becoming an increasing problem. Notifiable disease.

Clinical features Relapsing fever, rigors, abdominal pain, prostration, profuse perspiration, jaundice, hepatosplenomegaly, headache, vomiting, diarrhoea, increasing haemolytic anaemia. Infection with *P. ovale, P. vivax* and *P. malariae* tends to run a benign course but may relapse many years after the initial attack. *P. falciparum* produces a more serious illness and infection may lead to acute renal failure, hepatic failure, cerebral malaria and severe intravascular haemolysis leading to 'Blackwater fever'.

Investigations ● Always consider this diagnosis in a patient with PUO especially if there is any history of foreign travel ● Microscopy of thick and thin blood films looking for malarial parasites.

Management Bed rest, adequate hydration, paracetamol for headache. An acute attack may be treated with chloroquine, quinine dihydrochloride or amodiaquine. If chloroquine resistance is a problem maloprim (pyrimethamine/dapsone) or fansidar (pyrimethamine/sulphadoxine) can be used. Transfusion may be necessary in severe anaemia. Corticosteroids help to reduce haemolysis. Unfortunately the mortality remains high in complicated cases.

Prophylaxis This is important but is not a guarantee of protection and it is important to obtain accurate advice on drug resistant areas before travelling abroad. Chloroquine 300 mg weekly or proguanil 100–200 mg/day are effective prophylactic agents. If chloroquine resistance is a problem maloprim or fansidar 1 tablet/week can be used. Repellant creams or sprays, mosquito coils and nets are also an important aspect of malaria prophylaxis.

MEASLES

RNA paramyxovirus infection spread by droplets. Highly contagious, incubation period 7–14 days. Usually affects children. Biennial winter epidemics occur in temperate climates. One attack confers lasting immunity.

Clinical features

Catarrhal stage: fever, cough, coryza, conjunctivitis, Koplik's spots are present on the mucous membrane of the mouth (especially in the inside of the cheeks) and irritability. Most infectious during this stage.

Exanthematous stage: dark red macular or maculopapular rash behind the ears spreading to involve the face and trunk associated with increasing fever. The rash becomes confluent and blotchy.

Investigations ● Clinical diagnosis ● IgM and IgG antibodies can be measured.

Management Isolate from school for 10 days, paracetamol for pyrexia. Prevention is important by active immunization of children >1 year old who have not had the disease (→ Table 12.1, p 235). Passive immunization using immunoglobulin is possible in patients with severe malnutrition.

Complications Encephalitis, secondary bacterial otitis media, pneumonia (often with *Staph. aureus* or Gram-negative organisms in undernourished children), subacute sclerosing panencephalitis, croup, stomatitis, gastroenteritis and kwashiorkor.

RUBELLA (GERMAN MEASLES)

RNA togavirus spread by droplets. One attack confers immunity. Incubation period 18 days. Trivial disease in children but more severe in adults and may produce severe congenital abnormalities if it occurs during pregnancy (triad of blindness, deafness and cardiac defects together with hepatosplenomegaly, purpuric rash and cataracts).

Clinical features Faint pink macular rash on face spreading to trunk and limbs. Suboccipital lymphadenopathy, fever and myalgia.

Investigations • Viral isolation from throat swab • rising antibody titire.

> *Management* None. Prevent by active immunization of girls 11–13 years who lack serum antibodies to the disease. Offer termination if the disease occurs within the first sixteen weeks of pregnancy.

MUMPS

RNA paramyxovirus spread by droplets. Low infectivity rate although some cases may be subclinical. Incubation period 18 days.

Clinical features Fever, malaise, trismus, parotid gland swelling, orchitis in adult males, pancreatitis or oophoritis. Rarely encephalitis.

Investigations • Usually a clinical diagnosis. If doubt exists a rise in antibody titres or viral culture from saliva is diagnostic.

> *Management* Symptomatic only. Prednisolone for orchitis.

VARICELLA (CHICKEN POX)

DNA herpes virus spread by droplets or by direct contact with skin lesions. Highly infectious and usually affects children. One attack usually produces immunity but reactivation occurs and produces herpes zoster (shingles). Incubation period 14–21 days. May be disseminated in the immunocompromised host.

Clinical features Mild fever, characteristic rash on trunk spreading to the face and limbs (initially macular, then papular, vesicular and finally pustular). The rash appears in crops.

Investigations • Clinical diagnosis • Rising antibody titre.

Complications Secondary infection, pneumonia (leaves calcified scars on CXR), proliferative glomerulonephritis, demyelinating encephalitis.

> *Management* Varicella: symptomatic. If secondary skin infection occurs use topical chlorhexidine. Oral augmentin (1 tablet 8-hourly or flucloxacillin 500 mg 6-hourly may be needed). Human anti-varicella immunoglobulin can be given to the immunocompromised.

HERPES ZOSTER (SHINGLES)

Due to invasion of posterior root ganglia by varicella virus. The virus may lie dormant for many years and reactivation is often precipitated by other infection.

Clinical features   Severe pain in the distribution of the affected rosal nerve root. The skin then becomes erythematous before the characteristic vesicular scarring rash appears. The patient may be left with intractable neuralgia for many months. Myalgia, myelitis and encephalitis may occur. Involvement of the first division of the trigeminal nerve produces ophthalmic herpes with corneal vesicles and scarring.

Investigations   • Usually clinical • Confirmation by rising antibody titres.

> *Management*   Acyclovir halts the progression of the disease if given early enough and may reduce the incidence of post-herpetic neuralgia (800 mg orally or 5% cream topically 5 times daily for 7 days, or 5 mg/kg 8-hourly for 7 days given slowly as an infusion over 1 hour in severe infections). Topical 5% idoxuridine 6-hourly for 7 days is useful. Pain should be treated adequately eg regular coproxamol. Amitriptyline or carbamazepine may be useful for post-herpetic neuralgia if simple analgesics are not sufficient.

HERPES SIMPLEX (→ p 293)

INFECTIOUS MONONUCLEOSIS (GLANDULAR FEVER)

Due to infection with the Epstein-Barr virus, a herpes virus which also causes nasopharyngeal carcinoma and Burkitt's lymphoma. Mildly infectious and tends to spread by close contact eg kissing. Tends to affect young adults. Incubation period 4–5 weeks.

Clinical features   Fever, sore throat, malaise, cervical lymphadenopathy, petechial haemorrhages on the palate, maculopapular rash (especially if ampicillin is prescribed), hepatosplenomegaly, rarely meningitis, encephalitis, haemolytic anaemia, thrombocytopenia and pancarditis.

Investigations   • Initially a mild neutrophil leucocytosis followed by an atypical lymphocytosis (activated T lymphocytes). Similar atypical lymphocytes are seen in toxoplasmosis, CMV infection, lymphoma and leukaemia • Heterophile antibody is present and can agglutinate sheep RBCs (Paul-Bunnell reaction). Agglutination can be prevented by prior absorption with beef RBCs but not with guinea pig cells. The Monospot test is similar but easier and quicker to perform although not as specific ● EBV antibodies titres can be measured (IgM and IgG).

Management Symptomatic, rest, avoid alcohol, corticosteroids are rarely needed.

FUNGAL INFECTIONS

Classification   (→ Table 12.6)

> **Table 12.6**
> **Classification of fungal infections**
>
> *Superficial infections:*
> Dermatophytes   → Dermatology (p 294)
> Candidiasis   → Dermatology (p 295)
> Pityriasis versicolor → Dermatology (p 295)
>
> *Subcutaneous infections*
> Mycetoma (Madura's foot)
> Chromomycosis
>
> *Systemic infections*
> Histoplasmosis
> Aspergillosis
> Coccidioidomycosis
> Cryptococcus

MYCETOMA

Chronic infection of the deep soft tissues and bones. May affect the limbs, trunk or head. Due to eumycetes and actinomycetes both of which produce grains.

Clinical features Painless swelling at the site of impregnation. Sinuses, abscesses, scarring and deformity are produced.

Investigation   ● Microscopy and culture of pus or biopsy.

Management Largely unsuccessful for eumycetic infection. Actinomycetes may respond to penicillin, dapsone or streptomycin but amputation may be needed.

HISTOPLASMOSIS

Due to *Histoplasma capsulatum* or *duboisii*. Usually secondary to inhalation of spores.

Clinical features May be asymptomatic. Can mimic tuberculosis. Fever, anaemia, lymphadenopathy, endocarditis, hepatosplenomegaly, diarrhoea, cough and sputum.

Investigations ● CXR/AXR shows calcification in lungs, liver or spleen ● Tissue biopsy for microscopy and culture ● Delayed hypersensitivity skin tests ● Complement fixation test.

Management Amphoteracin on alternate days for up to one month. Adverse reactions (fever, headache, malaise, venous thrombosis) may be minimized by concurrent prednisolone therapy.

CRYPTOCOCCUS

Caused by *Cryptococcus neoformans*. Common in the immunocompromised eg HIV infection.

Clinical features Meningitis, pulmonary and gastrointestinal involvement.

Investigations ● Microscopy (Indian ink dye) and culture of biopsies or CSF ● Complement fixation test.

Management Amphoteracin plus 5-flucytosine.

ASPERGILLUS

Commonest respiratory mycosis in the UK and the cause of many diseases (→ Table 12.7). Aspergillus species also commonly present in the atmosphere. The demonstration of fungal hyphae in a sample of sputum is however always of diagnostic significance. Most cases are due to *Aspergillus fumigatus* but there are many other members of the genus (eg *Aspergillus clavatus*, *A. flavus* and *A.niger*).

Asthma
Usual symptoms of allergic asthma (→ p 66). Skin hypersensitivity may be present and *Aspergillus fumigatus* may be isolated from sputum. Treatment is of the underlying asthma.

Table 12.7
Diseases caused by aspergillus species

Asthma
Allergic bronchopulmonary aspergillosis
Aspergilloma
Extrinsic allergic alveolitis
Invasive aspergillosis
Otomycosis

Allergic bronchopulmonary aspergillosis

A rare but important complication of asthma. May be asymptomatic and discovered on routine CXR.

Clinical features   Fever and usual symptoms of asthma may occur. Occlusion of a major bronchus by tenacious sputum may cause lobar collapse. Repeated infection can produce bronchiectasis.

Investigations • CXR shows various transient abnormalities (collapse/consolidation, peripheral shadows, thickened bronchial wall markings) • peripheral blood film shows eosinophilia • serum precipitating antibodies to Aspergillus species may be present, early (20 min) and late (6 h) skin-test prick may be positive • Fungal spores/hyphae may be seen on sputum microscopy or grown on culture.

Management   Involves optimizing asthma therapy together with oral prednisolone (20–40 mg/d) reducing slowly to zero if possible. The rate of steroid reduction depends on the individual patient's response to therapy. A small proportion of patients with recurrent episodes of aspergillosis may need to be maintained on a small dose of oral prednisolone. The oral antifungal agent itraconazole may prove to be valuable in future.

Aspergilloma

Clinical features   May be asymptomatic. Forms in cavities produced by previous lung diseases (eg tuberculosis, abscesses or areas of pulmonary infarction). Haemoptysis can occur and may be severe. Usually due to *A. fumigatus*. May produce secondary invasion of the lung.

Investigations   • CXR (solid opacity within a cavity, often with a crescent of air between the fungal ball and the wall of the cavity) • Sputum culture may be positive especially if the aspergilloma communicates with a bronchus.

> **Management** This is largely unsatisfactory although itraconazole may be useful. Surgery may be needed. Corticosteroids should be avoided if possible.

Extrinsic allergic alveolitis

Clinical features Fever, malaise, breathlessness without wheeze six hours after exposure to the antigen (eg *A. clavatus* in Maltworker's lung or *Micropolyspora faeni/Thermoactinomyces vulgaris* in Farmer's lung), followed eventually by progressive exertional breathlessness if exposure continues.

Investigation ● Microscopy and culture of sputum (24-h specimen is most reliable), bronchial washings or transbronchial/open-lung biopsies ● Immediate and delayed (6 h) skin hypersensitivity reaction ● serum precipitins ● CXR may show micronodular shadowing ● Serology demonstrates precipitating antibodies eg *Aspergillus* ● Pulmonary function tests show a restrictive defect, reduced transfer factor for carbon monoxide and reduced lung volumes ● ABG analysis may show type I respiratory failure. Allergen provocation tests in association with pulmonary function tests and serial temperature measurement may be needed to establish the diagnosis.

> **Treatment** Avoid the precipitating antigen if possible. Courses of prednisolone may be required during the acute illness. Established pulmonary fibrosis/respiratory failure is extremely difficult to treat.

Invasive aspergillosis

Clinical features Usually occurs in the presence of immunosuppression and presents as a suppurative pneumonia which does not respond to conventional antibiotic regimes. It has a grave prognosis.

Investigation ● CXR shows widespread parenchymal infiltration with abscess formation ● Sputum microscopy and culture is required.

> **Management** This is with a combination of amphoteracin and flucytosine but is rarely successful unless given very early during the course of the illness.

GASTROENTERITIS

Presents with diarrhoea, vomiting and abdominal pain within 48 hours of the consumption of the infected food or drink.

Aetiology (→ Table 12.8)

Table 12.8
Causes of gastroenteritis

Bacteria	Salmonella typhimurium
	Shigella dysenteriae, flexneri, sonnei, boydii
	Clostridia perfringens, botulinum
	Staphylococcus aureus
	Campylobacter jejuni
	Escherichia coli
	Bacillus cereus
	Yersinia enterocolitica
	Vibrio cholerae
Viruses	Rotavirus
	Adenovirus
	Norwalk agent
Protozoa	Giardia lamblia
	Entamoeba histolytica

SALMONELLOSIS

Due to *Salmonella typhimurium* and is responsible for 75% of reported cases of food poisoning in UK. Common infective sources are poultry, milk, cream, cattle and pigs. Usually due to inadequate initial cooking or rewarming partially cooked food. Outbreaks are common and may involve many people. The organism produces its effect by both invasion and by toxins. Incubation period 12–48 hours.

Clinical features Usually mild diarrhoea which lasts a few days but may produce severe diarrhoea, abdominal pain, vomiting and dehydration and in debilitated patients is occasionally fatal.

Investigations ● Epidemiological help is needed to pinpoint the source ● Stool culture may remain positive for longer than 8 weeks in 30% of cases.

Management Prevention by strict hygiene of all food handlers and adequate cooking of all foods is vital. Antibiotics (amoxycillin, chloramphenicol or cotrimoxazole) should be limited to those few cases with systemic disease as acquired drug resistance via plasmids is a problem. Carrier states are rarely encountered. Notifiable disease.

CAMPYLOBACTER

Due to ingestion of contaminated poultry, milk or water.

Subclinical infection is common. Incubation period 12–48 hours.

Clinical features   Abdominal pain, diarrhoea (often bloody), rarely septicaemia, arthritis, pancreatitis and endocarditis. May mimic acute appendicitis or colitis.

Investigations   ● Stool and blood cultures.

> **Treatment**   Erythromycin 500 mg 6-hourly.

SHIGELLOSIS (BACILLARY DYSENTERY)

Usually spread by faecal-oral route under conditions of poor hygiene. Commoner in tropical climates. The organism produces colonic inflammation with toxin formation which results in profuse diarrhoea.

Clinical features   These range from subclinical to severe infection. Diarrhoea (occasionally bloody), fever, colicky abdominal pain and tenderness, tenesmus, lethargy, arthralgia and iritis.

Investigations   ● Stool culture.

> **Treatment**   Rehydration, adequate hygiene, codeine or loperamide for diarrhoea, antibiotics in severe cases (ampicillin 500 mg 6-hourly or cotrimoxazole 960 mg 12-hourly), but drug resistance can be a problem.

ESCHERICHIA COLI

Various strains exist which can produce gastroenteritis (usually in children).

Enterotoxigenic: produce heat labile and heat stable toxins producing watery travellers' diarrhoea with no inflammatory features.

Enteroinvasive: produce dysenteric-like illness with bloody diarrhoea.

Enteropathogenic: diarrhoea produced by unknown mechanism.

Clinical features   Usually acute onset diarrhoea occasionally associated with vomiting.

Investigations   ● Stool culture.

> **Treatment**   Rehydration and codeine or loperamide. Antibiotics are reserved for severe cases (cotrimoxazole).

YERSINIA

Due to ingestion of contaminated shellfish, water, milk or meat. Person to person spread may occur resulting in epidemics. Bowel invasion occurs.

Clinical features Abdominal pain, diarrhoea (usually watery and containing mucous but may be bloody), rashes, erythema nodosum and iritis. May mimic Crohn's disease of the terminal ileum and produce a seronegative arthropathy in individuals with HLA B27.

Investigations ● Stool culture.

> *Treatment* Antibiotics are rarely needed (chloramphenicol or tetracycline).

STAPHYLOCOCCUS AUREUS

Produces a heat stable enterotoxin which results in an episode of acute vomiting 1–6 hours after ingestion of contaminated meat or cream cakes. Treatment is symptomatic. IV rehydration may occasionally be needed.

CLOSTRIDIUM

Clostridium perfringens: is a common cause of food poisoning especially when inadequately cooked meat is allowed to cool slowly and then reheated. Incubation period 12–24 hours. Diarrhoea is present but vomiting is uncommon.

C. botulinum: produces an enterotoxin which acts on the CNS producing paralysis and eventually death due to respiratory failure in 50% of cases. Incubation period 12–72 hours. Vomiting and diarrhoea occur. An antitoxin should be given. Artificial ventilation may be needed.

C. difficile: is associated with pseudomembranous colitis. Treatment is with oral vancomycin 125 mg 6-hourly.

BACILLUS CEREUS

Spore bearing aerobic organism which may result in vomiting, abdominal pain and diarrhoea 1–5 hours after the ingestion of infected rice, milk and meat.

VIBRIO

Vibrio cholera (classical and El Tor biotypes) produces cholera in man. Common in tropical and subtropical countries under conditions of poor hygiene. The organism colonizes the small intestine with production of a powerful toxin but no bowel invasion occurs.

Clinical features The disease varies from the asymptomatic carrier state to that of severe painless diarrhoea associated with vomiting and muscle cramps. Hypovolaemic shock, uraemia and hypoglycaemia may occur.

Investigations ● Clinical diagnosis.

> ***Management*** Aggressive rehydration is vital using oral solutions containing sodium, glucose, potassium, chloride and bicarbonate (eg WHO solution), or iv replacement. Antibiotics are useful (tetracycline, cotrimoxazole or chloramphenicol). Cholera vaccine is of limited value and only lasts 3–6 months.

Vibrio parahaemolyticus can contaminate shellfish and produce profuse watery diarrhoea. Treatment is by rehydration and antibiotics (tetracycline or chloramphenicol).

VIRAL DIARRHOEA

Rotaviruses, adenoviruses and the Norwalk agent can all produce diarrhoea especially in children. They act by destroying gut villi. Management is by rehydration. Vaccines are being developed.

GIARDIASIS

Infection due to the flagellated protozoan *Giardia intestinalis (Giardia lamblia),* common in tropical areas and N. America. May be entirely asymptomatic or produce severe malabsorption.

Clinical features Acute diarrhoea, abdominal pain and distension, flatulence, lethargy, nausea and weight loss.

Investigations ● Demonstration of cysts on microscopy of fresh stool or trophozoites in jejunal aspirate.

> ***Management*** Metronidazole 400 mg tds for 14 days (avoid alcohol because of antabuse effect), or tinidazole 0.5–2.0 g as a single dose repeated after one week if necessary.

AMOEBIASIS

Due to infection with *Entamoeba histolytica*. Spread occurs by the ingestion of food contaminated by cysts. Trophozoites form in the colon with invasion of the bowel wall producing amoebic dysentery. Haematogenous spread may occur resulting in amoebic liver abscesses. Incubation period from 2 weeks to many years.

Clinical features

Amoebic dysentery: abdominal discomfort, episodes of diarrhoea alternating with constipation, blood stained mucus is often passed PR, rarely bowel perforation may occur or a localized amoebic granuloma ('amoeboma') may be mistaken for a colonic carcinoma.

Hepatic amoebiasis: lethargy, swinging pyrexia, sweating and tender hepatomegaly with referred shoulder-tip pain. The liver abscess may rupture catastrophically into the pleural, pericardial or peritoneal cavities.

Investigations • Identification of trophozoites by microscopy of fresh stool • sigmoidoscopy and biopsy reveals colonic ulceration • Hepatic amoebiasis can be diagnosed by US, radioisotope or CT scanning, and confirmed by serological tests (immunofluorescent antibody test).

Management

Amoebic dysentery: metronidazole 800 mg tds for 5 days or tinidazole 2 g daily for 3 days. Both should be followed by furamide 500 mg tds for 10 days to eliminate any luminal cysts.

Hepatic amoebiasis: treatment as above but aspiration may be needed if the abscess is large. Secondary bacterial infection may occur and should be treated with appropriate broad spectrum antibiotics. Cure is not always complete.

ACQUIRED IMMUNODEFICIENCY SYNDROME

First recognized in 1983 and due to a RNA retrovirus known as human immunodeficiency virus 1 (HIV-1). Other related viruses (HIV-2 and simian immunodeficiency virus) also produce immunosuppression. The origin of the virus is unknown but it may have come from Africa. The disease tends to affect certain well-known groups in society (homosexual men, iv drug abusers, haemophiliacs and blood recipients) but no group is spared and the incidence in the heterosexual population is increasing. The virus has lymphotrophic and neurotropic properties and produces remorseless destruction of the immune system. For classification and transmission → Tables 12.9 and 12.10.

Table 12.9
CDC Classification for HIV infection

Group 1	Acute infection	
Group 2	Asymptomatic infection	
Group 3	Persistent generalized lymphadenopathy	
Group 4	Other disease	
	Subgroup A:	constitutional disease (AIDS related complex) fever>1 month diarrhoea>1 month weight loss>10% body weight
	Subgroup B:	neurological disease dementia, myelopathy, peripheral neuropathy
	Subgroup C:	secondary infection pneumocystis carinii pneumonia, tuberculosis, herpes zoster, oral hairy leucoplakia, nocardiasis, candidosis, salmonella
	Subgroup D:	secondary cancers Kaposi's sarcoma, primary cerebral lymphoma, Non-Hodgkin's lymphoma

Table 12.10
Modes of transmission of AIDS

Sexual intercourse	Anal and vaginal
Contaminated needles	Intravenous drug abuse, needle stick injuries (very rare)
Contaminated blood and blood products	Transfusion
Contaminated organ and tissue donation	Bone marrow, organ transplant
Vertical mother to child	In utero, at birth

Clinical features (→ Table 12.11). The initial infection is usually asymptomatic but as progression occurs there is increasing evidence of immunodeficiency with recurrent common infections, increasing constitutional symptoms and finally opportunistic infections and the occurrence of unusual tumours. These lead to an early death.

Acute infection: occurs 4–6 weeks after infection and is usually asymptomatic. An influenza-like illness may occur with fever, myalgia, arthralgia, headache, nausea, sore throat, rash, transient

Table 12.11 Organ involvement in AIDS	
Lung	Pneumocystis carinii pneumonia Tuberculosis – typical and atypical Cytomegalovirus Bacterial pneumonia – Strep. pneumoniae, Staph. aureus, H. influenzae Fungi – invasive candidosis Lymphocytic interstitial pneumonitis Pulmonary Kaposi's sarcoma
GI tract	Oropharynx – candidosis, HSV, leucoplakia, Kaposi's sarcoma Stomach – Tuberculosis, Kaposi's sarcoma, cryptosporidium Small intestine – cryptosporidium, giardia, salmonella, campylobacter Large intestine – HSV, cryptosporidium, CMV, Kaposi's sarcoma, lymphoma
Liver/biliary tract	Atypical mycobacteria, HSV, histoplasmosis, toxoplasmosis, cryptosporidium
Skin	Kaposi's sarcoma, Non Hodgkin's lymphoma, atypical mycobacteria, folliculitis, seborrhoeic dermatitis, herpes zoster, HSV
Nervous system	Encephalopathy, transverse myelitis, peripheral neuropathy, myelopathy, dementia, depression, demyelination encephalitis, retinitis, focal intracranial lesion – toxoplasmosis, lymphoma abscess – cryptococcus, aspergillus, mycobacteria, candida

lymphadenopathy and rarely meningo-encephalitis. A period of asymptomatic infection then follows and this may last from a few months to many years.

Persistent generalized lymphadenopathy: nodes >1 cm diameter in 2 extrainguinal sites for >3 months. There is usually no evidence of any other symptoms or signs of disease at this time.

AIDS related complex: symptomatic disease with evidence of constitutional upset and minor opportunistic infections ($\rightarrow$ Table 12.12). This stage is one short of the fully developed AIDS.

Table 12.12 Features of AIDS related complex*	
Symptoms	Lethargy, malaise, fever, night sweats, weight loss >10%, diarrhoea >1 month
Signs	Oral candidiasis/leucoplakia, tinea, dermatitis/eczema/folliculitis, pityriasis versicolor, impetigo, molluscum contagiosum/warts, herpes simplex, herpes zoster, hepatosplenomegaly, PUO >2 months, persistent generalized lymphadenopathy
Investigations	HIV isolation, HIV antibody positive, lymphocytopenia, thrombocytopenia, anaemia, raised ESR, anergy to three common antigens ↓ CD4 lymphocyte count

* To qualify for a diagnosis of AIDS related complex (ARC) the patient must have 2 symptoms, 2 signs and 2 positive investigations.

AIDS: severe immunodeficiency due to HIV infection. There is evidence of life threatening opportunistic infections and/or unusual tumours (*pneumocystis pneumonia,* cerebral toxoplasmosis, CMV, cryptosporidiosis, cerebral lymphoma, non-Hodgkin's lymphoma, mycobacterial infection, Kaposi's sarcoma). Neurological problems (encephalopathy, myelopathy, neuropathy, encephalitis, demyelination and retinitis) are all common and may be present in up to 50% of cases.

Investigations • Detection of virus/viral antigen: time consuming, expensive and not generally available • Detection of antibody (HIV antibody test): seroconversion usually occurs about 2 months after exposure to the virus. Techniques include ELISA assays and Western blot • Lymphocytopenia <1.5

$\times 10^9/1$ • Reduced T4(CD4) Lymphocyte (helper/inducer) cell count $< 0.4 \times 10^9/1$ • Throbocytopenia $<150 \times 10^9/1$ • Anaemia • Raised ESR • Increased IgA level • Anergy to 3 recall antigens • Decreased HIV p24 antibody level • Increased HIV p24 antigen level.

Management No satisfactory antiviral drug has been produced yet and all the currently available drugs have important toxic adverse reactions.

Zidovudine (AZT): analogue of the nucleic acid thymidine. Acts by interrupting the transcription of viral RNA to DNA by inhibiting viral DNA polymerases. Half-life 1 hour and is able to penetrate the CNS. Metabolized in the liver. Adverse reactions include nausea, vomiting, bone marrow suppression and myalgia.

Other anti-HIV drugs are currently being developed and may have a role to play in the future (γ-interferon, ribavarin and deoxycytidine). An effective HIV vaccine is also being sought. The most important aspect of HIV control is the avoidance of possible risk factors and education with the adoption of 'safer sex' techniques ($\rightarrow$ Table 12.13).

Table 12.13
Safer sex guidelines

Avoid casual sexual contact with multiple partners
Avoid unprotected sexual intercourse with casual partners (use a condom)
Avoid high risk activities – anal sex, sex acts which draw blood
Regular venereological screening for high risk groups – prostitutes

KAPOSI'S SARCOMA

Commonest tumour in AIDS and is present in 25% of cases. May affect any organ although CNS involvement is rare. Usually multifocal at presentation and is locally invasive.

Clinical features Commonly affects the skin and presents as a firm, non-tender, non-pruritic, purple coloured lesion in the skin or subcutaneous tissue. May be initially mistaken for a bruise.

Investigations • Biopsy reveals spindle-shaped cells, intracellular clefts and extravasated RBCs.

> *Management* Unsatisfactory. Local radiotherapy is useful. Chemotherapy: α-interferon or vinblastine and bleomycin may be needed in rapidly advancing cases but this may provoke the development of opportunistic infections.

PNEUMOCYSTIS CARINII PNEUMONIA

Commonest life threatening opportunistic infection in AIDS and is the presenting feature in 50% of cases. Due to a protozoan.

Clinical features Gradually increasing breathlessness (may be over months), fever, lethargy, retrosternal chest discomfort, cough (worse on inspiration), night sweats, tachycardia, tachypnoea, occasionally cyanosis. Chest auscultation may reveal scanty crackles.

Investigations ● CXR shows typical bilateral, diffuse perihilar interstitial shadowing with relative sparing of the peripheral lung fields until late in the disease ● ABG reveals hypoxaemia and often hypocapnia. Hypoxaemia is most marked following exercise (using finger oximetry) ● Decreased KCO and abnormalities on gallium scanning are early features ● Sputum induced by hypertonic saline is useful ● Bronchoscopy with bronchoalveolar lavage and transbronchial biopsies may be needed to confirm the diagnosis and exclude other opportunistic infections.

> *Management* High-dose cotrimoxazole 4 tabs qid. The drug should be given iv initially followed by the oral preparation. Adverse reactions are common and include rashes, fever and BM suppression (use folinic acid supplements). Alternatively pentamidine 4 mg/kg/day can be used (slow intravenous infusion or via nebuliser) but this drug often produces hypoglycaemia and hypotension. If neither drug can be tolerated trimethoprim plus dapsone may be effective. Prophylaxis against further infections can be undertaken using cotrimoxazole 960 mg/day or 960 mg 3 times a week or using nebulized pentamidine 300 mg once per month (via a Mizer type system). Bronchospasm may be minimized by using nebulized salbutamol before pentamidine.

CRYPTOSPORIDIUM

Protozoan which may produce diarrhoea, malabsorption, weight loss, fever and abdominal pain.

Investigations • Stool culture (oocytes) • Small-bowel biopsy which can also exclude other causes of diarrhoea (*salmonella*, mycobacteria, *giardia*, *campylobacter*).

Management This is with spiramycin 1 g 6-hourly in combination with anti-diarrhoeal agents (codeine, loperamide) and adequate hydration.

NON-SPECIFIC URETHRITIS

Also known as non-gonococcal urethritis. Commonest sexually transmitted disease in the UK. Incubation period 7–21 days. Due to *Chlamydia trachomatis* in most cases but may be caused by *Ureaplasma urealyticum*, *Trichomonas vaginalis*, HSV and *Candida*. May be promoted by stress, alcohol or frequent change of sexual partner.

Clinical features Insidious onset and produces only mild discomfort (rather than the abrupt onset dysuria with gonococcal urethritis).

Investigation • By exclusion of gonococcal infection.

Management Tetracycline 500 mg qds for 5 days for each sexual partner.

SYPHILIS

Systemic infection due to the spirochaete *Treponema pallidum*. Incubation period 10–90 days. The time interval dividing early from late syphilis is two years. For classification → Table 12.14.

Table 12.14
Classification of syphilis infection

Congenital		
Acquired	Early	Primary
		Secondary
		Latent
	Late	Latent
		Tertiary
		Quaternary

Clinical features

Primary: small papule which erodes to form a small painless ulcer at the site of infection (chancre). Serous exudate from this ulcer is highly infectious. Painless, rubbery regional lymphadenopathy occurs.

Secondary: begins 1–4 months after healing of the primary chancre. Generalized, non-pruritic macular rash (may involve palms and soles), flat papular condylomata lata develop in moist areas (eg perianally), generalized painless lymphadenopathy, superficial ulceration on mucous membranes ('snail-track' ulcers), fever, arthritis, anterior uveitis, hepatosplenomegaly and meningitis may occur. The disease can then enter a latent stage which may last many years.

Tertiary: chronic infection which may appear 30 years after the primary stage and involves gumma formation in bones, skin and subcutaneous tissues. The disease may finally progress to the quarternary stage.

Quaternary stage: The main systems involved are cardiovascular and nervous systems (aortic dilatation, aortic valve incompetence, tabes dorsalis, Argyll Robertson pupils – small, irregular, unequal, do not react to light but respond to convergence and show an impaired response to mydriatics – general paralysis of the insane and meningovascular syphilis). The features of neurosyphilis are due to either endarteritis obliterans or to the formation of localized gummatae.

Congenital syphilis may result in spontaneous abortion, stillbirth or foetal abnormalities, failure to thrive, rash, iritis, bone and teeth involvement, VIII nerve deafness, tabes, paralysis and early death.

Differential diagnosis HSV, traumatic genital ulceration, drug eruption, lichen planus, viral warts, HSV, IM, AIDS, *condyloma acuminata* and yaws.

Investigations ● *T. pallidum* can be identified by dark ground microscopy of serum from primary chancre or secondary mucous patches ● Serological tests are positive 1 month after infection. VDRL is a non-specific test and may be falsely positive in infectious mononucleosis (IM), SLE, malaria and leprosy. It may also be negative in tertiary and quaternary cases. TPHA or FTA are more sensitive and specific. These tests can be carried out on blood or CSF. An antitreponemal IgG ELISA test is now available and is both sensitive and specific, titres <0.9 are negative, 0.9–1.1 are equivocal and values >1.1 are positive ● The CSF in neurosyphilis shows increased protein (gamma globulin fraction), lymphocytosis and positive serology.

Management   Penicillin (long acting im procaine penicillin 600 mg/day for 10–12 days in primary, 14–15 days in secondary, tertiary and latent cases and 21 days in quaternary). The Jarisch-Herxheimer reaction 6–12 hours after the first penicillin injection may occur and is a febrile episode due to release of endotoxin from dead spirochaetes. In cases of penicillin allergy tetracycline 500 mg/day for up to 28 days can be used. Contact tracing should also be undertaken.

GONORRHOEA

Due to Gram-negative intracellular diplococcus *Neisseria gonorrhoeae*. Incubation period 2–10 days.

Clinical features   Urethritis with dysuria and mucopurulent discharge (may be asymptomatic in 50% females), prostatitis, salpingitis, pelvic inflammatory disease, pustular/erythematous rash on limbs, arthritis, rarely endocarditis and meningitis. In male homosexuals pharyngitis or proctitis may be produced.

Differential diagnosis   *Chlamydia trachomatis*, ureaplasma urealyticus, Reiter's disease, or candidiasis.

Investigations   • Gram stain and culture of discharge, blood culture or joint aspirate.

Management   im procaine penicillin 2.4 mg + probenecid 1 g orally as single dose, or ampicillin 2 g + probenecid 1 g orally as single dose. If penicillin allergy exists cotrimoxazole 8 × 480 mg tablets as a single dose. If drug resistance is present cefotaxime can be used.

268

Abscess: collection of pus in a cavity >1.0 cm in diameter.

Angioedema: diffuse oedema which extends to the subcutaneous tissues.

Annular: ring like.

Arcuate: curved.

Atrophy: thinning due to diminution of all the layers of the skin and subcutaneous fat.

Bulla: circumscribed elevation of skin >0.5 cm diameter and containing fluid.

Circinate: circular.

Comedo: plug of keratin and sebum wedged in a dilated pilosebaceous orifice. Open comedones are blackheads.

Crust: flake composed of dried blood or tissue fluid.

Cyst: epithelial lined cavity containing fluid or semi-solid material.

Discoid: disc like.

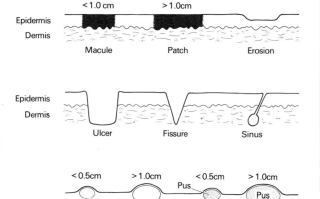

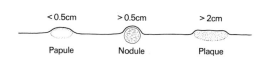

Fig. 13.1
Skin lesions.

Erosion: area of skin denuded by a complete or partial loss of the epidermis.

Erythema: area of reddened skin which blanches on pressure.

Excoriation: an ulcer or erosion produced by scratching.

Fissure: slit in the skin.

Gyrate: wave like.

Haematoma: swelling from gross bleeding in dermis or deeper structures.

Koebner phenomenon: the occurrence of skin lesions (eg psoriasis) at the site of skin trauma.

Lichenification: thickened skin with exaggerated skin lines.

Macule: small flat area of altered colour or texture <1.0 cm.

Nodule: solid palpable mass in the skin >0.5 cm in diameter.

Nummular: round or coin like.

Papilloma: nipple-like mass projecting from the skin.

Papule: small solid elevation of skin <0.5 cm diameter.

Patch: macule >1.0 cm in diameter.

Petechiae: pinhead sized macules of blood in the skin.

Plaque: elevated area of skin >2.0 cm diameter but without any depth.

Poikiloderma: combination of atrophy, reticulate pigmentation and telangectasia.

Purpura: large macule or papule of blood in the skin which does not blanch on pressure

Pustule: visible accumulation of pus in the skin.

Retiform and reticulate: net like.

Scale: a flake arising from the horny layer.

Scar: permanent replacement of normal skin structures by fibrous tissue as a result of healing.

Sinus: cavity or channel that allows the escape of pus or fluid.

Stria: a streak-like, linear, atrophic, pink, purple or white lesion due to changes in the connective tissue.

Telangiectasia: visible dilatation of cutaneous blood vessels.

Tumour: enlargement of the tissues by normal or pathological material or cells that form a mass usually >1.0 cm in diameter.

Ulcer: area of skin from which the whole of the epidermis and at least the upper part of the dermis has been lost.

Vesicle: circumscribed elevation of skin <0.5 cm in diameter and containing fluid.

Weal: elevated white compressible evanescent area produced by dermal oedema usually surrounded by a red axon mediated flare.

PSORIASIS

A chronic relapsing and remitting papulo-squamous skin disease which affects both sexes equally, may appear at any age and involve any part of the skin. The incidence is approximately 1–2% in the Caucasian population.

Clinical features Erythematous, scaly lesions commonly involving the extensor aspects of the knees, elbows and scalp. Each lesion is elevated, palpable and topped by greyish-white scales. If the lesions are rubbed pinpoint bleeding occurs from dilated superficial capillaries (Auspitz's sign).

Variants
Guttate: commoner in children, multiple small lesions mainly on the trunk.
Seborrhoeic: classical scalp lesions associated with lesions in the groins, axillae and inframammary regions.
Erythrodermic: extensive erythema leading to loss of thermoregulation and high-output cardiac failure.
Pustular: sterile pustules at the advancing edge of psoriatic lesions.

May be asymtomatic or pruritic. Usually runs a chronic course. Nail involvement is common – pits, ridges, onycholysis, subungual hyperkeratosis and discolouration. Mutilating seronegative psoriatic arthropathy may be present and involves the distal interphalangeal and sacroiliac joints. A higher incidence of arthropathy is seen in patients with nail changes. Scalp hair may be thin.

Differential diagnosis Reiter's disease, lichen planus, pityriasis rosea; seborrhoeic dermatitis and pityriasis rubra pilaris.

Investigation ● Clinical diagnosis ● If in doubt perform a skin biopsy.

Management

Topical: coal tar preparations (<1–20% ointment, paste or lotion) as antimitotic agent+/– salicylic acid as a keratolytic agent. These preparations are grey or black and tend to stain clothes and bedding and are unsuitable for use on the face and scalp. Alternatively anthralin or dithranol can be used as they are cosmetically more acceptable than tar. Scalp lesions are commonly treated with salicylic acid preparations (2–20%), light oils (olive oil) or tar shampoos.

Ultra violet light: commonly in association with systemic psoralens (PUVA) is now established for widespread disease but concern still exists over possible long-term adverse reactions (eg skin malignancy).

Cytotoxic drugs: methotrexate or hydroxyurea may be indicated in a small proportion of severely affected patients attending dermatology clinics.

Topical steroids: use is controversial with often only a short-lived response and more unstable disease when discontinued. Possible pituitary-adrenal axis suppression is also a drawback. The management of both nail changes and psoriatic arthropathy is largely unsatisfactory.

Retinoids: Analogs of vitamin A are currently showing much promise in severe cases but adverse reactions can prove troublesome eg hypercholesterolaemia, LFT abnormalities, ossification of the paraspinal ligaments, DISH syndrome (disseminated interstitial skeletal hyperostosis) and teratogenicity. Refinement of these agents, perhaps in combined modality therapy (eg with PUVA) may be successful.

LICHEN PLANUS

A condition of unknown aetiology characterized by intensely pruritic flat topped papules most commonly seen on the inner aspect of the wrists and elbows. The mucous membranes are usually affected and spontaneous resolution often occurs.

Clinical features Intensely itchy shiny red or purple papules on the skin. The lesions inside the mouth or on the genitalia may be asymptomatic. With time the skin lesions become violaceous and develop a fine white network on their surface (Wickham's striae). As in psoriasis, new lesions appearing at sites of trauma (Koebner's phenomenon) is a feature of the active disease.

Differential diagnosis Usually clearcut. Psoriasis, contact dermatitis or drug induced eruption.

Investigation • Clinical diagnosis • Occasionally a biopsy is required.

Management Systemic antihistamines, 1–2% menthol in calamine lotion, weak coal tar preparations or topical steroids may be required to combat the intense itch. Intradermal or even systemic steroids may be needed in severe cases. Vitamin A (retinoic acid) or the newer synthetic retinoids may also be useful.

PITYRIASIS ROSEA

A self-limiting disorder characterized by the development of asymptomatic erythematous macules on the trunk. Increased incidence in spring and autumn possibly due to viral infection.

Clinical features Herald patch: an isolated erythematous area on the trunk with a peripheral collar of fine scales followed by oval macules on the trunk ('Christmas-tree' distribution), thighs and arms. Purpuric lesions are rare. Usually remits spontaneously in 4–8 weeks.

Differential diagnosis Drug eruptions, pityriasis versicolor, secondary syphilis, guttate psoriasis.

Investigations ● Usually clinical ● Rarely a biopsy is needed.

Management Reassurance as the disease is self limiting. Topical antipruritic (eg 1–2% menthol in calamine or aqueous cream). Neither topical or systemic corticosteroids are usually indicated.

ECZEMA (DERMATITIS)

A chronic remitting pruritic cutaneous disorder which may be caused by a variety of genetic and environmental factors.

Exogenous: irritant, allergic contact and photodermatitis.

Endogenous: (constitutional) atopic, seborrhoeic, discoid (nummular), pompholyx gravitational (stasis).

Unclassified: asteatotic, neurodermatitis, juvenile plantar dermatosis.

Clinical features May be divided into acute, subacute and chronic phases. All three phases may coexist simultaneously.

Acute: redness and swelling, usually with an ill-defined border. Papules, vesicles, large blisters, crusting, white dermatographism and scaling may be present.

Subacute: erythema and crusting are present without the extreme oedema and exudation of acute reactions.

Chronic: less vesicular and exudative, more scaly, pigmented and thickened. More likely to be lichenified and have fissures. Asthma and rhinitis are often associated with the atopic form.

Differential diagnosis Psoriasis, fungal infections, scabies, lichen planus, angio-oedema, pityriasis rosea, drug reactions, head lice.

Investigations ● Usually clinical diagnosis.

● *Atopic:* patch testing, serum IgE levels, specific antigen detection (Radio Allergo Sorbent Test=RAST)

● *Contact:* search for any possible sensitizing antigen (patch test if necessary). Biopsy may be required. Exclude fungal infections by culture of scrappings.

Management

Acute: apply wet dressing impregnated with 1% ichthamol in calamine lotion or 1:8000 solution of potassium permanganate to weeping sites. Each soaking followed by a smear of corticosteroid cream or lotion. Preparations containing tar or ichthamol applied on top of the steroid reduce the quantity of steroid required. Systemic antihistamines can be used to control itch.

Subacute: steroid creams or lotions (dose depends on the severity of the attack).

Chronic: steroids in an ointment base, or ichthamol and zinc cream. Treat the associated dry skin with emollients (eg oilatum). Avoid perfumed soaps. Bacterial superinfection can often be controlled by the incorporation of antibiotics (eg neomycin) or antiseptics (eg vioform) into the steroid formulation. A short course of systemic corticosteroids may be needed in severe attacks. Avoid precipitating antigen if possible.

Complications Higher incidence of warts and fungal infections in the atopic form. Occasionally widespread viral infections (eg herpes simplex or vacinnia Kaposi's varicelliform eruption). Time may be lost from work or alternative employment may be necessary.

ACNE VULGARIS

A disorder characterized by comedones, papules, and pustules centered on the pilosebaceous follicles. Affects most teenagers, usual age of onset is between 12–14 years. Androgens stimulate sebum secretion. Genetic factors may be important. The role of *Corynebacterium acnes* is uncertain.

Clinical features Comedomes, papules and pustules on the forehead, nose, chin, upper chest and back. In severe cases the whole face may be involved and the lesions may heal with scarring. The skin is usually greasy.

Variants:

Tropical: affects young Caucasians in hot humid environments.

Steroid: patients on systemic steroids.

Chemical: due to contact with cutting oils or chlorinated hydrocarbons.

Infantile: rare, exclude androgen secreting tumour.

Differential diagnosis Drug eruptions (eg anti-epileptics and anti-tuberculous medication), rosacea and pyogenic folliculitis.

Investigation ● Clinical diagnosis.

Management

Local: regular cleansing with soap and water or anti-bacterial cleansers (eg chlorhexidine), benzoyl peroxide (begin with 2.5% solution), abrasive pastes, topical antibiotics (eg tetracycline, clindamycin), sulphur preparations, alcoholic solutions of aluminium chloride, cosmetic camouflage.

Systemic: antibiotics (eg tetracycline 250 mg 4 times a day for at least 4 months, may be needed for a year or two) but avoid in pregnancy. Tetracycline may produce stained teeth and dental hypoplasia in children. Hormonal treatment with a combined antiandrogen/oestrogen pill (2 mg cyproterone acetate and 0.035 mg ethinyloestradiol) may be useful in women only. Retinoids (eg 13-cis-retinoic acid) inhibit sebum excretion, the growth of *C. acnes* and acute inflammatory processes but are reserved for severe or resistant cases. There is little evidence to suggest that the avoidance of certain foods (eg chocolate) helps.

Physical: ultraviolet B radiation, local exision of cysts, intralesional injections of steroids, dermabrasion or collagen injections.

ROSACEA

The association of facial erythema, flushing, and acneform features in adults.

Clinical features Cheeks, nose, centre of forehead and chin are commonly affected with sparing of the periorbital and perioral areas. Intermittent flushing is followed by fixed erythema and telangiectasia. Papules, pustules and nodules but no comedones or seborrhoea occur. Rhinophyma and lymphoedema may be present. Ocular complications can occur (eg blepharitis, conjunctivitis, keratitis, corneal ulceration).

Investigation • Clinical diagnosis.

Management Systemic antibiotics (eg tetracycline 250 mg b.d. for 3–6 months) are the mainstay, topical agents are of doubtful help (eg 2% sulphur or 2% ichthamol), topical steroids should be avoided as rebound flare-ups occur. Sunscreens are useful. Severe rhinophyma may need surgery.

PEMPHIGUS

A group of conditions characterized by the formation of blisters in the epidermis. An antibody is directed against the intercellular substance of the epidermis. Acantholysis occurs in which individual keratinocytes lose their normal intercellular bridges and they may be seen floating freely in the resultant blister.

Varieties: vulgaris, foliaceus, vegetans and erythematosus.

Clinical features Painful mouth and genital ulcers followed by fragile skin blisters. Clinically normal skin may demonstrate the Nikolsky's sign – if lateral pressure is put on the skin surface with the thumb the epidermis appears to slide over the underlying dermis.

Investigations • Skin biopsy (immunoflurescent – IgG and C3 binding in intercellular area of epidermis) • circulating IgG intercellular antibodies.

Management Systemic steroids (may need 60–100 mg/d initially reducing slowly to a probable lifelong maintenance dose). Steroid sparing immunosuppressives (eg azathioprine or cyclophosphamide) or plasmaphoresis may be useful. Topical treatment is symptomatic to protect raw skin and prevent infection (eg ripple beds).

BULLOUS PEMPHIGOID

A chronic blistering disorder characterized by large tense blisters on an erythematous base. Commoner than pemphigus in the UK, may be associated with malignancy. The blister is subepidermal and as such they are relatively resilient and may remain intact for days.

Clinical features Itchy blisters with an eczematous base on the arms and thighs. Oral lesions are less common than in pemphigus.

Investigations • Skin biopsy, (immunoflurescent – linear band of IgG and C3 along the basement zone between the epidermis and the dermis) • circulating IgG antibodies.

Management Systemic steroids (begin with 60–100 mg/d but the dose can usually be reduced slowly and eventually stopped). Dapsone can also be a very useful single or adjuvant therapy.

DERMATITIS HERPETIFORMIS

An intensely itchy blistering condition associated with a gluten-sensitive enteropathy. M>F. Blisters are subepithelial but smaller than pemphigoid. Aggregations of leucocytes are present at the tips of dermal papillae ('microabscesses'). No circulating antibody to skin has yet been discovered.

Clinical features Intense burning itch on the affected sites (eg scalp, scapula, buttocks and elbows). Small blisters are quickly excoriated leaving raw lesions. Most patients have no evidence of malabsorption but a jejunal biopsy should be performed and reveals villous atrophy.

Investigations • Skin biopsy of surrounding uninvolved skin (immunofluroscent – granular deposits of IgA and C3 in the dermal papillae and superficial dermis) • jejunal biopsy • antibodies to muscle endomysium.

Management Gluten-free diet, dapsone or sulphapyridine (can both cause rashes, haemolytic anaemia, leucopenia, methaemoglobinaemia and peripheral neuropathy).

ERYTHEMA MULTIFORME

An erythematous disorder characterized by annular target lesions which may develop into blisters. Often of unknown aetiology (50%) but may be secondary to viral (eg herpes simplex or orf), fungal, parasitic or bacterial infection (eg mycoplasmal pneumonia), drugs, pregnancy, or malignancy.

Clinical features   Symptoms of an URTI followed by annular lesions on the palms, soles, legs and forearms. Lesions enlarge but clear centrally to form 'targets'. Blisters may occur. The Stevens-Johnson variant is the association of erythema multiforme with fever and mucous membrane involvement. Severe lesions in the tracheobronchial may produce asphyxia or corneal ulceration may lead to blindness. The lesions appear in crops.

Differential diagnosis   Urticaria, pemphigus, pemphigoid, dermatitis herpetiformis.

Investigations   ● Clinical diagnosis ● Skin biopsy ● Search for a cause: Tzanck smears, viral culture from scrapings, CXR, atypical pneumonia titres, autoantibodies and drug history.

Management   Identify and remove the cause if possible. Antihistamines; systemic steroids may be needed in Stevens-Johnson syndrome. Prevent secondary infection and dehydration. Acyclovir (200 mg 5 times daily orally for 5 days or 5–10 mg/kg 8-hourly iv for 10 days) if herpes simplex infection is present.

SKIN TUMOURS

An important factor in the aetiology of skin tumours is excessive exposure to sunlight (especially ultraviolet light in the UVB 280-320 nm part of the spectrum). The risk is higher in fair skinned Caucasians. Genetic factors may be important.

PREMALIGNANT CONDITIONS

Actinic keratoses (senile keratoses)
Multifocal scaly, hyperpigmented or ulcerated lesions. Use sunscreens eg 4% mexenone (Uvistat) prophylaxis. Cryotherapy, local exision or topical cytotoxic preparations (eg 5-fluouracil) for established lesions.

Kerato-acanthoma
May follow exposure to photosensitizing chemicals (eg tar or mineral oils) or after immunosuppresion. Grows rapidly as a papule which develops into a nodule and may rarely transform into a squamous carcinoma. Excise or curette and cauterize.

Intra-epithelial carcinoma (Bowen's disease)
Slowly expanding pink, scaly plaque with a sharply defined border. May develop into an invasive squamous carcinoma. Treat by excision or cryotherapy.

BENIGN CONDITIONS

Viral warts
Caused by human papilloma virus (HPV), typical appearance, treat by wart paint containing salicylic acid. If unsuccessful after 8–12 weeks try paint containing formaldehyde or glutaraldehyde. Cryotherapy or excision may be needed.

Squamous cell papilloma
Arises from keratinocytes and may form a horn-like excrudescence – excise or curette with cautery and check histology.

Seborrhoeic keratosis (basal cell papilloma or seborrhoeic wart).
Flat, raised, or pedunculated yellow or dark brown 'stuck-on' lesions, usually multiple. Leave alone or treat by excision, cryotherapy, or curettage.

Skin tags
Excise if cosmetically unacceptable.

Melanotic naevi
Unknown cause, may be congenital or acquired (junctional, compound, intradermal, Spitz, blue or dysplastic). May swell and become painful, depigment but rarely become malignant. Signs of possible malignant transformation: enlargement, itch, increased or decreased pigmentation, irregularity of edge or surface, asymmetry, ulceration, inflammation or bleeding. Excise and examine histologically if in any doubt.

MALIGNANT CONDITIONS

Basal cell carcinoma
Commonest skin cancer, usually of middle aged or elderly, invade locally but rarely if ever metastasize. Develop on sun damaged skin on the face or in scar tissue. Initially a red nodule which expands leaving a characteristic rolled edge with central ulceration 'rodent ulcer'. Treat by surgery or radiotherapy. Excellent prognosis.

Squamous cell carcinoma
Derived from keratinocytes, often on sun-exposed skin. Hyperkeratotic, ulcerated, rapidly expanding nodule. Metastatic spread to the local draining lymph nodes and beyond may occur. Excision or radiotherapy is required.

Cutaneous malignant melanoma
Derived from melanocytes, increased sun exposure is impor-

tant in the aetiology. Risk is highest in those with dysplastic naevi or congenital melanocytic naevi. A pre-existing naevus is seen histologically in 30%. F>M by a ratio of 2:1

Varieties ● lentigo maligna ● superficial spreading and ● nodular. Treat by excision and skin grafting. Histological analysis of the tumour allows microstaging – Breslow's method assesses the height from the granular cell layer to the deepest part of the tumour. Clark's method assesses the degree of penetration. The 5-year survival is 90% with shallow tumours (<1.0 mm) but worsens with increasing penetration. Regional node clearance is required in thicker tumours (2.0–3.5 mm). Adjuvant chemotherapy may be required in advanced tumours but is rarely curative. Campaigns to educate both doctors and patients to recognize melanoma at an early curable stage are vital.

Paget's disease of the nipple
Well-defined red and scaly plaque over and around the nipple due to invasion of the epidermis by cells from an underlying intraductal breast carcinoma. Biopsy to confirm the diagnosis, mastectomy may be required.

Cutaneous lymphoma
Most originate from T cells (unlike other forms of lymphoma) eg mycosis fungoides which occurs in middle age as a pruritic cutaneous plaque which may form a nodule or ulcerate. Biopsy reveals T cell lymphoid infiltration. May progress to involve local lymph nodes or metastasize. Treat with topical steroids, ultraviolet light, PUVA or radiotherapy. Responds poorly to systemic chemotherapy and treatment is aimed at controlling the disease rather than curing it.

URTICARIA

Recurrent transient cutaneous swellings and erythema due to fluid transfer from the vasculature to the dermis. Wide spectrum exists from trivial forms to life threatening angio-oedema with laryngeal involvement. Sometimes caused by an allergy but is often mediated by non-allergic methods.

allergens: may be contacted in a number of ways – ingestion, inhalation, instillation, insertion, injection, insect bites, infestations and infections.

physical: cold, solar, heat, cholinergic, dermatographism, delayed pressure.

inherited: hereditary angio-oedema, hypersensitivity.

> *pharmacological:* due to histamine release by various agents eg drugs, food, bites, inhalants, pollens, insect venoms, animal dander.
>
> *miscellaneous:* connective tissue disorders, hyperthyroidism, diabetes, pregnancy, intestinal parasites, neoplasia.
>
> *contact and idiopathic.*

Clinical features Sudden appearance of pink, annular, itchy weals which usually disappear over a few hours. In the acute form weals may cover most of the skin surface but in the chronic form only a few weals may develop each day. Angio-oedema affects the subcutaneous tissues and may produce swelling of the tongue, laryngeal mucosa, airways, periorbital, perioral and genital mucosa.

Differential diagnosis Erythema multiforme, urticarial vasculitis, dermatitis herpetiformis, pemphigoid, erysipelas.

Investigations ● History is vital (including all drugs) ● FBC ● urinalysis ● LFTs ● CXR ● sinus X-rays ● MSU ● stool examination ● ANF, complement and C1 esterase inhibitor level ● autoantibodies.

> **Management** Eliminate the cause if possible, antihistamines (eg terfenidine 60 mg 2×day), systemic steroids should only be used in acute cases, topical agents (eg menthol 1–2% in calamine lotion) are useful in relieving itch. Subcutaneous adrenaline and maintenance of the airway may be lifesaving in acute cases. Methylprednisolone, trasylol, danazol, stanozolol and fresh plasma may all be needed in angio-oedema. Salicylates, benzoates and azo-dyes (widely used as food additives) should also be avoided as they are well recognized histamine releasing agents.

ICHTHYOSIS

> A disorder of keratinization characterized by excessive dry and scaly skin. *Varieties:* vulgaris (autosomal), nigricans (sex linked), lamellar, Refsum's syndrome, epidermolytic hyperkeratosis, acquired (secondary to Hodgkin's disease, lymphoma, leprosy, malabsorption, poor diet or sarcoidosis).

Clinical features Excessively dry scaly skin, accentuated skin creases. Appears in the first few years of life in the inherited forms and persists throughout life. Can be severely handicapping.

Investigations Usually none are required.

DISORDERS OF SKIN PIGMENTATION

ALBINISM

A condition characterized by a lack of melanin production by melanocytes in the epidermis, the eye and hair bulb. Autosomal recessive in inheritance.

Clinical features Lack of normal pigmentation, poor tolerance of sunlight, photophobia and rotatory nystagmus.

Management Avoid sun exposure, use sun barrier creams, watch for the development of skin tumours.

VITILIGO

Islands of skin depigmentation secondary to loss of normal melanocyte function. Possible genetic association (link with autoimmune disorders eg thyroid disease, Addison's disease, diabetes mellitus and pernicious anaemia).

Clinical features Sharply demarcated patches with relative lack of skin pigmentation commonly affecting the dorsum of the hands, wrists, knees, neck and around body orifices. Koebner's phenomenon is present. May improve spontaneously.

Investigations • Usually obvious but exclude fungal infection • Leprosy should be excluded by biopsy if considered relevant.

Management Artificial tanning creams, cosmetic masking creams or PUVA in selected patients. Avoid sunburn.

CHLOASMA

Hormonally stimulated increase in pigmentation mainly affecting the face in pregnancy or when taking the OCP.

Clinical features Increased pigmentation.

> *Management* Self-limiting condition. Use cosmetic masking creams.

HAIR DISORDERS

> The scalp contains approximately 100 000 hairs, we shed 100 hairs each day and each hair grows for about 1000 days.

ALOPECIA

Localized hair loss can be divided into two types:

Non scarring: alopecia areata, androgen, hair pulling habit, scalp ringworm, traction alopecia.

Scarring: burns, radiodermatitis, aplasia cutis, carbuncle, sarcoid, basal cell carcinoma, SLE, lichen planus.

Aetiololgy ($\rightarrow$ Table 13.1)

Table 13.1
Causes of diffuse hair loss

Androgenic (male pattern baldness)
Telogen effluvium (post partum, fever, 'stress')
Syphilis
Endocrine (eg hypo/hyperthyroidism)
Nutritional (eg iron deficiency)
SLE
Drug induced (eg cytotoxics, anticoagulants, ethionamide,
                carbimazole, excess vitamin A)
Alopecia areata
Trichotillomania
Hair shaft defects (eg pilo torti, monilethrix)

Alopecia areata

Characterized by either localized or generalized sudden loss of hair from the scalp or other body sites. May be a genetic link. Commoner in Down's syndrome. Two subgroups exist: ● atopic tendency ● associated autoimmune disease eg vitiligo, diabetes. No scarring occurs. Hairs plucked from the margin of the affected area are often broken leaving behind remnants that resemble 'exclamation marks' which are diagnostic. The nails are often pitted and ridged. Excluded fungal infection by scraping and the use of Wood's light. Most cases are self limiting but occasionally UVB light, intralesional steroids, topical minoxidil or wigs are useful.

HIRSUITISM

Excess growth of androgen dependant hair in a male pattern (eg beard area, abdominal wall, around the nipples). May cause marked psychological distress.

Aetiology (→Table 13.2).

Table 13.2 **Causes of hirsuitism**	
Adrenal	Cushing's syndrome, virilizing tumours, congenital adrenal hyperplasia
Pituitary	Acromegaly
Ovarian	Polycystic disease, virilizing tumours, gonadal dysgenesis
Turner's syndrome	
Iatrogenic	Due to androgenic drugs
Idiopathic	Target organ hypersensitivity

Investigations • Exclude an underlying remediable cause. • Check menstrual history • Perform tests of endocrine function as indicated (eg diurnal cortisol levels, ACTH, dexamethasone suppression test, testosterone, glucose tolerance test with GH measurement, abdominal US, LH, FSH).

Management Treat any remediable cause as indicated. Remove excess hair by shaving, bleaching, depilatory cream or waxing.

NAIL DISORDERS

Beau's lines
Transverse ridges due to temporary interference with nail growth eg following severe illness. Usually self limiting.

Koilonychia
Loss of the normal nail contour resulting in a flat or depressed surface. Nails are brittle. Reputed to be associated with iron deficiency anaemia.

Paronychia
Inflammation of the nail fold, may be bacterial (*staphlococcal, Pseudomonas* or *Proteus*), or fungal (Candida). Exacerbated by immersion in water. Treat with appropriate antibiotic (eg flucloxacillin, nystatin or amphoteracin).

LEG ULCERATION

VENOUS

Accounts for 70–80% of lower limb ulceration. Due to incompetence of valves resulting in an increase in capillary pressure, capillary damage, fibrosis and a poorly nourished skin which is easily damaged by even minor trauma.

Clinical features Often affects obese women with a history of varicose veins and DVTs. Ulcer forms over the medial malleolus, is usually pain free and the surrounding skin is discoloured due to extravasated blood.

Differential diagnosis Exclude diabetes, sickle cell disease, RA, malignancy, syphilis.

> *Management* Weight reduction, supportive elastic stockings, protective dressings, leg elevation, clean the ulcer and dress with paraffin tulle (plain or impregnated with 0.5% chlorhexidine) or apply an absorbant dressing (eg granuflex or seaweed based). If infected apply a dressing containing eg potassium permanganate (1 in 10 000). Use diuretics if cardiac failure exists. Systemic antibiotics are reserved for spreading infections and the choice depends on swab results. Analgesia as required. Avoid systemic steroids.

ARTERIAL

Usually painful, M>F, often in association with poor peripheral circulation. Punched out in appearance and may be associated with diabetes, atherosclerosis, RA, Bucrgcr's disease and connective tissue diseases. Varicose veins are usually absent.

> *Management* Symptomatic, topical therapy as for venous ulceration, rest and warmth, sympathectomy. Systemic vasodilators are of limited use.

LYMPHOEDEMA

> Swelling of the limbs which is firm, pits poorly and is often longstanding.

Aetiology (→ Table 13.3, p 286)

Table 13.3
Causes of lymphoedema

Primary
Due to a developmental defect in the lymphatic system.

Secondary

Recurrent lymphangitis	Erysipelas
Lymphatic obstruction	Filariasis, tumour, tuberculosis
Lymphatic destruction	Tumour, radiation therapy, surgery
Unknown aetiology	Yellow nail syndrome, rosacea

Clinical features Swelling of one or more limb which may not appear until puberty or adulthood.

Management Elevation, compression bandages, diuretics and antibiotics if infection is present. Surgery is occasionally needed.

VASCULITIS

A pathological inflammatory process based primarily on blood vessel walls (mainly small and medium-sized vessels) resulting in nodules, purpura and ulceration. The different types are listed in Table 13.4.

Table 13.4:
Types of vasculitis

Predominant cell type in infiltrate	Clinical condition
Lymphocyte	Lupus pernio Chillblains SLE Erythema nodosum
Polymorph	Henoch-Schönlein purpura Polyarteritis nodosa
Granuloma formation	Pyoderma gangrenosum Temporal arteritis Erythema induratum Wegener's granulomatosis

ERYTHEMA NODOSUM

A lymphocytic vasculitis predominantly affecting the lower limbs. F>M = 5:1.

Clinical features   Painful, palpable, dusky blue-red lesions on the calves, shins and forearms, malaise, fever and arthralgia.

Aetiology   Streptococcal infections, drugs (eg sulphonamides OCP), sarcoidosis, viral and chlamydial infections, tuberculosis, ulcerative colitis, Crohn's disease, Bechet's disease, yersinia, mycoplasma, rickettsia, fungi (eg coccidioidomycosis) leprosy.

Differential diagnosis   Trauma, cellulitis, abscess, phlebitis.

Investigations   ● FBC ● ESR ● CXR ● throat swab ● ASO ● Mantoux test ● Kveim test ● acute and convalescent viral titres.

Management   Mainly symptomatic as the disease is usually self limiting. Antibiotics if due to a bacterial infection, bed-rest, NSAID for analgesia. Systemic steroids are not usually needed.

POLYARTERIS NODOSA

A rare, severe, generalized disease characterized by necrotizing polymorph arteritis.

Clinical features   Febrile, malaise, weight loss, abdominal pain, chest pain, skin ulceration, subcutaneous nodules, purpura, gangrene, splinter haemorrhages, livido reticularis, myalgia, neuropathy, hypertension and signs of renal failure.

Differential diagnosis   ● Panniculitis ● Wegener's granulomatosis ● SLE ● RA, tissue infarction.

Investigations   ● FBC ● ESR ● gammaglobulins ● RF, cryoglobulins, HBsAg may be positive ● Biopsy of involved organs (eg skin or kidneys). These investigations often yield non-specific results.

Management   Systemic steroids and steroid sparing immunosuppressives (eg azathioprine or cyclophosphamide) but the mortality remains high.

PYODERMA GANGRENOSUM

Clinical features   Characterized by large and rapidly spreading ulcers with a blue, indurated, undermined or pustular margin. Due to underlying thrombosis and vasculitis. Associated with RA, ulcerative colitis, Crohn's disease, monoclonal gammopathy or myeloma.

Investigations ● look for the underlying disease.

> *Management* Systemic corticosteroids (eg prednisolone 60–100 mg/d reducing slowly to zero). Dress with sofratulle.

TEMPORAL ARTERITIS (giant cell arteritis)

Affects large vessels of head and neck, most commonly in elderly people and is associated with polymyalgia rheumatica.

Clinical features Tender, pulseless temporal arteries in association with severe headaches. Necrotic ulcers may appear on the scalp and blindness may occur due to involvement of the retinal arteries.

Investigations ● Elevated ESR ● C-reactive protein in active disease.

> *Management* Systemic corticosteroids without delay.

WEGENER'S GRANULOMATOSIS

Granulomatous vasculitis of unknown aetiology.

Clinical features Fever, malaise, weight loss, nasorespiratory symptoms (eg hearing loss, rhinitis, haemoptysis, sinusitis), skin lesions (ulcers or papules). arthralgia, haematuria, eye, heart, lung and nerve involvement.

Investigations ● Antineutrophil cytoplasmic antibody ● elevated KCO ● CXR ● biopsy of nasal mucosa, lung or kidney.

> *Management* Cyclophosphamide alone or with corticosteroids.

HENOCH-SCHÖNLEIN PURPURA

Vasculitis which may be an allergic reaction to ingested drugs or bacteria and is associated with fever, lethargy, renal and gastrointestinal disease.

Clinical features Multiple purpuric lesions on the limbs and buttocks, fever, malaise, arthralgia, abdominal pain and haematuria. May be a preceding streptococcal sore throat.

Investigations ● Normal platelet count ● exclude connective tissue diseases and other forms of vasculitis ● May need renal biopsy ● Urinalysis.

Management Usually symtomatic as the disease is self limiting. Steroids for severe systemic disease.

BACTERIAL INFECTIONS

IMPETIGO

A superficial infection caused by either streptococci or staphylococci. Highly contagious, especially under conditions of poor hygiene.

Clinical features Thin-walled blisters which burst rapidly leaving areas of exudation and yellowish crusting, usually on the face.

Investigations ● Swab lesions and send for culture.

Management Remove crusts, apply topical antibiotics (eg fucidin), systemic antibiotics for severe cases (eg erythromycin, flucloxacillin, penicillin V). May complicate eczema or acne and may rarely lead to glomerulonephritis.

ERYSIPELAS

Cutaneous streptococcal infection with a sharply demarcated edge, commonly on the face.

Clinical features Fever, malaise, shivering followed by the development of a red skin eruption with a well defined advancing edge. Infecting organism gains entry through a small abrasion.

Investigations ● Swab but do not delay treatment.

Management Penicillin V or erythromycin.

CELLULITIS

Inflammation of the skin involving deeper tissues than erysipelas.

Clinical features Raised, hot, tender area of skin with a less well demarcated margin than erysipelas. Organism enters through an abrasion. Fever and rigors may occur.

Management Systemic antibiotics (eg penicillin V or erythromycin).

CUTANEOUS TUBERCULOSIS

Lupus vulgaris
Firm skin nodule occurring after primary infection in people with a high degree of natural immunity. F>M.

Clinical features Discrete reddish, brown nodule which may invade deeper tissues and scar. Malignant change may occur.

Investigations • diascopy (pressure with a slide) shows characteristic 'apple jelly' appearance • biopsy reveals tuberculoid granulomata.

Scrofuloderma
Cutaneous tuberculosis with involvement of the lymphatic system.

Clinical features Fistulae, abscesses and scars most commonly occurring in the neck.

Investigations • Biopsy and culture

Erythema nodosum (→ vasculitis p 287).

Erythema induratum (Bazin's disease)
Cutaneous tuberculosis with deep ulcerating nodules on the calves.

Tuberculides
Recurring crops of firm dusky ulcerating papules usually at the knees or elbows.

Management (→ Table 12.5, p 244).

LEPROSY

Infection due to *Mycobacterium leprae*.

Clinical features Depend on the degree of immune response of the patient. If high resistance exists the tuberculoid form occurs, if low resistance exists the lepromatous form occurs. The borderline form lies between the two ends of the spectrum.

Tuberculoid

Organisms hard to find, non-infectious, localized lesions and positive lepromin test. Well formed granulomata invade the dermis from within the nerve trunks. Anaesthetic depigmented plaque or macule. Palpable enlarged nerves.

Lepromatous

Many organisms, infectious, generalized lesions and negative lepromin test. Macules, papules, nodules and ulceration occurring at sites where tissue temperature is low (eg nostrils and nasal septum leading to collapse of the nasal bones).

Borderline

Some organisms, slightly infectious, scattered lesions and intermediate resistance.

Investigations ● Biopsy ● Ziehl-Neelsen stain and culture of skin or sensory nerve ● The lepromin test is of no use in diagnosing the condition but is useful in determining the form of disease which is present (eg negative in lepromatous and positive in tuberculoid).

> ***Management*** Combination of dapsone, rifampicin and clofazimine. Drugs may have to be continued for life in the lepromatous form. Two forms of lepra reactions may occur during treatment.
>
> *Type I:* (in tuberculoid and borderline) lesions become increasingly inflamed and painful and paralysis may occur.
>
> *Type II:* (in lepromatous) immune complex mediated vasculitis eg erythema nodosum.

VIRAL INFECTIONS

WARTS

Benign cutaneous tumours due to the human wart virus (human papilloma virus – HPV). Transmitted by direct contact.

Varieties: common wart (verruca vulgaris), plantar wart (verruca plantaris), anogenital, mosaic and planar.

Clinical features Raised, multiple, hyperkeratotic nodules which may develop into clusters. Demonstrate Koebner's phenomenon and may be resistant to treatment. May enlarge rapidly during pregnancy or may be large and persistent if malignancy (eg leukaemia) coexists. Some forms of genital warts may predispose to cervical carcinoma.

Differential diagnosis Plantar corns, granuloma annulare, amelanotic melanoma • molluscum contagiosum, condyloma lata, periungual fibromata of tuberose sclerosis.

Investigations • Usually clinical • Can be identified by EM • If in doubt always biopsy.

> *Management* Usually improve spontaneously, salicylic acid paint (12–20%) for 3 months, cryotherapy with liquid nitrogen or carbon dioxide, paint containing glutaraldehyde or formaldehyde. Podophyllin in soft paraffin may be useful in genital warts (not in pregnancy).

VARICELLA (CHICKENPOX)

Cutaneous infection caused by herpes varicellae.

Clinical features Malaise followed by the appearance of crops of itchy centripetal papules which develop into clear vesicles whose contents become pustular. The lesions crust then fade leaving scars. Rarely pneumonitis, secondary infection or haemorrhagic lesions.

Investigation • Usually clinical • Examine by smear and EM.

> *Management* Symptomatic, topical calamine lotion, resolution usually occurs in 7–10 days, acyclovir can be used in severe attacks or hyperimmune globulin in the immunocompromised.

HERPES ZOSTER (SHINGLES)

Cutaneous infection caused by herpes varicellae.

Clinical features Usually reactivation of virus which has remained dormant in a dorsal root ganglion since an earlier episode of chickenpox. Pain in a dermatome followed by malaise, pyrexia and a linear erythematous blistering band along this dermatome. Post-herpetic neuralgia may develop. Ramsay Hunt's syndrome is involvement of the geniculate ganglion with blistering of the external auditory meatus. The ophthalmic division of the trigeminal nerve with subsequent damage to the eye may occur. Zoster may become disseminated in the immunocompromised and may prove fatal.

Investigation • Usually clinical • If in doubt send blister fluid for culture and EM.

> *Management* Symtomatic for mild cases, systemic acyclovir for early severe infections. The management of post-

herpetic neuralgia is unsatisfactory but carbamazepine may
be helpful.

HERPES SIMPLEX

Cutaneous infection due to herpes virus hominis. Two types
have been isolated: Type 1 causes 'cold sores', Type 2 causes
genital lesions.

Clinical features

Type 1: febrile illness with painful ulcerated blistering perioral lesions and cervical lymphadenopathy which last for up to
a week and resolve spontaneously. The eye may also be involved.

Type 2: produces painful genital lesions.

Investigation • Usually clinical • If in doubt take a thick smear
and send for culture and EM • Check acute and convalescent
antibody titres.

Management Symptomatic, topical acyclovir or 5-idoxu-
ridine applied 5–6 times daily. Systemic acyclovir can be
used in severe infections. Antibiotics for secondary infections.

MOLLUSCUM CONTAGIOSUM

Cutaneous lesion caused by the pox virus.

Clinical features Elevated, smooth red papules seen on the
face, neck and trunk. The lesions have a characteristic central
punctum.

Investigation • Usually clinical • Examine debris expressed
from the lesions under microscopy and identify large swollen
epidermal cells.

Management Destructive measures which induce an inflammatory reaction eg squeezing, piercing or curetting the
lesions or applying liquid nitrogen or carbon dioxide.

ORF

A rapidly growing cutaneous lesion due to a pox virus. Usually
secondary to contact with sheep.

Clinical features Red papule which develops rapidly one week
after infection and commonly affects the finger. The lesion
may grow to 10 mm in diameter and may ulcerate. Fever,
lymphadenopathy and erythema multiforme may occur.

Management Spontaneous recovery occurs and confers immunity but if secondary infection occurs systemic antibiotics are required.

FUNGAL INFECTIONS

Two main groups of fungi affect man: dermatophyte – ringworm; candida – thrush, candidiasis.

DERMATOPHYTE INFECTIONS

Produce athlete's foot , tinea corporis, nail infections and scalp ringworm. Invade keratin only and do not penetrate living tissue, the resulting inflammation is due to metabolic products produced by the fungus or to delayed hypersensitivity. Three genera exist:

- Microsporum – nail and skin infections
- Trichophyton – nail, skin and hair infections
- Epidermophyton – skin and nail infections

Clinical features

Athlete's foot (tinea pedis): usually affects toe webs with soggy scaling. Itching may be prominent.

Ringworm (tinea corporis): itchy erythematous rash on the axillae or groins with a raised advancing edge.

Tinea infection of the nails: produces yellow discolouration with crumbling and subungual hyperkeratosis.

Scalp infections: can produce boggy swelling, pustules, kerion and scarring alopecia. Epidemics may occur in schools, public baths and swimming pools.

Investigations ● Microscopic examination of skin or nail scrapings ● Culture and examination under UV Wood's light revealing green fluorescence.

Management

Local: topical antifungal agents eg miconazole or clotrimazole.

Systemic: used for tinea infections of the scalp and nails or for skin infections which have failed to respond to topical therapy eg griseofulvin (500 mg daily for up to 18 months) but adverse reactions such as nausea, vomiting, rashes and headache may occur and it should be avoided in pregnancy, porphyria and liver disease.

CANDIDA

Normal commensal of the gastrointestinal tract but may become pathological in the immunocompromised or diabetic.

Clinical features Napkin dermatitis in infants and intertrigo affecting the submammary folds, groins and axillae in the elderly, present as shiny red areas and are characterized by satellite lesions with occasional fissures. Commonly seen on hands chronically immersed in water. May also affect mucous membranes producing raised white patches which leave raw bleeding areas if scraped. Itchy balanitis or vulvovaginitis associated with a white vaginal discharge may occur. Chronic paronychia may affect the nails. If candidiasis is generalized immunosuppression should be suspected (eg AIDS).

Investigation • Swab affected areas and send for microscopy and culture • Exclude diabetes mellitus.

Management Eliminate predisposing factors eg poorly fitting dentures, keep hands dry, topical amphotericin or nystatin (eg mouthwashes, pessaries or lozenges).

PITYRIASIS VERSICOLOR

A fungal infection of the skin due to malassezia furfur which is usually asymtomatic.

Clinical features Fawn coloured or depigmented areas with brawny scaling. Usually affects the upper trunk. Reinfection may occur.

Investigation • Usually clinical but microscopic examination of scrapings is useful • Pale yellow fluorescence under Wood's light.

Management Topical application of 2.5% selenium sulphide applied for 12 hours at weekly intervals for 3 weeks.

CUTANEOUS INFESTATIONS

SCABIES

A persistent and intensely itchy skin eruption due to the mite *Sarcoptes scabei*.

Clinical features Severe itch especially after bathing and at night. Classically affects the finger webs, fingers, wrists, elbows, areolae, genital area and periumbilical skin. Papules, linear burrows and pustules.

Investigation ● Extract the acarus from its burrow.

Management 1% gamma benzene hexachloride GBH or 25% benzyl benzoate BB applied to the entire body for a 24-hour period. One application of GBH is usually sufficient but BB may need to be applied up to 3 times. The entire family has to be treated. Crotamiton cream controls the itch. Launder all clothes and sheets.

CUTANEOUS MANIFESTATIONS OF SYSTEMIC DISEASES

Many diseases have a cutaneous component and these are listed in Table 13.5.

Table 13.5
Cutaneous manifestations of systemic diseases

Diabetes mellitus	Necrobiosis lipoidica, granuloma annulare, candida infections, staphylococcal infections, diabetic dermopathy, vitiligo, pruritus, eruptive xanthomas, neuropathic ulcers, tight waxy skin on fingers, atherosclerosis
Addison's disease	Buccal pigmentation
Acromegaly	Seborrhoea, soft tissue hypertrophy
Hypothyroidism	Alopecia, coarse broken hair, xeroderma, oedema, pruritus
Hyperthyroidism	Alopecia, pruritus, pretibial myxoedema, exophthalmos
Cushing's syndrome	Obesity, buffalo hump, acne, striae, oedema, moon face
Sarcoidosis	Erythema nodosum, lupus pernio, plaques, nodules, papules, scars, granulomata
Renal disease	Dry skin, pruritus, yellow pigmentation, 'half-and-half' nails

Table 13.5 (contd)

Porphyria	Photosensitivity, blisters, skin fragility, pigmentation, hypertrichosis, hirsuitism
Hyperlipidaemias	Xanthelasmata, xanthomata-tendinous, tuberous, planar, eruptive
Scurvy (vitamin C deficiency)	Bleeding gums, purpura, poor wound healing
Pellagra (nicotinic acid deficiency)	'3 Ds': diarrhoea, dermatitis, dementia, erythema after sunlight
Tuberous sclerosis	Shagreen patch, adenoma sebaceum, periungual fibromata
Neurofibromatosis	Cutaneous neurofibromata, axillary freckling, cafe-au-lait spots
Graft-v-host disease	Acute: morbilliform rash, skin desquamation, toxic epidermal necrolysis Chronic: pigmentation, vesicles
Malignancy	Acne, flushing, jaundice, acanthosis nigricans, erythema gyratum repens, necrolytic migratory erythema, dermatomyositis, generalized pruritus, superficial thrombophlebitis
Liver disease	Spider naevi, bruising, palmar erythema, pigmentation in PBC, xanthelasma, scratch marks, jaundice, oedema, finger clubbing, leukonychia, 'paper-money skin'

DRUG ERUPTIONS

Always be aware of the possibility of a drug related aetiology with any rash (consider all the medications that a patient is taking including over the counter preparations) (→ Table 13.6, p 298).

Management Withdraw the offending drug. In severe ana-phylactoid reactions emergency administration of subcuta-neous adrenaline (0.5 ml of 1 in 1000 solution given slowly may be life saving. Systemic antihistamines (eg 10 mg of ⟶

chlorpheniramine iv), systemic corticosteroids (100–200 mg of hydrocortisone iv followed by oral prednisolone 40–60 mg/d). The steroids can be reduced slowly to zero over 7–10 days. Nebulized salbutamol (5 mg) is needed if wheeze is present. Soothing topical therapy eg calamine lotion or 1–2% menthol in calamine cream may be helpful. Report possible drug eruptions to the Committee for Safety in Medicine (CSM).

Table 13.6
Drug reactions

Reaction	Likely drug
Urticaria	Salicylates
Toxic erythema	Sulphonamides
	Ampicillin
Acne, gingival hyperplasia	Phenytoin
Erythema multiforme	Sulphonamides
Erythema nodosum	OCP, sulphonamides
Vasculitis, purpura	NSAIDs, heparin
	Phenytoin
Psoriasis	Lithium, β-blockers
Toxic epidermal necrolysis	Phenylbutazone,
	Allopurinol
Photosensitivity	Phenothiazines
	Tetracycline
Alopecia	Cytotoxics
	Warfarin
SLE-like syndrome	Antibiotics
	Hydralazine
Exfoliative dermatitis	Gold, isoniazid
Blistering disorder	Barbiturates
	Penicillamine
Pustules	Bromide

14

Clinical chemistry

LIVER FUNCTION TESTS

The term liver function tests is used to incorporate bio-chemical analytes which reflect hepatobiliary disease rather than purely hepatic function. Abnormalities in the analytes measured are common and do not always indicate liver damage as other disorders such as septicaemia and cardiac failure may cause derangement. One of the commonest classifications of liver disorders is based on jaundice (ie obstructive vs. hepatocellular) and the first step in differen-tiation is based on whether the LFTs indicate an hepatitic or obstructive pattern.

Hepatitic damage
Biochemically this is characterized by abnormality in serum transaminase levels. The two most commonly measured are aspartate (AST or SGOT) and alanine (ALT or SGPT). The latter is more specific for liver damage. High levels occur in hepatic injury, due to leakage from hepatocytes.

Aetiology: includes hepatitis (viral, autoimmune or alcohol), paracetamol poisoning, drug hypersensitivity (eg hydralazine, isoniazid, methyldopa), circulatory failure, Wilson's disease.

Cholestasis
Obstruction of the biliary tree produces a rise in serum alkaline phosphatase. This enzyme is also raised with bone disease, puberty and pregnancy, although isoenzyme analysis can confirm the tissue of origin. In most situations abnormalities in hepatic alkaline phosphatase are accompanied by raised gamma glutamyl transpeptidase (GGTP) levels. Abnormal GGTP levels with a normal alkaline phosphatase often indicate alcohol abuse. The highest levels of alkaline phosphatase are seen with incomplete biliary obstruction.

Aetiology: includes

- Gallstones (choledocholithiasis)

- Pancreatic cancer

- Primary biliary cirrhosis

- Sclerosing cholangitis

- Metastatic liver disease.

Hepatic failure
The liver has considerable functional reserve and failure occurs only after major damage has taken place. The biochemical abnormalities that accompany liver failure are hypoalbuminae-mia, coagulopathy and jaundice. Clinical features of encepha-lopathy and ascites frequently coexist.

Isolated hyperbilirubinaemia

The commonest cause of hyperbilirubinaemia, which is usually minor, is Gilbert's syndrome which affects 3–5% of the population. The bilirubin in this condition is unconjugated, is increased by fasting and stress and is unaccompanied by any other abnormality in LFTs.

Other liver associated analytes

- α fetoprotein: raised in hepatocellular carcinoma

- Ferritin: extremely high in haemochromatosis

- Caeruloplasmin: low or absent in Wilson's disease

- α_1-antitrypsin: low or absent in α_1-antitrypsin deficiency

- IgG: raised in CAH

- IgM: raised in PBC

- IgA: raised in alcoholic liver disease.

ACIDOSIS

Acidosis, the presence of excessive hydrogen ions in body fluids, can be divided into two varieties: respiratory and metabolic. ($\rightarrow$ Fig. 14.1, p 302).

Respiratory acidosis

This occurs due to accumulation of CO_2 secondary to reduced respiratory clearance. Causes include COLD, sedatives, CVA, chronic lung disease, airway obstruction, severe acute asthma and neuromuscular disease.

Clinical features Include confusion, vasodilatation with warm peripheries, papilloedema and asterixis.

Management Improve ventilation by treatment of bronchospasm or airways obstruction, reversal of sedation or neuromuscular relaxants. Intubation and artificial ventilation may be required in severe acute cases.

Metabolic acidosis

This is due to reduction in bicarbonate ions in body fluids usually due to neutralization of bicarbonate by acids such as lactic acid ($\rightarrow$ Table 14.1, p 302) or ketones or exogenous substances such as salicylates, ethylene glycol or ethanol. In such circumstances an increased anion gap (Na-(Cl+HCO$_3$)>12 mmol/l exists. In certain circumstances metabolic acidosis exists with a normal anion gap and is due to loss of HCO_3 from the renal or GI tract.

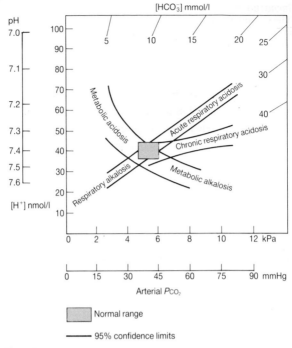

Fig. 14.1
Acid base diagram.

Table 14.1 Causes of lactic acidosis	
Group A	Shock due to any cause, respiratory failure, poisoning with cyanide or carbon monoxide; profound anaemia
Group B	Diabetes mellitus, hepatic failure, severe infection, malignant neoplasm (lymphoma, leukaemia), fits, drugs (biguanides, streptozotocin, salicylate, isoniazid, fructose, sorbitol), toxins (ethanol, methanol), congenital enzyme defects

Clinical features Hyperventilation, shock, nausea, vomiting, anorexia and coma.

> *Management* Correct the underlying abnormality such as diarrhoea, ketoacidosis, or renal failure by treating dehydration with iv fluids and instituting dialysis or insulin therapy whichever is appropriate. In only a minority of situations where acidosis is severe (pH<7.1) should bicarbonate treatment (1.26%) be considered and only the minimum administered to correct the acidosis (ie pH>7.2). During the administration of HCO_3 the serum K^+ falls and should be closely monitored. Administration of 8.4% HCO_3 is indicated only during cardiac arrest.

ALKALOSIS

Respiratory ventilation over and above that required to remove CO_2 will result in respiratory alkalosis by reducing $PaCO_2$. The causes are listed in Table 14.2. A mixed picture of metabolic acidosis and repiratory alkalosis is common in sepsis, salicylate poisoning and hepatic failure.

Table 14.2
Causes of respiratory alkalosis

Hysterical overbreathing
Assisted ventilation – overventilation
Lobar pneumonia, pulmonary embolism
Meningitis, encephalitis
Poisoning with salicylate
Hepatic failure

Clinical features Rapid deep respiration, tetany, paraesthesia particularly perioral and peripheral, light-headedness and collapse.

> *Management* This should be directed towards the cause. Sedation or rebreathing into a paper bag should be considered in those with psychogenic hyperventilation.

Metabolic

An increase in serum HCO_3 usually occurs due to loss of acid from the stomach or renal tract. Volume contraction due to excessive diuretic administration results in alkalosis as does hypokalaemia by increasing HCO_3 reabsorption. Excessive mineralocorticoids, either endogenous or exogenous results in metabolic alkalosis.

Clinical features Usually non-specific. Tetany, neuromuscular excitability, lethargy and delirium occur in acute, severe cases.

> *Management* Again treat the underlying cause eg pyloric obstruction, potassium supplementation or stop overzealous diuretic administration. Occasionally administration of acidic fluids containing ammonium chloride 70 mmol/l may be indicated.

HYPERCALCAEMIA

> The physiologically important calcium in blood is the ionized form but this is rarely assayed. The total calcium when associated with hypoalbuminaemia should be corrected by adding 0.1 to the calcium every 5 g/l the albumin is below 40 g/l).

Aetiology Over 90% of cases are due to primary hyperparathyroidism or malignancy, eg squamous cell bronchial carcinoma. Most tumour-related hypercalcaemia is caused by a peptide with PTH-like activity, although bone metastases and rarely ectopic PTH may be responsible. Other causes of hypercalcaemia include sarcoidosis, thyrotoxicosis, Addison's disease, milk-alkali syndrome, Paget's disease (if immobilized), iatrogenic (vitamin D therapy and drugs eg thiazides).

Clinical features Often asymptomatic, discovered on biochemical screening, weakness, constipation, confusion, anorexia, renal colic, polyuria, nocturia, polydipsia and proximal myopathy.

Investigation • Ionized calcium if available • serum calcium and albumin • skeletal survey • isotopic bone scan • 24-hour urinary calcium • PTH assay • parathyroid US or selective cervical vein canalization with PTH assay and • screen for malignancy.

> *Management* Mild hypercalcaemia responds well to oral phosphate 1–2 g/day. Moderate or severe hypercalcaemia should be treated with iv fluids (6–8 l/d); potassium supplements are usually required. Additional therapy with iv frusemide, prednisolone 20–40 mg/day, mithramycin and phosphates may be needed. Treatment of the underlying disease may reverse the hypercalcaemia.

HYPERKALAEMIA

A serum potassium above 5.5 mmol/l represents a medical emergency and may be due to impaired potassium excretion eg acute renal failure, potassium sparing diuretics in those with renal impairment, hypoaldosteronism, adrenal insufficiency excessive potassium intake in those with renal impairment or imbalance in internal potassium balance eg diabetic ketoacidosis, haemolysis and rhabdomyolysis.

Clinical features Often asymptomatic. Muscle weakness may be present but the most important features are cardiac with arrhythmias and conduction defects leading to asystole.

Investigations • Serum potassium • ABG analysis • ECG • creatinine clearance and • urinary potassium excretion • Low urinary excretion in those with hyperkalaemia suggests renal failure, normal excretion hypoaldosteronism and high excretion tissue potassium leakage.

Management

- 10 ml 10% calcium gluconate iv

- Insulin 10 U in 100 ml 10% dextrose over 1 hour

- Rectal or oral calcium resonium 15 g tid

- 100 ml 1.26% HCO_3 over 60 minutes iv

- Acute haemodialysis may be indicated to control hyperkalaemia particularly in those with renal failure.

Identification and treatment of the cause, such as removal of spironolactone in those with moderate renal impairment is essential.

HYPOKALAEMIA

A serum potassium <3.5 mmol/l may result from excessive renal loss eg diuretic therapy or magnesium deficiency, GI loss eg diarrhoea, vomiting, metabolic imbalance such as occurs in alkalosis, insulin therapy or in periodic paralysis, and endocrine causes such as hyperaldosteronism, Bartter's syndrome, Cushing's syndrome (severe hypokalaemia with ectopic ACTH).

Clinical features Muscular weakness, polyuria, ECG changes with U-waves and flattened T-waves, ileus.

Investigations • Serum potassium, 24-hour urinary potassium (if low suggests low intake or GI losses cf a high output which indicates a renal cause or hyperaldosteronism) • ECG.

Management Treat the underlying cause such as vomiting, discontinue diuretic therapy or supplement with KCl or a potassium sparing diuretic. If hypokalaemia is severe, or if vomiting precludes oral oral potassium supplements, iv KCl should be administered but at a rate not to exceed 20 mmol/hour.

HYPONATRAEMIA

This is commoner than hypernatraemia and is defined as a serum sodium <135 mmol/l. It indicates a relative excess of body water and can be divided into three types: • hypervolaemic: CCF, cirrhosis, nephrotic syndrome. In these urinary sodium is low (<10 mmol/l) • hypovolaemic: diarrhoea, blood loss followed by crystalloid replacement. In these situations renal sodium is low compared with primary renal causes eg excess diuretic therapy, osmotic diuresis or adrenal insufficiency where urinary sodium is high (>20 mmol/l) • normovolaemic: inappropriate ADH secretion (SIADH) eg malignancy (especially small cell bronchial carcinoma), respiratory disease, eg pneumonia, CNS disease, eg encephalitis, drugs eg opiates, chlorpropamide, tricyclics and nicotine, adrenal insufficiency and myxodema may cause normovolaemic hyponatraemia.

Clinical features Confusion, lethargy, anorexia, seizures and coma, if severe.

Investigations • Assess circulation for signs of dehydration including erect and supine BP • skin tugor and central pressure if indicated • serum and 24-hour urinary sodium levels • CXR • drug history.

Management Determine state of hydration and likely cause. Hypovolaemia responds to saline infusion whilst water restriction is appropriate in hypervolaemic states and with SIADH. Albumin infusion may be useful in cirrhosis and nephrotic syndrome. Demeclocycline, 0.9–1.2 g daily initially, which results in nephrogenic diabetes insipidus may be indicated in those with resistant SIADH. In severe hyponatraemia associated with coma or seizures controlled infusion of hypertonic saline to raise plasma sodium by 0.5 mmol/l/hour is indicated; too rapid infusion may result in central pontine myelinolysis.

HYPERNATRAEMIA

A serum sodium >150 mmol/l results from a deficiency of body water relative to total body sodium.

Aetiology

- Renal water loss eg DI, osmotic diuresis
- Extrarenal water loss eg burns, hyperventilation
- Adrenal disease eg Conn's and Cushing's disease
- Excess sodium administration or lack of water intake (eg unconscious patient).

Clinical features Confusion, seizures and coma. When hypernatraemia is severe cerebral thrombosis or haemorrhage may occur.

Investigations • Serum, 24-hour urinary and spot urinary sodium • Plasma and urine osmolality • CVP monitoring may be useful particularly in measuring fluid replacement • Consider DI, Cushing's and Conn's disease.

Management In normovolaemic or hypervolaemic states loop diuretic therapy in conjunction with the slow administration of 5% dextrose should be undertaken to correct plasma osmolality. In hypovolaemic states fluid replacement with dextrose-0.45% saline is appropriate. Treatment of patients with cranial diabetes insipidus require iv/im vasopressin followed by intranasal desmopressin whilst those with nephrogenic DI require sodium restriction and thiazide diuretics.

HYPERLIPIDAEMIA

This is a common disorder and is defined as an increase in serum cholesterol and/or triglyceride beyond the reference range in the population. Lipid is carried in blood as: chylomicrons, large triglyceride rich molecules transporting fat from the intestine to adipose tissue and muscle; VLDL (very low density lipoproteins), smaller particles which transport endogenous triglyceride from the liver; LDL (low density lipoprotein) cholesterol rich particles derived from VLDL once triglyceride has been removed via IDL (intermediate density lipoprotein) and HDL (high density lipoprotein), small particles which carry cholesterol from peripheral cells to the liver.

Definition Hyperlipidaemia is usually defined according to the various abnormalities in the proportions of chylomicrons, VLDL, LDL and HDL (→ Table 14.3, p 308).

Table 14.3
Definition of hyperlipidaemia

Type	Name	Lipoproteins elevated	Diet
I	Hyperchylomicro-naemia	chylomicrons	↓ fat
IIa	Familial hypercholesterolaemia	LDL	↓ cholesterol ↓ saturated fat
IIb	Mixed hyperlipidaemia	LDL+VLDL	↓ cholesterol ↓ saturated fat ↓ weight ↓ carbohydrate
III	Broad B disease	IDL	as for IIb
IV	Familial hypertriglyceridaemia	VLDL	↓ carbohydrate ↓ weight
V	I+IV	chylomicrons+VLDL	↓ carbohydrate ↓ weight

Types IIa, IIb and IV are common and important risk factors for the development of atheroma. Type IIa may be primary or secondary to hypothyroidism, nephrotic syndrome or cholestasis. It results in corneal arcus, tendon and tuberous xanthomata. Type IIb is common in association with diabetes mellitus and produces corneal arcus and xanthelasma. Type IV may be primary or secondary to diabetes mellitus, obesity and alcoholism and produces eruptive cutaneous xanthomata. Type III is rare but notable for its association with palmar xanthomata. Many drugs eg thiazides and β-blockers are associated with hyperlipidaemia.

Management Treatment of the underlying disease eg thyroxine replacement in hypothyroidism, improvement of diabetic control, reduction in alcohol intake is of value. In all patients who are obese weight reduction must be achieved. Dietary advice should be given and smoking must be stopped. Drug therapy is indicated in severe cases. Nicotinic acid, cholestyramine and colestipol reduce cholesterol and triglycerides. Probucol lowers LDL and HDL and is used for resistant cases. Bezafibrate lowers LDL and triglycerides whilst increasing HDL. Many new drugs such as gemfibrozil and acipimox are available and their place in therapy requires clarification.

15

Medical emergencies

This should be recognized in a patient who has collapsed and in whom the carotid or femoral pulses are absent. The brain suffers irreversible damage within minutes of circulatory failure and throughout resuscitation an adequate cardiac output should be maintained.

Management

- DC cardioversdion should be undertaken at the earliest opportunity once VF is recognized, although this is often delayed until resusitation equipment arrives.

- A precordial thump may restart cardiac rythmn.

- Place the patient supine and elevate the legs.

- Initiate cardiac massage at a rate of one beat per second.

- Start artificial ventilation by mouth to mouth ventilation or more commonly, after insertion of an oropharyngeal airway, by means of an ambu bag. One ventilation per 4–5 cardiac massages is recommended.

- Insert an iv line and administer 100 ml 8.4% $NaHCO_3$, followed by 10 ml/minute.

- Establish ECG monitoring.

- If VF defibrillate with 200 or 400J followed by iv lignocaine 100 mg over 2 minutes and a lignocaine infusion. If this is unsuccessful drugs to consider include practolol 10 mg iv, propranolol 1–2 mg iv, phenytoin 100 mg and bretylium tosylate 5 mg/kg.

- If asystole administer 5 ml 1:10 000 iv adrenaline via a central line. If unsuccessful give 0.6 mg atropine and 10 ml 10% calcium gluconate iv. Continue cardiac massage throughout. Intracardiac adrenaline and/or calcium occasionally is effective where iv administration fails.

- If electromechanical dissociation ie no output with a normal ECG give calcium gluconate 10% 10 ml and consider pericardial tamponade.

- If complete heart block give 0.6 mg atropine followed by isoprenaline (2 mg per 500 ml 5% dextrose) administered at an infusion rate to produce a response. If none consider emergency pacing.

- Atrial fibrillation rarely produces the picture of cardiac arrest but when present should be treated by cardioversion (400J), verapamil 5 mg by slow iv infusion or digoxin 0.75 mg by iv infusion, depending upon the clinical state.

KETOACIDOSIS

This is a true medical emergency with a mortality of 10–20% and may present in a known diabetic or those previously unknown to be diabetic.

Clinical features These are dominated by ● dehydration characterized by tachycardia, hypotension and dry, slack skin ● acidosis with deep rapid respiration (air hunger) and ● ketosis with vomiting, fetor and abdominal pain ● Drowsiness is common but unlike hypoglycaemia coma is uncommon ● Precipitating features such as infection eg pneumonia, MI or surgery may be obvious.

Investigations ● Blood glucose ● U+Es and ● blood gases.

Management

● Establish iv line.

● Administer 1000 ml normal saline over 1 hour, followed by 1000 ml over 2 hours and 500 ml 2-hourly thereafter. The CVP should be monitored in elderly patients and those with IHD.

● Start iv insulin infusion of 4–8 units /hour.

● Monitor urine output

● Administer iv potassium depending upon blood results. Even when the initial blood potassium is high 20 mmol/l of fluid replaced will be required to maintain normokalaemia and more is frequently required. Continuous ECG monitoring is useful.

● Bicarbonate replacement to correct the acidosis is rarely required. If the arterial pH is below 7 a slow infusion 100 mmol NaHCO$_3$ (1.26%) over 4–6 hours may be given. Extra potassium supplements will be required. Bicarbonate therapy has been associated with cerebral oedema and many authorities discourage its use.

● In comatose patients, where vomiting is prominent or a succussion splash is present, a nasogastric tube should be passed to empty the stomach since gastric paresis and ileus are common.

● Once the blood glucose is below 15 mmol/l 5% dextrose should be substituted for iv saline to avoid hypernatraemia.

● The precipitating cause of ketoacidosis should be sought. This may be obvious from the history eg omission of insulin but is commonly due to infection. Sputum culture, a CXRMSU, and blood cultures should be taken. Routine administration of broad-spectrum antibiotics eg ampicillin 500 mg qid are recommended by some authorities.

Constant monitoring of clinical condition, blood pressure, electrolytes and blood glucose is essential. Complications to avoid are cerebral oedema (due to too rapid lowering of blood glucose, injudicious use of bicarbonate or excess hypotonic fluids), hypoglycaemia and hypokalaemia. Cerebral oedema is a significant cause of mortality, particularly in children, as is aspiration pneumonia if a nasogastric tube is not inserted. Return to subcutaneous insulin should be delayed until the bowel sounds have reappeared and the patient has been able to tolerate light solid food without vomiting.

ACUTE SEVERE ASTHMA (→ p 67)

EPILEPTIC FIT (→ p 156)

ANAPHYLAXIS

This occurs in the clinical setting of the introduction, usually in the form of an injection, of antigen in patients already hypersensitive to the allergen eg penicillin, antisera or insect sting.

Clinical features Rapid onset (within minutes) of laryngeal spasm, pruritus, nausea and vomiting, hypotension, urticaria, cyanosis and dyspnoea.

Management Adrenaline 500–1000 μg im and an antihistamine such as chlorpheniramine 10 mg slow iv infusion. In those with severe reactions systemic steroids eg hydrocortisone 200 mg iv followed by further steroids is indicated. In hereditary angioneurotic oedema due to Cl esterase deficiency (an autosomal dominant trait) FFP followed by danazol 200–800 mg/day prophylaxis is effective.

PULMONARY EMBOLISM

This is due to the passage of a venous thrombosis usually from the deep veins in the leg or pelvis to the pulmonary artery. In many situations obvious DVT is absent. The diagnosis often relies on a high degree of clinical suspicion.

Clinical features Collapse, hypotension, sweating and tachycardia. Haemoptysis if present is suggestive.

Investigations ● ABG analysis usually demonstrates hypoxia and hypocapnia ● CXR is often normal although classically reveals wedge shaped collapse, bilateral abnormalities or a pleural effusion ● A ventilation/perfusion scan usually reveals numerous mismatched ventilation perfusion abnormalities ● ECG may show R heart strain, RBBB or a S1, Q3, T3 pattern ● Pulmonary angiography is occasionally required and is the 'gold standard' investigation.

Management ● in those with adequate systemic perfusion: iv administration of heparin at approximately 1000 units/hour with subsequent titration to keep the thrombin time 2–3× normal and oxygen 40–60% ● in those with profound hypotension thrombolytic agents such as streptokinase may be useful or in the profoundly ill surgical consultation for pulmonary artery embolectomy should be considered ● inotropic support with dobutamine 2.5–10 µg/kg/minute and dopamine 2–5 µg/kg/minute should be used in those with shock.

Oral anticoagulants, usually warfarin, should be started after 3–5 days of heparin and continued for 6 months (or lifelong in recurrent PE disease).

Prophylaxis against pulmonary emboli in those at risk eg post-MI should be with subcutaneous heparin 5000 units tid and T.E.D. support stockings. In those with recurrent PE despite anticoagulation the insertion of an IVC umbrella should be considered.

HYPOGLYCAEMIA

The biochemical definition of hypoglycaemia is a blood glucose <2.2 mmol/l although symptoms may begin at higher blood sugar levels. Causes include diabetes treated with excessive insulin or sulphonylureas, liver failure, hepatoma and Addison's disease.

Clinical features Sweating, tremor, confusion, tachycardia, and, if prolonged, coma, focal CNS signs including hemiparesis or, most serious, cerebral cortical infarction.

Investigations Immediate diagnosis and treatment is important ● A blood glucose on finger-prick testing should be obtained wherever possible and a sample taken for laboratory confirmation.

Management should not be delayed waiting for the blood glucose result. If the patient is conscious 20–30 g of readily absorbable carbohydrate (lucozade, milk) should be given orally. If the patient is unable to take oral fluid iv glucose in the form of 50% dextrose (50 ml) should be administered through a large venflon. Glucagon 0.5–1 mg im raises the blood sugar more slowly than iv glucose and should only be used in those where iv access is difficult or by relatives while awaiting medical attention. In unusual situations where iv access cannot be obtained and glucagon is unavailable or contraindicated (eg sulphonylurea induced hypoglycaemia) glucose should be administered via an nasogastric tube.

Recurrent hypoglycaemia is common in diabetics taking long-acting insulin preparations or sulphonylureas and hospital admission is required for monitoring in such cases.

HYPOTHERMIA

This is particularly likely to occur in the elderly, alcoholics and in those unexpectedly exposed to low temperature eg immersion in cold water. The diagnosis may be missed unless low reading thermometers are used in those at risk who have a low reading on an ordinary mercury thermometer. Risk factors include hypothyroidism, pituitary and adrenal insufficiency, CVA and drug/alcohol abuse.

Clinical features Cold peripheries, hypotension, pallor, confusion, cyanosis, coma, respiratory depression and bradycardia.

Investigations ● Rectal temperature using a low-reading thermometer ● U+Es, FBC ● ABG (metabolic acidosis) ● CXR and ECG (J waves may be present) ● Overdosage with drugs eg antidepressants, benzodiazepines should be considered.

Management Maintain an adequate airway, administer oxygen, iv fluids, monitor blood potassium and cardiac rhythm. If the arterial pH <7.2 consider NaHCO$_3$ 1.26% administration. Rewarming can usually be achieved by passive means by wrapping the patient in a space blanket in a warm room. Failure to rewarm passively should suggest hypothyroidism. Persistent hypotension on rewarming may result in renal failure requiring peritoneal or haemodialysis. Pneumonia is a common complication and many would advocate prophylactic antibiotics eg iv cefuroxime 750 mg tid and metronidazole 500 mg tid. Resuscitation of patients with hypothermia complicated by asystole should be continued until the patient has been rewarmed to normal temperatures. Rapid rewarming of patients by warm water baths is appropriate when they have been exposed to profound low temperatures, eg immersion in cold water.

POISONING

GENERAL MEASURE

The conscious level of the patient must be assessed immediately (eg by the Glasgow coma scale) and treatment such as assisted ventilation instituted where appropriate. Gastric lavage, to remove the poison, should only be undertaken in those who have a gag reflex and where tablets have been taken within the previous four hours with the exception of aspirin and tricyclic antidepressants which may remain within the stomach for many hours. Under no circumstances should lavage be undertaken as a punative procedure. If lavage is undertaken large volumes of fluid (many litres) may be required and should be continued until the returned fluid is clear. No more than 300 ml of water should be administered at each individual washout. The induction of vomiting with ipecacuanha (30 ml for adults and 10–20 ml for children) is an effective alternative.

In all cases irrespective of the agent implicated special attention should be paid to the patients BP, HR, respiratory rate and temperature and wherever appropriate support in the form of iv fluids, positive inotropes and assisted ventilation provided. Constant vigilance for changes in the concious level and clinical state must be maintained.

Whenever the treatment for a poisons patient is unclear advice should be sought from the regional poisons centre (for phone numbers → p 344).

Aspirin

Clinical features Hyperventilation, vomiting, dehydration, tinnitus, sweating, deafness and restlessness.

Investigation • Measure salicylate levels (levels above 3.6 mmol/l indicate significant poisoning) • blood gases • U+Es • metabolic acidosis • hypokalaemia are usual.

Management Gastric lavage if tablets were taken within 6 hours, establish an iv line and administer 1–2 l of dextrose/saline containing 20 mmol of KCl per 500 ml bag. In severe cases the addition of 500 ml 1.26% bicarbonate accelerates salicylate excretion. If renal failure coexists peritoneal or haemodialysis is effective in removing the poison. Just as in diabetic ketoacidosis careful monitoring of fluids and electrolytes is essential. Oral activated charcoal should be given in severe poisoning.

Paracetamol

Clinical features Usually non-specific although nausea and vomiting are common. Late adverse reactions due to liver damage such as hypoglycaemia, jaundice, hypotension, metabolic acidosis, renal failure and a bleeding tendency may occur in those after serious poisoning.

Investigation • Blood paracetamol levels which must be interpreted with the time since tablet ingestion (Fig. 15.1) • Serious hepatic damage can be anticipated from the drug blood level in relation to the time after overdosage • A prothrombin time at 36 hours after overdosage greater than 36 seconds indicates a high risk of developing hepatic failure.

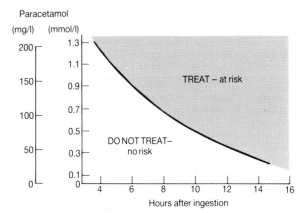

Fig. 15.1
Paracetamol venous blood levels following overdose.

Management Administration of N-acetylcysteine (150 mg/kg in 200 ml 5% dextrose over 15 min followed by infusion of 50 mg/kg in 5% dextrose 4-hourly) is effective in reducing hepatotoxicity if commenced within 16 hours of overdosage. Administration of N-acetylcysteine after 16 hours may still offer some benefit. iv dextrose should be maintained to prevent hypoglycaemia. Renal failure in those that develop hepatic failure is common and may require haemodialysis. If fulminant hepatic failure develops appropriate intensive care is indicated and for those in whom death is likely (eg

PTT >100s and creatinine >300 µmol/l or pH <7.3) consideration of hepatic transplantation is appropriate.

Benzodiazepines

Clinical features Drowsiness, confusion, ataxia, respiratory depression and hypotension. The combination of benzodiazepine and alcohol poisoning is common and has synergistic effects (eg hypotension).

Management The benzodiazepine antagonist, flumazenil, will reverse many of the sedative effects of the benzodiazepines but is short acting and repeated administration may be necessary. It should be administered by slow iv injection or infusion (eg 200 µg over 15 s followed by 100 µg per min as required to produce reversal). General supportive measures are also required in the majority.

Tricyclic antidepressants

Clinical features Many resemble anticholinergic overdosage with dry mouth, dilated pupils, urinary retention, absent bowel sounds, hypotension, hyperreflexia, convulsions, extensor plantar reflexes, cardiac conduction defects and arrhythmias. Reduced conciousness is common but deep coma is rare.

Management Gastric lavage should be undertaken in those where poisoning has occurred within the previous 12 hours because gastric stasis slows absorption. Treatment otherwise is largely supportive with iv fluids, anticonvulsants where required, sedation for delirium and urinary catheterization for retention. Although cardiac arrhythmias are common anti-arrhythmic drugs should be avoided where possible. Administration of 40 mmol $NaHCO_3$ by infusion over 20 minutes may control many arrhythmias. The administration of physostigmine salicylate 1–3 mg by slow iv injection may reverse some of the CNS affects and may improve cardiac stability. When respiratory depression is profound assisted ventilation may be indicated.

16

Pre and postoperative care

Many procedures which are common in hospital require special preparation and/or after care. The outline below is only a general guide and varies in different places and with variations of the procedure.

Table 16.1
Pre and postoperative care

	Pre	Per	Post
Endoscopy			
Upper GI	Fast >6 h. Consent. PTR for ERCP	Diazepam (dose titrated). Atropine 0.6 mg Pharyngeal Xylocaine spray. Pethidine if procedure, e.g. stricture dilatation	Fast 2 h. Close attention to respiration until awake. CXR if procedure, e.g. dilatation. Amylase if abdominal pain after ERCP
Broncho-scopy	Fast >6 h. Consent	Atropine 0.6 mg. Diamorphine (dose titrated). Oxygen (nasal cannulae) Pharyngeal Xylocaine spray	Fast 4 h. Close attention to respiration until awake. CXR if transbronchial biopsy
Colono-scopy	Colon prepared with laxatives and oral fluids only for 36 h. Consent	Diazepam (dose titrated)	Respiratory observation if sedated until awake
Ultrasound	Fast >6 h. Full bladder usually	—	—

Table 16.1 (*contd*)

	Pre	Per	Post
Surgery under GA	Fast >6 h. Consent. Often atropine 0.6 mg im. Enema if lower bowel operation. Shaving appropriate area. Consider DVT prophylaxis	GA	TPR every 15 min for 2 h, then 30 min for 2 h then 1-hourly for 12 h. Fluid balance operation recorded. Wound check
Liver/renal biopsy	Consent	Local anaesthesia	BP & HR every 15 min for 1 h, 30 min for 2 h and 1-hourly 6 h. Analgesia, e.g. Temgesic S.L. although beware masking complications
Pleural aspiration and biopsy	Consent	Local anaesthesia	TPR hourly for 4 h. CXR
Central line insertion	Consent	Local anaesthesia	CXR
Paracentesis	Consent	Local anaesthesia	If > 3 l removed administer colloid usually albumin 500 ml per 1–2 l. BP & HR hourly for 12 h ± CVP U & E & creatinine daily for 3 days

Table 16.1 (*contd*)

Special Cases

Diabetes mellitus
Minor procedure e.g. endoscopy. Admit to hospital the previous day and check diabetic control, fast overnight, omit morning insulin or oral hypoglycaemics and put first on list. Ensure blood glucose is 7–10 mmol/l. Give short acting insulin only with lunch, then normal evening insulin dose.

Major procedure, e.g. laparotomy. Fast overnight. Preop. put up iv line administering 5% dextrose 4-hourly. Preop containing 10 units soluble insulin per 500 ml, check blood glucose before and hourly during procedure. Postoperatively short acting insulin only should be administered to cover each meal until on normal diet.

Antibacterial prophylaxis for patients with prosthetic valves
For gastrointestinal procedures prophylaxis for patients with valve lesions other than prosthetic valves is not now considered necessary. Just before induction amoxycillin 1 g iv or im plus gentamicin 120 mg iv or im, followed by oral amoxycillin 500 mg 6 hours later. If hypersensitive to penicillin or received penicillin twice or more in the previous month gentamicin as above plus iv vancomycin 1 g over one hour before induction.

Jaundice
In jaundiced patients before surgery any anaemia should be corrected and the prothrombin time corrected either with vitamin K in cholestatic jaundice or FFP in those with hepatocellular dysfunction. Prophylactic antibiotics, either cefotaxime or gentamicin and ampicillin should be given before biliary tract surgery. Postoperative renal failure can largely be avoided if sepsis is excluded before surgery and adequate hydration and urine output is maintained throughout and after surgery. Diuretics such as frusemide or mannitol are indicated if urine output falls despite satisfactory hydration.

Table 16.1 (contd)

Children
Most procedures done under GA before the age of 16, and
parental consent necessary.

Consent
Just getting the patient to sign the 'consent form' is not
adequate and not medicolegally valid. The procedure should
be explained fully and the major complications discussed,
preferably in front of a witness. This should be recorded in
the notes, dated and signed.

17

Drug usage

SKIN

Urticaria
Aspirin
Penicillin
Sulphonamides

Erythema multiforme
Barbiturates
Chlorpropamide
Codeine
Phenytoin
Phenylbutazone
Sulphonamides
Tetracycline
Thiazides

Bullae
Allopurinol
Barbiturates
Penicillin
Phenylbutazone
Phenytoin
Sulphonamides

Dermatitis
Barbiturates
Gold
Penicillin
Phenylbutazone
Phenytoin
Quinidine

Fixed drug eruption
Barbiturates
Captopril
Phenolphthalein
Quinine
Salicylate
Sulphonamides

Non-specific rash
Allopurinol
Ampicillin
Barbiturates
Phenytoin

Hyperpigmentation
ACTH
Busulphan
Gold
Oral contraceptives
Phenothiazines

Erythema nodosum
Oral contraceptives
Penicillin
Sulphonamides

HAEMATOLOGICAL

Agranulocytosis
Captopril
Carbimazole
Chloramphenicol
Cytotoxics
Gold
Indomethacin
Phenylbutazone
Phenothiazines
Propylthiouracil
Sulphonamides
Tolbutamide
Tricyclic antidepressants

Aplastic anaemia
Chloramphenicol
Cytotoxics
Gold
Phenylbutazone
Phenytoin
Sulphonamides

Thrombocytopenia
Aspirin
Carbamazepine
Carbenacillin
Chlorpropamide
Chlorthalidone
Digitoxin
Frusemide
Indomethacin
Methyldopa
Phenylbutazone
Phenytoin
Quinidine
Quinine
Thiazides

Megaloblastic anaemia
Cotrimoxazole
Folate antagonists
Oral contraceptives
Phenobarbitone
Phenytoin
Primidone
Triamterene
Trimethoprim

Haemolytic anaemia
Aspirin
Cephalosporins
Chlorpromazine
Dapsone
Insulin
Isoniazid
Levodopa
Mefenamic acid
Methyldopa
Penicillin
Phenacetin
Procainamide
Quinidine
Rifampicin
Sulphonamides

Lymphadenopathy
Phenytoin
Primidone

CARDIOVASCULAR

Arrhythmias
Adriamycin
Anticholinesterases
Atropine
Digitalis
Lithium
Phenothiazines
Propranolol
Procainamide
Quinidine
Sympathomimetics
Tricyclic antidepressants
Thyroxine
Verapamil

Hypotension
Citrated blood
Calcium antagonists
Diuretics
Levodopa

Morphine
Nitroglycerin
Phenothiazines

Hypertension
ACTH
Corticosteroids
MAOI + sympathomimetics
Oral contraceptives
Phenylbutazone
Sympathomimetics
Tricyclic antidepressants with sympathomimetics

Worsening of angina
α-blockers
β-blocker withdrawal
Ergotamine
Hydralazine
Methysergide
Oxytocin
Thyroxine
Vasopressin

Cardiomyopathy
Adriamycin
Daunorubicin
Lithium
Phenothiazines
Sulphonamides
Sympathomimetics

Pericarditis
Hydralazine
Methysergide
Procainamide

Thomboembolism
Oral contraceptives

Anaphylaxis
Dextran
Demeclocycline
Iodinated contrast media or drugs
Iron dextran
Insulin
Penicillin

RESPIRATORY

Asthma
Aspirin and other NSAIDs
β-blockers
Cholinergic drugs

Cephalosporins
Streptomycin

Respiratory depression
Aminoglycosides
Hypnotics
Opiates
Polymixins
Sedatives

Pulmonary oedema
Contrast media
Heroin
Hydrochlorthiazide
Methadone

Pulmonary infiltrates
Amiodarone
Bleomycin
BCNU
Busulfan
Cyclophosphamide
Melphalan
Methysergide
Nitrofurantoin
Procarbazine

GASTROENTEROLOGY

Peptic ulcers
Aspirin and other NSAIDs
Ethacrynic acid
Phenylbutazone
? steroids

Nausea and vomiting
Digitalis
Ferrous sulphate
Levodopa
Oestrogen
Opiates
Potassium chloride

Diarrhoea
Antibiotics (especially
  clindamycin and
  linocomycin)
Colchicine
Digitalis
Magnesium containing
  drugs
Methyldopa

Constipation
Aluminium containing drugs

Barium sulfate
Calcium carbonate
Ferrous sulphate
Ganglionic blockers
Ion exchange resins
Opiates
Phenothiazines
Tricyclic antidepressants

Malabsorption
Antibiotics
Ion exchange resins
Colchicine

Pancreatitis
Azathioprine
Corticosteroids
Ethacrynic acid
Frusemide
Opiates
Oral contraceptives
Sulphonamides
Thiazides

HEPATIC

Cholestasis
Anabolic steroids
Androgens
Chlorpropamide
Erythromycin estolate
Gold
Oral contraceptives
Phenothiazines

Hepatitis
Allopurinol
Aminosalicylic acid
Erythromycin estolate
Halothane
Isoniazid
Ketoconazole
Methotrexate
Methoxyflurane
Methyldopa
Monoamine oxidase
  inhibitors
Nitrofurantoin
Phenytoin
Propylthiouracil
Rifampicin
Salicylates
Sulphonamides

Tetracycline
Valproate

RENAL

Urinary retention
Anticholinergics
Disopyramide
Monoamine oxidase
  inhibitors
Tricyclic antidepressants

Nephrotic syndrome
Captopril
Gold
Penicillamine
Probenecid

Tubular necrosis
Aminoglycosides
Amphotericin
Cephaloridine
Colistin
Cyclosporin
Iodinated contrast media
Polymyxins
Sulphonamides
Tetracycline

NEUROLOGICAL

Extrapyramidal
Haloperidol
Levodopa
Methyldopa
Metoclopramide
Oral contraceptives
Phenothiazines
Reserpine
Tricyclic antidepressants

Peripheral neuropathy
Chlorpropamide
Chloroquine
Clofibrate
Demeclocycline
Disopyramide
Ethambutol
Hydralazine
Isoniazid
Metronidazole
Nitrofurantoin
Nalidixic acid
Perhexiline

Procarbazine
Phenytoin
Tolbutamide tricyclic
  antidepressants
Vincristine

Fits
Amphetamines
Isoniazid
Lithium
Lignocaine
Nalidixic acid
Penicillins
Phenothiazines
Physostigmine
Theophylline
Tricyclic antidepressants
Vincristine

MUSCULOSKELETAL

Osteoporosis
Corticosteroids
Heparin

Myopathy
Amphotericin B
Carbenoxolone
Chloroquine
Clofibrate
Corticosteroids
Oral contraceptives

METABOLIC

Hypercalcaemia
Antacids
Thiazides
Vitamin D

Hyperglycaemia
Chlorthalidone
Corticosteroids
Diazoxide
Ethacrynic acid
Frusemide
Growth hormone
Oral contraceptives

Hyponatraemia
Corticosteroids
Chlorpropamide
Cyclophosphamide
Diuretics
Vincristine

Hyperkalaemia
Amiloride
Corticosteroid withdrawal
Cytotoxics
Lithium
Potassium salts
Succinylcholine
Spironolactone
Triamterene

Hypokalaemia
Amphotericin B
Corticosteroids
Diuretics
Insulin
Laxatives

SYSTEMIC

Gynaecomastia
Cimetidine
Digoxin
Isoniazid
Methyldopa
Oestrogens
Spironolactone
Testosterone

Fever
Amphotericin B
Antihistamines
Barbiturates
Bleomycin
Cephalosporins
Methyldopa

Penicillin
Phenytoin
Procainamide
Quinidine
Sulphonamides

Lupus-like syndrome
Acebutolol
Hydralazine
Isoniazid
Procainamide

MISCELLANEOUS

Cataracts
Busulfan
Chlorambucil
Corticosteroids
Phenothiazines

Deafness
Aminoglycosides
Aspirin
Bleomycin
Chloroquine
Ethacrynic acid
Frusemide
Quinine

Precipitate porphyria
Barbiturates
Chlordiazepoxide
Chlorpropamide
Oestrogens
Oral contraceptives
Sulphonamides

ADVERSE REACTIONS OF COMMONLY PRESCRIBED DRUGS

This list is not exhaustive and the reader is referred to the BNF for further details.

ACE inhibitors   Dry cough, loss of taste, marrow suppression, hyperkalaemia, renal impairment, rash, hypotension (especially following first dose).

Allopurinol   Rash, fever, GI upset, hepatotoxicity.

Aminoglycosides   Vestibular damage, nephrotoxicity, pseudomembranous colitis.

Aminophylline   Tachycardia, palpitations, headache, GI upset, arrhythmias, convulsions.

Amitriptyline Dry mouth, sedation, difficulty with micturition, tachycardia, hypotension, tremor, confusion, black tongue, jaundice, marrow suppression.

Aspirin GI irritation, bronchospasm (especially in a patient with nasal polyps), Reye's syndrome (do not prescribe to children <12 years).

Benzodiazepines Drowsiness, confusion, ataxia, dependence.

β-Blockers Bradycardia, heart failure, peripheral vasoconstriction, bronchospasm, GI upset, fatigue, nightmares.

Carbamazepine Dizziness, ataxia, headache, diplopia, GI upset, constipation, rash, marrow suppression.

Chlorpromazine Extra-pyramidal symptoms, tardive dyskinesia, drowsiness, confusion, depression, dry mouth, constipation, difficulty with micturition, blurred vision (anti-muscarinic effects), marrow suppression, tachycardia, hypotension, jaundice.

Cimetidine Rash, dizziness, gynaecomastia, confusion, alopecia, arthralgia, myalgia, interstitial nephritis.

Corticosteroids Hypertension, sodium and water retention, hypokalaemia, muscle weakness (mineralocorticoid effects), diabetes mellitus, osteoporosis, euphoria, depression, peptic ulceration, increased risk of infection, Cushing's syndrome, growth suppression, thinning of skin, bruising (glucocorticoid effects), adrenal suppression, withdrawal effects.

Digoxin Anorexia, nausea, vomiting, arrhythmias, visual disturbance, heart block, hypokalaemia predisposes to toxicity, gynaecomastia.

Diltiazem Bradycardia, first degree heart block, hypotension, headache, rashes.

Frusemide Hyponatraemia, hypokalaemia, hypotension, hyperuricaemia, gout, hyperglycaemia, rashes, marrow suppression, tinnitus, pancreatitis.

Glipizide GI upset, rashes, marrow suppression, hypoglycaemia.

Heparin Haemorrhage, thrombocytopenia, osteoporosis.

Insulin Local reactions and fat hypertrophy at injection site, hypoglcaemia.

Levodopa (L-DOPA) Anorexia, nausea, vomiting, agitation, postural hypotension, red discolouration of body fluids, psychosis, abnormal involuntary movements.

Lithium GI upset, polyuria, polydipsia, weight gain, oedema, blurred vision, drowsiness, ataxia, dysarthria, convulsions, goitre, coma, tremor.

Metoclopramide Extra-pyramidal effects, hyperprolactinaemia, tardive dyskinesia, diarrhoea.

Nifedipine Headache, flushing, dizziness, oedema, depression.

NSAID Nausea, GI bleeding, rashes, bronchospasm, tinnitus, fluid retention, renal failure.

Opioid analgesics Nausea, vomiting, constipation, drowsiness, respiratory depression, hypotension, dry mouth, hypothermia, dependance.

Oral contraceptive pill Hypertension, migraine, stroke, hepatoma.

Paracetamol Acute pancreatitis, rashes, liver damage following overdosage.

Penicillin Hypersensitivity reactions (urticaria, angio-oedema, fever, arthralgia, anaphylactoid shock), diarrhoea, rashes.

Phenytoin Nausea, vomiting, confusion, headache, tremor, insomnia, ataxia, dysarthria, nystagmus, hirsuitism, acne, SLE-like syndrome, rashes, marrow suppression, megaloblastic anaemia, rickets, osteomalacia.

Ranitidine Bradycardia, heart block, rarely gynaecomastia, rashes, dizziness, confusion.

Salbutamol Tremor, headache, tachycardia, hypokalaemia.

Streptokinase Nausea, vomiting, bleeding, allergic reactions, anaphylaxis.

Thiazide diuretics Hypokalaemia, hypomagnesaemia, hyponatraemia, hypercalcaemia, hyperuricaemia, gout, hyperglycaemia, rashes, photosensitivity, marrow suppression, impotence

Valproate Nausea, ataxia, weight gain, alopecia, jaundice, thrombocytopenia, amenorrhoea, rashes, pancreatitis.

Verapamil Constipation, nausea, flushing, headache, hypotension, bradycardia, heart block.

Warfarin Haemorrhage.

MECHANISMS OF DRUG INTERACTIONS

There are many mechanisms by which the effects of one drug can be altered by the prior or concurrent administration of a second drug:

- Opposing pharmacological effects.
- Similar pharmacological effects.

- Alteration of gastric absorption.

- Alteration of pH.

- Alteration of gastrointestinal motility.

- Interference with metabolism: enzyme induction
  enzyme inhibition.

- Displacement from site of protein binding.

- Interference with excretion.

Table 17.1 contains a list of possible drug interactions but is by no means exhaustive and the reader is referred to the BNF for more detailed information.

Body surface area may be calculated from Figure 17.1 to allow the dose of a particular drug to be calculated, eg cytotoxic drugs.

Table 17.1
Drug interactions

Affected drug	Interacting drug	Result of interaction
ACE inhibitors	Potassium sparing diuretics	Hyperkalaemia
	Alcohol	Enhanced hypotension
Allopurinol	Thiazide diuretics	Enhanced toxicity
Aminoglycosides	Frusemide	Increased risk of ototoxicity
Aminophylline	Cimetidine, erythromycin	Decreased metabolism with enhanced toxicity
Amitriptyline	Alcohol	Increased sedation
	OCP	Reduced effect
Antihistamines	Alcohol	Increased sedation
Azathioprine	Allopurinol	Increased cytotoxicity
Barbiturates	Alcohol	Increased CNS depression
Benzodiazepines	Opioid analgesics, antidepressants, antihistamines, cimetidine	Enhanced sedation

Table 17.1 (contd)

Affected drug	Interacting drug	Result of interaction
β-blockers	Alcohol, sympathomimetics, verapamil	Enhanced hypotension
	Ergotamine	Enhanced vasoconstiction
Calcium-channel blockers	Amiodarone	Increased bradycardia
	Quinidine	Hypotension
Carbamazepine	Erythromycin, isoniazid	Increased toxicity
Cephalosporins	Loop diuretics	Increased nephrotoxicity
	Alcohol	Disulfiram-like action
Chlormethiazole	Cimetidine	Increased sedation
Cimetidine	Antacids	Reduced absorption
Contraceptive (OCP)	Rifampicin, Tetracylines	Reduced contraceptive effect
Corticosteroids	Carbenoxalone	Hypokalaemia
	Aminoglutethamide	Enhanced metabolism
Co-trimoxazole	Cyclosporin	Increased nephrotoxicity
	Methotrexate	Increased antifolate effect
Digoxin	Diuretics	Toxicity increased by hypokalaemia
	Antacids	Reduced absorption
	Phenytoin, rifampicin	Increased metabolism
Erythromycin	Benzodiazepines	Increased sedation
Frusemide	Thiazides	Hypokalaemia
Heparin	Aspirin, dipyridamole	Increased anticoagulant effect
Iron	Antacids	Reduced absorption
L-DOPA	Phenothiazines	Antagonism
	Metoclopramide	Extra-pyramidal effects

Affected drug	Interacting drug	Result of interaction
Lithium salts	Diuretics	Sodium depletion
	Haloperidol	Extra-pyramidal effects
	Antidepressants	CNS toxicity
	Diltiazem, verapamil	Nephrotoxicity
MAOIs	Alcohol, tyramine	Hypertensive crisis
Methyldopa	NSAID, diuretics	Hypotension
	Corticosteroids	Antagonism of hypotension
Metoclopramide	Lithium	Extra-pyramidal effects
Metronidazole	Alcohol	Disulfiram-like effect
Metformin	Alcohol	Lactic acidosis
Mianserin	Alcohol, anxiolytics	Enhanced effect
NSAID	Probenecid	Reduced excretion
	Antacids	Reduced absorption
	Haloperidol	Drowsiness
	Diuretics, ACE inhibitors	Nephrotoxicity
Opioid analgesics	Anxiolytics, cimetidine	Sedation
Penicillins	Antacids	Reduced absorption
	Probonocid	Reduced excretion
Phenothiazines	Alcohol	Sedation
	Rifampicin	Increased metabolism
	Metoclopramide	Extra-pyramidal effects
Phenytoin	Cimetidine, isoniazid, aspirin, amiodarone	Increased toxicity due to decreased metabolism
	Carbamazepine, alcoholism	Increased metabolism
Sulphonylureas	Alcohol, β-blockers	Hypoglcaemia
	Rifampicin	Increased metabolism
Tetracylines	Antacids	Decreased absorption
	Phenytoin	Increased metabolism

Table 17.1 (contd)

Table 17.1 (*contd*)

Affected drug	Interacting drug	Result of interaction
Thyroxine	Phenytoin, fenclofenac	Falsely low total serum thyroxine level due to binding protein displacement
Valproate	Aspirin Antidepressants Other antiepileptics	Enhanced effect Antagonism Increased metabolism
Warfarin	Barbiturates, carbamazepine, rifampicin	Reduced anticoagulant effect due to increased metabolism
	Cimetidine, amiodarone, alcohol	Increased effect due to inhibition of coumarin metabolism
	Sulphonamides	Increased effect due to displaced protein binding

DRUG TREATMENT OF COMMONLY ENCOUNTERED INFECTIONS

The likely infecting organism and its antibacterial sensitivity will usually suggest an appropriate antibiotic but other factors (eg age, pregnancy, breast feeding, ethnic origin, severity of illness, history of allergy, renal or hepatic impairment) also influence the choice of antibiotic.

Samples (eg sputum, urine and blood) should be taken before an antibiotic is started.

The antibiotic dose may vary depending on age, weight, renal and hepatic function and severity of illness. Drug levels (eg aminoglycosides) should be monitored to allow optimal peak and trough levels to be achieved.

Duration of treatment depends on the nature of the infection and also on the response to therapy.

The BNF (or equivalent) should be referred to for up-to-date information on drug dosages, adverse reaction, interactions and routes of administration.

Table 17.2
Drug treatment of commonly encountered infections.

Infection	Bacterial pathogen	Antibacterial agent
Arthritis	*Staphylococcus aureus*	Flucloxacillin 500 mg qds
		Fusidic acid 500 mg tds
	Haemophilus influenzae	Ampicillin 500 mg qds
	Neisseria gonorrhoeae	Ampicillin
		Ciprofloxacin 500 mg bd
Aspiration pneumonia/ lung abscess	Oral streptococci	Penicillin 0.6–2.4 g/d in 2–4 divided doses
	Anaerobes	Metronidazole 400 mg tds
	Coliforms	Aminoglycoside*
	Staphylococcus aureus	Flucloxacillin
Bacillary dysentery	*Shigella* spp.	Ampicillin
		Cotrimoxazole 960 mg bd
		Ciprofloxacin 200 mg bd
Bronchitis	*Streptococcus pneumoniae*	Ampicillin
		Amoxycillin 250 mg tds
	Haemophilus influenzae	Cotrimoxazole
Burns	*Streptococcus pyogenes*	Penicillin
		Erythromycin 500 mg qds
	Pseudomonas spp.	Aminoglycoside*
		Azlocillin 2 g tds
		Ceftazidime 2 g bd
		Ciprofloxacin
Cellulitis	*Streptococcus pyogenes*	Penicillin
		Erythromycin
	Staphylococcus aureus	Flucloxacillin
Cholecystitis/ cholangitis	Coliforms	Ampicillin
		Aminoglycoside*
Endocarditis	*Streptococcus viridans*	Penicillin + aminoglycoside*
	Streptococcus faecalis	Ampicillin + aminoglycoside*
	Staphylococcus aureus	Flucloxacillin + aminoglycoside*

Table 17.2 (contd)

Infection	Bacterial pathogen	Antibacterial agent
Enteric fever	*Salmonella* spp.	Chloramphenicol 500 mg qds Cotrimoxazole Amoxycillin
Meningitis	*Neisseria meningitidis* *Streptococcus pneumoniae* *Haemophilus influenzae* *Listeria* spp.	Penicillin Chloramphenicol Penicillin Chloramphenicol Ampicillin + aminoglycoside*
Pneumonia lobar	*Streptrococcus pneumoniae*	Penicillin Erythromycin
broncho	Coliforms	Cotrimoxazole Amoxycillin
cavitating	*Staphylococcus aureus* *Klebsiella* spp.	Flucloxacillin Fusidic acid Aminoglycoside* + cephalosporin 1–2 g qds
atypical	*Legionella* spp. *Mycoplasma* *Coxiella* spp. *Chlamydia* spp.	Erythromycin Erythromycin Tetracycline 500 mg qds Tetracycline
Osteomyelitis	*Staphylococcus aureus*	Flucloxacillin
Pseudo-membranous colitis	*Clostridium difficile*	Vancomycin 125 mg qds
Pyelonephritis	Coliforms	Cotrimoxazole Amoxycillin
Salpingitis/ pelvic inflammatory disease	*Neisseria gonorrhoeae* Anaerobes	Penicillin Metronidazole
Syphilis	*Treponema pallidum*	Procaine penicillin

Table 17.2 (*contd*)

Infection	Bacterial pathogen	Antibacterial agent
Urinary tract infection	Coliforms	Cotrimoxazole Amoxycillin

* The dose of aminoglycoside depends on age, sex, weight and renal function and should be monitored by both trough and peak blood levels.

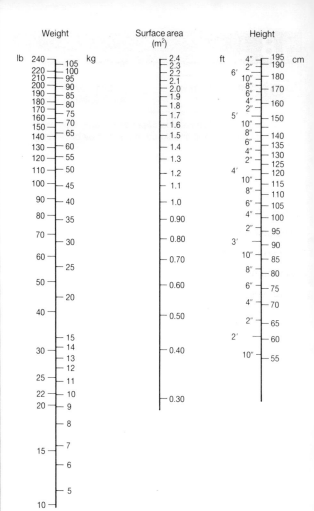

Fig. 17.1
A normogram for surface area from height and weight.

18

Notes for housemen

DEATH

The resident should certify the death as soon as possible after the death has occurred. The time of death should be recorded. The patient should be pulseless, heart sounds should be absent for one minute, apnoeic for one minute and pupils should be fixed and dilated. There should be no response present to a painful stimulus. These examination findings should be documented in the case notes, which should be signed and dated.

After certifying the death the consultant and the GP should both be informed. The relatives should be informed and seen. A death certificate can be issued if the cause of death is not in any doubt. If there is any doubt a post mortem examination should be requested. If there is any evidence of violence, neglect, injury, poisoning, alcohol intoxication, suicide or if the death occurred during surgery or anaesthesia the death must be reported to the Procurator Fiscal or Coroner and a death certificate must not be issued unless permission is granted to do so.

If the patient is being supported on a ventilator tests of brain death may have to be performed ($\rightarrow$ Table 18.1). Two doctors (one of whom must be a consultant and the other at least a senior registrar) should carry out the tests on two occasions usually 24 hours apart. An EEG recording is not required in the UK. Brain death is defined as death of the brainstem. Conditions which may mimic or complicate this diagnosis have to be excluded ($\rightarrow$ Table 18.2).

The importance of possible organ donation from patients maintained on a ventilator should be remembered.

Table 18.1
Tests of brainstem function

Fixed, unreacting pupils
Absent corneal reflex
Absent gag reflex to bronchial stimulation.
Absent vestibulo-ocular reflex (no eye movement in response to slow injection of 20 ml of iced water into each external auditory meatus. Ensure that the tympanic membranes can be visualized).
Absent cranial nerve motor response
Absent respiratory effort to hypercapnia (disconnect patient from ventilator and allow $PaCO_2$ to rise to at least 6.7 kPa).

Table 18.2
Conditions which should be exluded before brain death can be certified

Hypothermia (<35 C)
Drug intoxication
Hypoglycaemia
Acidosis
Electrolyte imbalance

CHECKLIST FOR DISCHARGE

- Liaise with nursing staff and patient's relatives re discharge date.

- Organize discharge ambulance transport if required.

- Send discharge letter to pharmacy at least 24 hours before planned discharge date to allow drugs to be dispensed.

- Liaise with social worker, home help supervisor, district nurse, occupational therapist and physiotherapist re discharge date.

- Inform GP of planned discharge date.

- Ensure that a follow-up appointment has been made (if required) and that the patient has been informed of the date and time of the appointment. Book any ambulance transport which may be needed for clinic attendance.

PAIN CONTROL

- Reassure the patient.

- Treat the underlying pathology (eg prolapsed intervertebral disc, metastatic disease).

- Become familiar with a few drugs rather than using a large number of different drugs.

- Give regular doses of analgesics to control pain rather than prn doses.

- Try oral medications before using parenteral drugs if possible.

- Treat associated conditions (eg nausea, constipation, depression).

- Use complementary treatment (eg local heat, radiotherapy, regional local anaesthesia).

Table 18.3
Drugs used to control pain

Analgesic	Adverse reactions
Mild pain	
Paracetamol 0.5–1 g 6–8-hourly	Dangerous in overdosage
Aspirin 300–900 mg 4–6-hourly	Gastric erosions, bronchospasm (avoid in asthma)
Moderate pain	
Dihydrocodeine 30–60 mg 4–6-hourly	Constipation
Coproxamol (dextropropoxyphene hydrochloride+paracetamol) 1–2 tabs 6–8-hourly	CNS and respiratory depression, dangerous in overdosage
Cocodamol (codeine phosphate+ paracetamol) 1–2 tabs 6–8-hourly	Constipation
NSAIDs (eg ibuprofen 1.2–1.8 g daily in 3–4 divided doses after food)	GI discomfort/bleeding, fluid retention
Severe pain	
Diamorphine 5–10 mg 4–6-hourly	Nausea, constipation, respiratory depression, cough depression, hypotension, dependency
Morphine 10–20 mg 4–6-hourly	As for diamorphine
Pethidine 50–150 mg 4–6-hourly	As for diamorphine

POISONS INFORMATION SERVICE

Belfast 0232 24053

Birmingham 021 554 3801

Cardiff 0222 709901

Dublin 010 3531 379964 or 010 3531 379966

Edinburgh 031 229 2477 or 031 228 2441, (Viewdata)

Leeds 0532 430715 or 0532 432799

London 071 635 9191 or 071 407 7600

Newcastle 091 232 5131

USEFUL TELEPHONE AND BLEEP NUMBERS

Registrar _____

SHO _____

House officer _____

Senior registrar _____

Consultant _____

Consultant _____

Consultant _____

Consultant _____

Consultant _____

Consultant _____

Chemical chemistry _____

Haematology _____

Accident and emergency _____

BTS _____

Bacteriology _____

Pathology _____

X-ray _____

Porters _____

Virology _____

Nursing officer _____

Administrator _____

Anaesthetist _____

Social worker _____

Dentist _____

Pharmacy _____

Cardiology _____

Chest physician _____

Dermatology _____

Gastroenterology _____

Gynaecology _____

Renal medicine _____

Neurology _____

ENT _____

Paediatrics _____

Index

M

R

V

U

BIOCHEMICAL VALUES

Venous blood: adult reference values

Analyte	Reference values	
Acid phosphatase (unstable enzyme)	0.1–0.4 i.u./l	
Alanine aminotransferase (ALT) (glutamic-pyruvic transaminase (GPT))	10–40 i.u./l	
Alkaline phosphatase	40–100 i.u./l	
Amylase	50–300 i.u./l	
α₁-Antitrypsin	2–4g/l	
Ascorbic acid—serum	23–57 µmol/l	0.4–1.0 mg/dl
—leucocytes	1420–2270 µmol/l	25–40 mg/dl
Aspartate aminotransferase (AST) (glutamic-oxaloacetic transaminase (GOT))	10–35 i.u./l	
Bilirubin (total)	2–17 µmol/l	
Caeruloplasmin	1–2.7 µmol/l	
Calcium (total)	2.12–2.62 mmol/l	
Carbon dioxide (total)	24–30 mmol/l	
Chloride	95–105 mmol/l	
Cholesterol (fasting)	3.6–6.7 mmol/l	
Copper	11–24 µmol/l	
Creatinine	55–150 µmol/l	
Creatinine clearance	90–130 ml/min	
Creatine kinase (CK) —males	30–200 i.u./l	
—females	30–150 i.u./l	
Ethanol —marked intoxication	65–87 mmol/l	
—coma	>109 mmol/l	
Ferritin —males	6–186 µg/ml	
—females	3–162 µg/ml	
α-Fetoprotein	2–6 units/ml	
γ-Glutamyl transferase (γ-GT)—males	10–55 i.u./l	
—females	5–35 i.u./l	
Glucose (fasting)	3.9–5.8 mmol/l	
Immunoglobulins (Ig): IgA	0.5–4.0 g/l (40–300 i.u./l)	
IgG	5.0–13.0 g/l (60–160 i.u./l)	
IgM —males	0.3–2.2 g/l (40–270 i.u./l)	
—females	0.4—2.5 g/l (50–300 i.u./l)	
Iron—males	14–32 µmol/l	
—females	10–28 µmol/l	
Iron binding capacity (total)	45–72 µmol/l	
Iron binding capacity (saturation)	14–47%	
Lactate	0.4–1.4 mmol/l	
Lactate dehydrogenase (LDH)	100–300 i.u./l	
Lead	0.5–1.9 µmol/l	
Magnesium	0.75–1.0 mmol/l	
5' Nucleotidase	1–11 i.u./l	
Osmolality	285–295 mOsm/kg	
Phosphatase *see* acid and alkaline		
Phosphate	0.8–1.4 mmol/l	
Potassium	3.3–4.7 mmol/l	
Proteins—total	62–82 g/l	
—albumin	36–47 g/l	
—globulins	24–37 g/l	
—electrophoresis (% of total)		
albumin 52–68		
globulin α₁ 4.2–7.2		
α₂ 6.8–12		
β 9.3–15		
γ 13–23		
Sodium	132–144 mmol/l	
Triglyceride (fasting)	0.6–1.7 mmol/l	
Urate—males	0.12–0.42 mmol/l	
—females	0.12–0.36 mmol/l	
Urea	2.5–6.6 mmol/l	